You Code It!
A Case Studies Workbook

You Code It!
A Case Studies Workbook

Shelley C. Safian, MAOM/HSM, CCS-P, CPC-H, CHA

Herzing College
Orlando, Florida

McGraw-Hill
Higher Education

Boston   Burr Ridge, IL   Dubuque, IA   New York   San Francisco   St. Louis
Bangkok   Bogotá   Caracas   Kuala Lumpur   Lisbon   London   Madrid   Mexico City
Milan   Montreal   New Delhi   Santiago   Seoul   Singapore   Sydney   Taipei   Toronto

McGraw-Hill
Higher Education

YOU CODE IT! A CASE STUDIES WORKBOOK
Published by McGraw-Hill, a business unit of The McGraw-Hill Companies, Inc., 1221 Avenue
of the Americas, New York, NY, 10020. Copyright © 2009 by The McGraw-Hill Companies, Inc.
All rights reserved. No part of this publication may be reproduced or distributed in any form
or by any means, or stored in a database or retrieval system, without the prior written consent
of The McGraw-Hill Companies, Inc., including, but not limited to, in any network or other
electronic storage or transmission, or broadcast for distance learning.

Some ancillaries, including electronic and print components, may not be available to customers outside the United States.

This book is printed on acid-free paper.

2 3 4 5 6 7 8 9 0 QPD/QPD 0 9 8

ISBN   978-0-07-337402-4
MHID   0-07-337402-4

Vice President/Editor in Chief: *Elizabeth Haefele*
Vice President/Director of Marketing: *John E. Biernat*
Senior sponsoring editor: *Debbie Fitzgerald*
Managing developmental editor: *Patricia Hesse*
Executive marketing manager: *Roxan Kinsey*
Lead media producer: *Damian Moshak*
Media producer: *Marc Mattson*
Director, Editing/Design/Production: *Jess Ann Kosic*
Senior project manager: *Rick Hecker*
Senior production supervisor: *Janean A. Utley*
Designer: *Marianna Kinigakis*
Senior photo research coordinator: *Carrie K. Burger*
Media project manager: *Mark A. S. Dierker*
Outside development house: *Wendy Langerud*
Interior and cover design: *Pam Verros, pv design*
Typeface: *10.5/13 Melior*
Compositor: *Lachina Publishing Services*
Printer: *Quebecor World Dubuque Inc.*
Credits: The credits section for this book begins on page 509 and is considered an extension of
the copyright page.

The names of the facilities, health care professionals, and patients have all been changed to
protect the privacy and confidentiality of all concerned in these patient records. Any similari-
ties to actual persons or places are purely coincidental. These cases are to be used for educational purposes only.

The Internet addresses listed in the text were accurate at the time of publication. The inclusion of a Web site does not indicate an endorsement by the authors or McGraw-Hill, and
McGraw-Hill does not guarantee the accuracy of the information presented at these sites.

www.mhhe.com

About the Author

Shelley C. Safian, Chair of the Allied Health Department at Herzing College, is also the Senior Assistant Professor for the Medical Billing and Insurance Coding program. She is currently teaching coding and medical office administration at both Herzing College–Winter Park (Orlando), Florida, as well as Herzing College Online.

Safian is a Certified Coding Specialist-Physician-based (CCS-P) from the American Health Information Management Association (AHIMA) and a Certified Professional Coder–Hospital (CPC-H) from the American Academy of Professional Coders (AAPC). She also holds a National Certified Insurance Coding Specialist (NCICS) designation, as well as that of Certified HIPAA Administrator (CHA).

Safian completed her Graduate Certificate in Health Care Management in June 2005 at Keller Graduate School of Management. The University of Phoenix awarded her Master of Arts/Organizational Management degree in 2002.

Herzing College–Winter Park honored Safian by naming her 2007 Teacher of the Year, and she was awarded the Faculty Scholarship Award–First Runner Up for the Herzing College System.

Safian is a volunteer AHIMA Mentor, working with health information management students from all across the country, and sits on the AHIMA Classification Practice Council. She attends local chapter meetings of the Central Florida Health Information Management Association (CFHIMA) whenever her schedule permits and encourages her students to join her at the Florida Health Information Management Association (FHIMA) Annual Convention every year.

McGraw-Hill Higher Education published *Insurance Coding & Electronic Claims for the Medical Office* by Safian in July 2005. Her second, third, and fourth books, *The Complete Procedure Coding Book*, *The Complete Diagnosis Coding Book*, and *You Code It! A Case Studies Workbook* will be published simultaneously in February 2008.

Shelley C. Safian

Contents

Preface

A rather unique aspect of working in the health care industry is the fact that everyone who works in it will, at some point, become one of its customers. As a larger portion of the population of the United States moves into their older stage of life, the number of customers (patients) will continue to increase. The longer the human body lives, the more maintenance and repair it needs—the services of both preventive and therapeutic health care.

Every time a patient and a health care professional meet, the details of this meeting, known as an encounter, must be documented. Certain details must be reported to government agencies for statistical purposes, such as determining which type of research should be funded and prioritized, which preventive measures should be promoted to the public, or which type of care should be paid for by certain programs. Coders and health information managers are the professionals who interpret the information from the physicians, therapists, radiologists, and so forth, and report the data, in code, so that the agencies can process and work with it.

In addition, these same codes are used to gain payment—reimbursement from insurance carriers and other third party payers—to cover the expense of health care received by patients from their providers. Of course, all the professionals working in health care (physicians, nurses, medical assistants, health information managers) want to—deserve to—be paid for their expertise and hard work.

Coders are in high demand. According to the Bureau of Labor Statistics, the demand for health information management professionals will increase 40 to 50% by the year 2012. Every type of health care facility needs coders: hospitals, doctor's offices, nursing homes, assisted living facilities, clinics, laboratories, radiology centers, and more.

This workbook has been created to make the journey of entering the health information management workforce a little less scary by providing extensive, hands-on practice for those learning coding. The cases in this book are real patient charts from physician's offices and hospitals in different parts of the country. (Of course, the names have been changed to protect privacy.)

THE AUDIENCE

This book is written to enable the practice of all types of work involved in health care coding: ICD-9-CM, CPT, and HCPCS Level II for both outpatient and inpatient.

WHAT MAKES THIS BOOK SPECIAL?

This book contains actual patient charts from virtually every medical specialty for the practice of coding in almost any type of facility.

The author is a classroom instructor who wants to see her students succeed in their chosen health information management careers. This textbook has been created from her experiences, interacting with students learning coding and watching and evaluating their challenges in learning this demanding skill.

Responding to the comments and recommendations of these students, as well as classroom instructors, the author has created a student-friendly workbook presenting case studies for the practice of abstracting health care professionals' documentation and accurately translating the facts into the best, most accurate codes.

ACKNOWLEDGMENTS

Every book is created by a team, and I, as the author, am only a small part. I wish to thank every member of my team.

Thank you to the students of Herzing College, for without them I would not have the input, the direction, or the motivation to write this book. As if that weren't enough, they also served as testers, using this manuscript as their text to ensure this book works to help students learn in the best possible manner.

Thank you to the administration of Herzing College, especially Tammy Files and Drew Warren, who encouraged me, supported me, and gave me the opportunities to teach and share with my students.

Thank you to my team at McGraw-Hill Higher Education. The professionals in the editorial, marketing, production, and media departments are a pleasure to work with. You all have really helped make this the best book it can be, especially Roxan, Pat, Wendy, Rick, and certainly Ben, who started it all.

And thank you to April Waye, without whom I would not even know what coding was!

OVERVIEW

You Code It! Workbook: Features and Benefits

Overall Chapter Structure

This textbook is written to prepare students to work with actual patient records in any type of health care facility.

Layer 1. Preparation

The first chapter reviews methodologies for the **abstracting** of physician's notes and operative reports.

Layer 2. Practice, Practice, Practice

The rest of the chapters provide opportunities for students to practice coding from actual patient records. Divided by medical specialty, the records in this book can be used by students at any point in their education. Students learning each particular code set can use this book to practice only diagnosis coding or procedure coding. Faculty members can break out particular specialties to reinforce coding concepts such as using the records from Chapter 14, oncology, when teaching students how to code neoplasms,

MORRIS, SHALLERT & ASSOCIATES
Allergy & Immunology
975 CENTRAL AVENUE • SOMEWHERE, FL 32811 • 407-555-4321

PATIENT: HAYES, LEONARD
ACCOUNT/EHR #: HAYELE001
Date: 09/15/08

Attending Physician: Suzanne R. Shallert, MD

This 55-year-old male comes in with a complaint of bilateral hearing loss and allergy symptoms. He states that his hearing loss has been going on for several years, but he feels the right ear is worse than the left. He does admit to using Q-tips. He was seen by his primary care physician back in August and was told he had no wax impactions. He has had no otorrhea or tinnitus. He has no history of ear surgery, recent skull trauma, or noise exposure.

The review of systems, past medical history, family history, and social history are per the new patient history sheet dated September 15th.

PE: BP 100/62. HR: 68 T 98.3. The patient is a well-developed, well-nourished male in no apparent distress. Voice is normal. Face: symmetrical with normal salivary glands, and normal facial strength. Pinnae, external auditory canals, and tympanic membranes were normal with no evidence of middle ear effusion, acute infection, or cerumen impaction. The external nose was normal. Nasal cavity has no polyps or purulent drainage. The septum was essentially straight.

Oral cavity shows no masses or lesions. Normal mucosa. Lips, teeth, and gums are normal. The true vocal cords were mobile bilaterally with no nodules, polyps, or neoplasms in the larynx or hypopharynx. No lymphadenopathy, masses, or thyromegaly.

Audiogram: This revealed essentially normal hearing throughout the frequencies with 100 percent discrimination on the right and 96 percent on the left. Tympanograms were Type A bilaterally.

Impression: Perception of auditory loss; however, no evidence of significant hearing loss by audiogram. Allergic rhinitis that has responded well to allergy shots in the past.

Suzanne R. Shallert, MD

SRS/pw   D: 09/15/08 09:50:16   T: 09/17/08 12:55:01

You Code It!

What are the best, most accurate codes?

_____

_____

_____

Chapter 2   Allergy and Immunology Cases and Patient Records

or Chapter 7, endocrinology, when instructing students on the official guidelines for coding diabetes mellitus. Those learning procedure coding, both inpatient and outpatient, can practice evaluation and management (E/M) coding from almost any chapter and anesthesia coding from any of the operative reports included throughout the book. Certain chapters, such as Chapter 10, on gerontology, or Chapter 16, on orthopedics, lend themselves well to simulate the need for coding from the HCPCS Level II code set as well. Advanced coding students can use the cases in this book to practice coding complete charts.

Feature: You Code It! Case Studies

Benefit: Every chapter provides the reader with case studies to practice both the knowledge cluster and the coding process for virtually every medical specialty. Instructors can use these to reinforce and test students' learning progress of diagnosis and procedure coding individually or together to simulate real-world experiences.

Important Note

This workbook is designed to be used in conjunction with International Classification of Diseases, ninth revision, Clinical Modification, Volumes 1, 2, and 3 (ICD-9-CM), Current Procedure Terminology (CPT), and/or HCPCS Level II code books.

REVIEWERS

I would also like to thank the many instructors who provided detailed recommendations for improving chapter content throughout the review process.

Bobette Anderson
MedVance Institute of Ft. Lauderdale
Lauderdale Lakes, FL 33312

Norma Bird, MEd, BS, CMA
Idaho State University
Pocatello, ID 83209

Barbara Desch
San Joaquin Valley College–Visalia Campus
Visalia, CA 93391

Linda Eggersgluess
Ridgewater College
Hutchinson, MN 55350

Carolyn H. Greene
Virginia College at Birmingham
Birmingham, AL 35209

Robin Kern, BSN
Moultrie Technical College
Moultrie, GA 31788

Naomi Kupfer, CMA
Heritage College
Las Vegas, NV 89133

Norma Mercado, MAHS, RHIA
Austin Community College
Austin, TX 78702

Debra A. Slusarczyk BHS, RHIT
Camden County College
Woodbury, NJ 08096

Nona K. Stinemetz, LPN
Vatterott College, Des Moines Campus
Des Moines, IA 50321

Jim Wallace, MHSA
Director, Mental Health Billing
Stars Behavioral Health Group
Long Beach, CA 90810

To the Student

YOUR CAREER

This class introduces you to skills you will need in order to work in the health information management profession. A fundamental part of an insurance coding and medical billing specialist's job is to work with the insurance companies that will reimburse your health care facility for the services and treatments you provide to your patients. You may be employed by a hospital, clinic, doctor's office, health maintenance organization, mental health care facility, insurance company, government agency, or long term care facility. This career is challenging, interesting, and one of the ten fastest growing allied health occupations.

HOW CAN I SUCCEED IN THIS CLASS?

If you're reading this, you're on the right track.

> *"You are the same today that you are going to be five years from now except for two things: the people with whom you associate and the books you read."* Charles Jones

Right now, you're probably leafing through this book feeling just a little overwhelmed. You're trying to juggle several other classes (which probably are equally as intimidating), possibly a job, and on top of it all, a life.

These helpful hints have been designed specifically to help you focus. They're here to help you learn how to manage your time and your studies to succeed.

START HERE

It's true—you are what you put into your studies. You have a lot of time and money invested in your education. Don't blow it now by putting in only half of the effort this class requires. Succeeding in this class (and life) requires

- Making a commitment—of time and perseverance
- Knowing and motivating yourself
- Getting organized
- Managing your time

This text will help you learn how to be effective in these areas, as well as offer guidance in

- Getting the most out of your lecture
- Thinking through—and applying—the material

- Getting the most out of your textbook
- Finding extra help when you need it

Making a Commitment—of Time and Perseverance

Learning—and mastering—takes time, and patience. Nothing worthwhile comes easily. Be committed to your studies and you will reap the benefits in the long run.

Consider this: Your college education is building the foundation for your future—a future in your chosen profession. Sloppy and hurried craftsmanship now will only lead to ruin later.

Side note: A good rule of thumb is to allow two hours of study time for every hour you spend in lecture.

For instance, a three-hour lecture deserves six hours of study time. If you commit time for this course daily, you're investing a little less than one hour per day, including the weekend. Study time includes writing reports, completing practice problems, reading textual material, and reviewing notes.

Knowing and Motivating Yourself

What type of a learner are you? When are you most productive? Know yourself and your limits and work within them. Know how to motivate yourself to give your all to your studies and achieve your goals. Quite bluntly, you are the one who benefits most from your success. If you lack self-motivation and drive, you are the first person that suffers.

Knowing yourself—there are many types of learners and no right or wrong way of learning. Which category do you fall into?

Visual learner—you respond best to "seeing" processes and information. Particularly focus on text illustrations and charts and course handouts, and check to see if there are animations on the course or text website to help you. Also, consider drawing diagrams in your notes to illustrate concepts.

Auditory learner—you work best by listening to—and possibly tape recording—the lecture and by talking through information with a study partner.

Tactile/kinesthetic learner—you learn best by being "hands on." You'll benefit by applying what you've learned during lab time. Think of ways to apply your critical thinking skills in application ways.

Identify your personal preferences for learning and seek out the resources that will best help you with your studies. Also, learn by recognizing your weaknesses and try to compensate/work to improve them.

Getting Organized

It's simple, yet it's fundamental. It seems, the more organized you are, the easier things come. Take the time before your course begins to look around and analyze your life and your study habits. Get organized now and you'll find you have a little more time—and a lot less stress.

- **Find a calendar system that works for you**. The best kind is one that you can take with you everywhere. To be truly organized, you should integrate all aspects of your life into this one calendar—school, work, leisure. Some people also find it helpful to have an additional monthly calendar posted by their desk for "at a glance" dates and to have a visual of what's to come. If you do this, be sure you are consistently synchronizing both calendars so as not to miss anything. *More tips for organizing your calendar can be found in the time management discussion.*

- By the same token, **keep everything for your course or courses in one place**—and at your fingertips. A three-ring binder works well because it allows you to add or organize handouts and notes from class in any order you prefer. Incorporating your own custom tabs helps you flip to exactly what you need at a moments notice.

- **Find your space**. Find a place that helps you be organized and focused. If it's your desk in your dorm room or in your home, keep it clean. Clutter adds confusion and stress and wastes time. Or perhaps your "space" is at the library. If that's the case, keep a backpack or bag that's fully stocked with what you might need—your text, binder or notes, pens, highlighters, Post-its, phone numbers of study partners (a good place to keep phone numbers is in your "one place for everything calendar").

A helpful hint—add extra "padding" into your deadlines for yourself. If you have a report due on Friday, set a goal for yourself to have it done on Wednesday. Then, take time on Thursday to look over your project again, with a fresh eye. Make any corrections or enhancements and have it ready to turn in on Friday.

Managing Your Time

Managing your time is the single most important thing you can do to help yourself. And it's probably one of the most difficult tasks to master.

You are in college taking this course because you want to succeed in life. You are preparing for a career. In college, you are expected to work much harder and to learn much more than you ever have before. To be successful, you need to invest in your education with a commitment of time.

We all lead busy lives. But we all make choices as to how we spend our time. Choose wisely and make the most of every minute you have by implementing these tips:

- **Know yourself and when you'll be able to study most efficiently.** When are you most productive? Are you a late nighter? Or an early bird? Plan to study when you are most alert and can have uninterrupted segments. This could include a quick, five-minute review before class or a one-hour problem-solving study session with a friend.

- **Create a set study time for yourself daily.** Having a set schedule for yourself helps you commit to studying and helps you plan instead of cram. Find—and use—a planner that is small enough that you can take it with you—everywhere. This can be a $2.50 paper calendar or a more expensive electronic version. They all work on the same premise—**organize all of your activities in one place.**

- Less is more. **Schedule study time using shorter, focused blocks with small breaks.** Doing this offers two benefits:

  1. You will be less fatigued and gain more from your effort.

  2. Studying will seem less overwhelming and you will be less likely to procrastinate.

- **Plan time for leisure, friends, exercise, and sleep.** Studying should be your main focus, but you need to balance your time—and your life.

- Make sure you **log your projects and homework deadlines** in your personal calendar.

- **"Plot" your assignments on your calendar or task list.** If you have a large report, for instance, break down the assignment into smaller targets. Set a goal for a first draft, second draft, and final copy.

- Try to **complete tasks ahead of schedule.** This will give you a chance to review your work carefully before you hand it in (instead of at 1 A.M., when you are half awake). You'll feel less stressed in the end.

- **Prioritize!** In your calendar or planner, highlight or number key projects; do them first, and then cross them off when you've completed them. Give yourself a pat on the back for getting them done!

- **Review your calendar and reprioritize** daily.

- Try to **resist distractions by setting and sticking to a designated study time** (remember your commitment and perseverance!). Distractions include friends and surfing the Internet.

- **Multitask when possible.** You may find a lot of extra time you didn't think you had. Review material or organize your term paper in your head while walking to class or doing laundry.

Side note: Plan to study and plan for leisure. Being well balanced will help you focus when it is time to study.

Tip: Try combining social time with studying or social time with mealtime or exercise. Being a good student doesn't mean you have to be a hermit. It does mean you need to know how to budget your time smartly.

- **Learn to manage or avoid time wasters.**

Don't

- **Let friends manage your time.**

Tip: Kindly ask, "Can we talk later?" when you are trying to study; this will keep you in control of your time without alienating your friends.

- **Get sucked into the Internet.**

It's easy to lose hours in front of the computer surfing the web. Set a time limit for yourself and stick to it.

Do

- **Use small bits of time to your advantage**.

Example: Arrive to class five minutes early and review notes. Review your personal calendar for upcoming due dates and events while eating meals or waiting for appointments.

- **Balance your life**.

Sleep, study, and leisure are all important. Keep each in balance.

Getting the Most Out of Lectures

Believe it or not, instructors want you to succeed. They put a lot of effort into helping you learn and preparing their lectures. Attending class is one of the simplest, most valuable things you can do to help yourself. But it doesn't end there—getting the most out of your lectures means being organized. Here's how:

Prepare Before You Go to Class

You'll be amazed at how much more comprehensible the material will be when you preview the chapter before you go to class. Don't feel overwhelmed by this already. One tip that may help you is to plan to arrive to class 5–15 minutes before the lecture. Take your text with you and skim the chapter before lecture begins. At the very least, this will give you an overview of what may be discussed.

Be a Good Listener

Most people think they are good listeners, but few really are. Are you? Following are obvious but important points to remember:

- You can't listen if you're talking.
- You aren't listening if you're daydreaming.
- Listening and comprehending are two different things. If you don't understand something your instructor is saying, ask a question or jot a note and visit the instructor after hours. Don't feel dumb or intimidated; you probably aren't the only person who "doesn't get it."

Take Good Notes

- Use a standard-size notebook or, better yet, a three-ring binder with loose-leaf notepaper. The binder will allow you to organize and integrate your notes and handouts, integrate easy-to-reference tabs, and so on.
- Use a standard black or blue ink pen to take your initial notes. You can annotate later using a pencil, which can be erased if need be.
- Start a new page with each lecture or note-taking session (yes—you can and should also take notes from your textbook).
- Label each page with the date and a heading for each day.
- Focus on main points and try to use an outline format to take notes to capture key ideas and organize subpoints.

- Review and edit your notes shortly after class—at least within 24 hours—to make sure they make sense and that you've recorded core thoughts. You may also want to compare your notes with a study partner's later to make sure neither of you has missed anything.

Get a Study Partner

Having a study partner has so many benefits. First, he or she can help you keep your commitment to this class. By having set study dates, you can combine study and social time, and maybe even make it fun! In addition, you now have two sets of eyes and ears and two minds to help digest the information from the lecture and the text. Talk through concepts, compare notes, and quiz each other.

An obvious note: Don't take advantage of your study partner by skipping class or skipping study dates. You obviously won't have a study partner—or a friend—very long if it's not a mutually beneficial arrangement!

Helpful hint: Take your text to lecture, and keep it open to the topics being discussed. You can take brief notes in your textbook margin or reference textbook pages in your notebook to help you study later.

How to Study for an Exam

- Study, don't simply reread material.
- Be an active learner.
- Finish reading all material—text, notes, handouts—at least three days prior to the exam.
- Be an active participant in class; ask questions.
- Apply what you've learned; think through scenarios rather than memorize your notes.
- Three days prior to the exam, set aside time each day to do self-testing, to practice problems, and to review notes.
- Create an "I don't know this yet" list. Focus on strengthening these areas and narrow your list as your study.
- Create your own study tools, such as index card flash cards and checklists, and practice writing short essays if this is how your instructor tests.

Very important: Be sure to sleep and eat well before the exam.

Getting the Most Out of Your Textbook

McGraw-Hill and the author of this book have invested their time, research, and talents to help you succeed, as well. The goal is to make learning—for you—easier.

Here's how:
- Use the chapter objectives to guide you through the material presented.
- Review the key terms and definitions, and make certain you understand them.
- Read and jot down the important notes.

- Use the memory tips.
- Practice critical thinking skills.
- Practice coding using the sample cases and examples.
- Read chapter summaries.
- Complete chapter reviews.
- Explore the online learning center activities.

How to Abstract Notes

INTRODUCTION

The most efficient and effective way to code an encounter between a health care professional and a patient is to review the physician's notes for that encounter. When the coder can read exactly what the physician saw, heard, and observed in his or her own words, there is less confusion and miscommunication. The more accurate the communication between the attending physician and the professional coding specialist, the more accurate the codes will be—ensuring accurate reimbursement.

THE SEVEN STEPS OF CODING

There is a seven-step process for coding a health care encounter in the approved manner. As you gain experience, it will take less time. However, remember that time is not the number one consideration—no matter what anyone says—accuracy is the most important factor.

The steps are as follows:

1. Read through the superbill and the physician's notes for the encounter completely, from beginning to end. Make a copy of the pages relating to the visit, so that you can write on the copy without marking the originals.

≪≪ CODING TIP

Documentation is your watchword. You must have the information *in writing*. If it is not written down (or in a computer document), then as far as you are concerned, it never happened, and therefore, you cannot code it.

1

Query

To ask.

2. Reread through the physician's notes, and highlight key words regarding diagnoses and procedures directly relating to the encounter. Pulling out the _key words_ is also called **abstracting** physician's notes.

3. Make a list of any questions you have regarding unclear or missing information necessary to code the encounter. **Query** the health care provider who treated the patient. _Never assume._ Code only what you know from actual documentation. If the physician answers one of your questions verbally and promises to write it in the chart later, do _not_ code it until you receive the updated chart. It is not an issue of trusting the physician. It is the law that you must have the documentation to back up every code you submit on a claim form.

   Note: In class, your instructor is the person to query about anything you need to code an encounter properly.

EXAMPLE

The documentation indicates that the physician performed a posterior vestibuloplasty on Marion Jones. You pull out the key words: vestibuloplasty and posterior. However, when you look up the procedure in the CPT book, you see that there are two codes to choose from:

   40842 Vestibuloplasty; posterior, unilateral

   40843 Vestibuloplasty; posterior, bilateral

You must query the physician to find out whether the procedure was done unilaterally (one side) or bilaterally (both sides). Make certain the physician answers your question _and_ writes the answer down in the chart and initials it. Now, you know which code is the best, most appropriate code.

4. Code any diagnoses as stated by the physician. When there is no confirmed diagnosis to provide medical necessity for a procedure performed, code the patient's signs and/or symptoms describing why the patient came to see the health care provider for the encounter. Use the best, most appropriate code or codes available based on the documentation.

5. Code the procedure(s) as stated in the notes describing what the provider did for the patient. Use the best, most appropriate code(s) available based on the documentation.

6. Link every procedure code to at least one diagnosis code shown on the same claim form to document medical necessity. Not only is this required, but it is an excellent way to confirm that all your procedure codes are justified by a diagnosis code.

7. Double-check your work by back coding. It means that you look up the code you have chosen in the tabular (numeric) listing and reread the code description and the original notes to make certain they apply. This will help you catch innocent typos, accidentally missing a fourth or fifth digit, or other relevant notation.

Following the above steps will help you code precisely, resulting in a greater number of your claims being paid quickly, at the highest earned reimbursement rate.

THE CODING PROCESS

Many physician's offices are specialized. So you will most likely end up working with a limited number of sections within the International Classification of Diseases, ninth revision, Clinical Modification (ICD-9-CM) and Current Procedural Terminology (CPT) books.

Working for a specialized physician will make the entire process of coding from the huge coding books less intimidating. However, because most of you do not know the type of health care facility that you will be working in and some of you will go to work in a hospital or clinic that typically sees a wide range of illnesses and injuries, our learning here covers the entire array.

The best place to begin the coding process is with the physician's notes and the superbill for the encounter. Abstract, or pull out, the key words relating to the reason *why* the patient came to see the physician for the visit to get the best diagnosis codes and *what* the physician did for the patient to get to the best procedure codes.

Remember, the key words may be identified directly as the diagnosis, or you may need to find the patient's signs and symptoms (often called the patient's *chief complaint*). The procedure provided may be labeled as such, or you may need to read through the complete notes to identify everything that was done for the patient during the encounter.

Once you have identified the related key words abstracted from the notes, turn to the alphabetic index of the appropriate book: ICD-9-CM or CPT. You will use the alphabetic index to guide you to the correct page or category in the tabular (numerical) volume. Then you need to carefully read the code descriptions, beginning at the top of the subheading, so you can make certain that you find the best code, to the highest level of specificity, according to the physician's notes for a particular encounter, and within the directions of the book.

When you begin, you will find that looking for a diagnostic or procedural key word in the alphabetic index may not be as easy as it sounds. Sometimes, however, you find the code right away, and it's a snap!

EXAMPLE

Dr. Kinner diagnoses Alvira Gomez with polyphagia. Turn to the alphabetic index in ICD-9-CM and find Polyphagia 783.6.

Sometimes, you have to really look a little further.

EXAMPLE

Dr. Carlton removed a splinter from Jaleel Waters's finger.

Look in the alphabetic index in CPT under *removal:*

Removal

    Foreign Bodies

        Finger 26075–26080

Then in the tabular (numerical) listing, you see:

26075 Arthrotomy, with exploration, drainage, or removal of loose or foreign body; metacarpophalangeal joint, each

That looks great until you get to the word, *joint.* The splinter was not removed from the joint but from the finger . . . the flesh portion. Look again in the alphabetic index; only this time, you will need to look under:

Removal

    Foreign Body

        Skin

        With debridement 11010–11012

In the tabular (numerical) listing, you see:

11010 Debridement including removal of foreign material associated with open fracture(s) and/or dislocation(s); skin and subcutaneous tissues.

No, that isn't correct either, because there is no mention that Jaleel had a fracture or dislocation. However, read down the column below these codes and see:

11040 Debridement; skin, partial thickness

The term *debridement* means to remove debris. So this, finally, is a good code.

No, you didn't miss anything. Code 11040 is not listed in the alphabetic index anywhere under Removal. To find it in the alphabetic index, look under Debridement, skin, partial thickness. However, for a beginning coder, this is a difficult leap to make from the words the physician used in the notes.

Sometimes, it is like looking for a contact lens on a carpet—you have to really look carefully and think about what the facts are. Jaleel's case is a good example of the fact that, in some cases, determination and perseverance are a coder's best traits. The entire coding process will require you to use your reading skills, your analysis skills, your interpretation skills, and your medical dictionary, to figure it all out. The good news is that it will get easier as you gain more experience and practice.

EXAMPLE

Darlene Samanski broke a drinking glass in her hand. She was pretty certain she got all the glass out and cleaned the wound well, but, two days later, it was still hurting. She went to Dr. Mahoney, who removed several tiny shards of glass left in the wound.

You have to think about this and realize that the glass is actually a foreign body. In addition, you must figure out that the glass is not actually in Darlene's hand; it is in her soft tissue. Now, you will be able to find this in the alphabetic index:

Foreign Body, In, Soft Tissue (residual) 729.6

Other times, you may have to use alternate terms from those used in the notes to find the correct listing. A medical dictionary will help you with this.

Remember, accuracy is the *most* important issue here. It is not a race. You need to be careful and meticulous.

DIAGNOSIS AND MEDICAL NECESSITY

The International Classification of Diseases, ninth revision, Clinical Modification is a directory of every diagnosis, or reason, that a health care provider would spend time with, and/or provide a service to, a patient. Diagnosis codes are very important because they provide the information about why the physician provided a particular service or treatment. These codes establish **medical necessity**. Every procedure code reported must be accompanied by a diagnosis code that justifies that specific procedure. Some examples of diagnoses are a broken ankle, diabetes, or the flu.

Medical necessity

The assessment that the provider was acting according to standard practices in providing a procedure or service for an individual with a specific diagnosis.

PROCEDURES (SERVICES AND TREATMENTS)

In the process of translating procedures (services and treatments) in health care into codes, you might use any of the following volumes:

- CPT—Current Procedural Terminology
- HCPCS—Healthcare Common Procedure Coding System, Level II
- ICD-9-CM, Volume 3—International Classifications of Diseases, ninth revision, Clinical Modification, Volume 3 Procedures

Current Procedural Terminology (CPT), fourth edition, is used for reporting procedures, treatments, and services provided to outpatients—such as an x-ray, a vaccination, or the removal of a cyst—as well as physician's services provided almost anywhere.

The Healthcare Common Procedure Coding System, Level II (HCPCS, which is pronounced "hick-picks") lists codes used to identify the provision of **durable medical equipment (DME)**, medications, and certain other services not listed in the CPT book. Items coded from the HCPCS book might include a wheelchair, crutches, or a unit of blood for a transfusion.

International Classification of Diseases, ninth revision, Clinical Modification, Volume 3 (ICD-9-CM Vol. 3) is used for reported procedures, treatments, and other services provided to an inpatient, one who has been admitted into a hospital and stays overnight in this acute care facility. Codes are used from this volume to reimburse the hospital for its expenses. The physician's, or surgeon's, services are typically reported from CPT, by the physician's office coder, even though the services were provided in a hospital.

Durable medical equipment (DME)

Items that are used in the care and treatment of a patient that can either last a long time or can be used again and again.

ACCURACY

Each set of numbers and letters means something so specific that a code number just one digit off could mean something totally unrelated. Everyone can make an error occasionally transposing two numbers when writing, or typing, a sequence. You will be thinking 1-7-1, and accidentally write down 711. Instead of your just dialing the wrong phone number, that difference could cause the claim to be rejected, denied, or pulled for investigation, resulting in your office having to deal with delayed payment, or no payment at all, for the work it did. That is why it is critical to be careful and accurate when coding. *Always* double-check your codes.

EXAMPLE

301.7 Antisocial personality disorder (a neurosis)

307.1 Anorexia nervosa (an eating disorder)

EXAMPLE

30520 Septoplasty or submucous resection, with or without cartilage scoring, contouring or replacement with graft . . . *nose surgery*

DIFFERENT STYLES OF MEDICAL NOTES

SOAP Notes

No, SOAP notes do not have anything to do with the importance of washing your hands before seeing a patient. These notes are written in an outline format using four sections: subjective, objective, assessment, and plan. The term SOAP is an acronym for the four section titles.

*S*ubjective is the first section and will include the reason for the patient's visit today (chief complaint), status regarding current medications and/or treatments, history (family, problem-focused, and/or social), and an itemization of the symptoms.

*O*bjective, section two, will contain the results of any physical examination performed including vital signs, height/weight, etc., physician's observations, and the results of any diagnostic testing related to the concern at hand.

*A*ssessment is the diagnosis, or the physician's conclusions. If there is no definitive diagnosis, the coder must reread the objective portion of the notes to look for positive test results (such as a statement reading, "X-ray showed lateral fracture of the tibia") for coding a diagnosis. If there is no confirmed diagnosis as a result of the testing, then the patient's symptoms must be coded.

*P*lan, the last part of the notes, will document the physician's orders for the patient. These may include diagnostic tests to be done in the future, procedures to be performed ("Colonoscopy scheduled to be done in one week"), recommendations for lifestyle changes ("Patient is advised to quit drinking alcoholic beverages as soon as possible"), and follow-up care ("Recheck CBC in two weeks").

Many physicians like SOAP notes because they are more orderly and tend to be more thorough. With this format, they are reminded to address each portion, as they are dictating, or writing, to document all aspects of the encounter with the patient.

Figure 1-1 is an example of SOAP notes taken from a family practitioner. See if you can relate what each of the four terms means to the content of each paragraph or section.

Narrative Notes

Some physicians prefer to dictate their notes using the narrative format, as shown in Figure 1-2. It means that they tell the story of the encounter with the patient, including all the details. This is typed and presented in paragraph format.

Generally, it seems that family physicians, who may plan more time between appointments and have a wider scope of interest with regard to their patient's health (the whole body), tend to prefer SOAP notes, whereas specialists, who see their patients in sequenced appointments

««« CODING TIP

In Figure 1-1, an example of SOAP notes, you will notice the acronym MRN that stands for medical record number. At the bottom, under the physician's signature, you will see the date the notes were dictated (identified by the *D*), the date the notes were transcribed (identified by the *T*), and the initials of the medical transcriptionist (which in this case are *nk*).

PROGRESS NOTE

PT NAME:	YORK, MARY LOU
DATE:	03/03/08
DOB:	05/27/88
MRN:	05003579

S: This Pt is a 19-year-old white female, G0, LMP 2/18, not sexually active, not on any birth control that presents today with two main complaints. The first complaint is she feels a lump in her right groin. The second complaint is a vaginal discharge, no odor or itching, just feels irritated.

O: Pelvic exam revealed the external genitalia to be within normal limits. The vagina was without lesions. Scant discharge seen. Wet mount neg for Trichomonas, clue cells or hyphae. Increased bacteria in the background noted. Inspection of the rt groin revealed no abnormality. The Pt was asked to point out the area of abnormality and this felt to be dilated areas within one of the vessels in the groin. These were less than the size of a pea and did not feel like lymphadenopathy. Similar areas were felt on the lt side as well. The patient was reassured.

A: Possible nonspecific vaginitis

P: 1. Cleocin vaginal cream qhs times seven nights.
   2. Follow up in one month for reinspection of the rt groin.
   3. Otherwise follow up with us prn. She verbalized understanding.
   4. All questions were answered. She will follow up with us prn or for her yearly Pap smear.

Harold Donnelson, M.D.

D: 03/03/08
T: 03/08/08 nk

Figure 1-1 Example of SOAP Notes.

with more regularity and for a more singular focus (one particular part of the body and often one concern), tend to prefer the narrative notes. It may be because specialists typically will not have vital signs taken and documented with each visit, unless they are applicable to the problem, as well as the fact that each consecutive visit with a specialist is a follow-up to the original concern.

However, it is the physician's personal preference. For the coder and biller in the office, the only difference will be that SOAP notes' outline format can make it easier and faster to find the diagnosis, whereas the narrative format would require a more thorough reading of the entire encounter.

Procedure Notes

Procedure and operative reports, as shown in Figure 1-3, contain different types of information than standard office visit documentation. That is why these reports take on a different format.

PROGRESS NOTE

PT NAME: GROGANZI, ALFRED
DOB: 07/13/85
MRN: 06002795

Date: 09/08/07

[Office Visit] This patient is coming along well since his colonoscopy. He is having minimal problems. Examination reveals mild colitis. He was told I would not put him on any type of treatment at this time. The patient doesn't want to take steroids, he is not having enough problems to warrant steroids. We will see him again in three months. ks

Date: 12/18/07

[Office Visit] This patient is getting along exceptionally well. He was scoped up to 40 cm and has colitis up this far. However the worst of it is in the last ten centimeters. The patient will be given another course of Flagyl to see if we can get this to resolve. We will check him in three weeks. ks

Date: 01/09/08

[Office Visit] This patient is in today and he still has his colitis. It is getting worse. We will start him on some Rowasa. We will give him one a night for three weeks. We will see him after that and see how he is getting along. He will probably have to take it for six weeks before we will see a difference. ks

Suzanne Esperanza, M.D.

Figure 1-2   Example of Narrative Notes.

For extensive procedures that need operative support, such as those usually done in same-day surgical centers, the attending physicians may use an indications, procedure, impression, and plan (IPIP) outline format for their reports. In these cases, time is not typically spent discussing things with the patient or any other evaluation and management services. Often, the patient comes in, the procedure is performed, and the patient goes home. Follow-up will be done when the patient sees the physician in the office for the next appointment.

The sections on these reports include:

Indications: A statement of the diagnosis that is the reason for the procedure

Procedure: A step-by-step accounting of what was done during the procedure

Impression: The physician's impression of the results or findings of the procedure

Plan: The action to be taken for the patient's continued treatment

Hospital operative reports are similar, but will typically include a preoperative diagnosis and a postoperative diagnosis, along with a

PROGRESS NOTE

PT NAME: CASSIDY, CAROLINE
DOB: 07/13/85
MRN: 06002795
Date: 07/29/08
Procedure Performed: Colonoscopy

Physician: Morris Samson, M.D.
Indications: History of colitis

PROCEDURE: The patient was given no premedication at her request and the Olympus PCF-130 colon-oscope was used. The mucosa of the rectum was essentially normal apart from some mild nonspecific edema. Photographs and biopsies were obtained. The remainder of the rectum was normal. The sigmoid was normal as was the descending colon, splenic flexure, transverse colon, hepatic flexure, right colon and cecum. No evidence of polyps, tumors, masses, or inflammation. The scope was then withdrawn, these findings confirmed. The procedure was terminated and the patient tolerated it well.

IMPRESSION: Normal colonic mucosa through the cecum.

PLAN: Await results of rectal biopsies.

Morris Samson, M.D.

Figure 1-3   Example of Physician's Procedure Notes.

report of what was done during the procedure and what the findings were. Take a look at Figure 1-3.

LET'S CODE IT! _____

Let's go over a couple of the cases, and review the notes together.

Case #1. Sierra White

COMMUNITY HEALTH CENTER
A Complete Health Care Facility
159 CENTRAL AVENUE • SOMEWHERE, FL 32811 • 407-555-4321

PATIENT: WHITE, SIERRA
ACCOUNT/EHR #:   WHITSI001

Date: 09/16/08

Attending Physician: James I. Cipher, MD

S: This new Pt is a 25-year-old female who was involved in a 2 car MVA while driving on the job. She is complaining about some neck pain. She has tingling into her right hand and both feet. She states that her arm hurts when she tries to pull it overhead. She apparently was told, by a friend, that she should likely need to see a spine doctor, but somehow she came to see me first. PMH is remarkable for kidney trouble. Past bronchoscopy, laparoscopy and kidney stone surgery, otherwise noncontributory as per the medical history form completed by the patient and reviewed at this visit.

O: Ht 5′5″ Wt. 179 lb. R 16. Pt presented in a sling. She was told to use it by the same friend. She states if she does not use it her arm does not feel any different, so I had her remove it. She states that she has not had any prior injury to this area, and has no previous problems with her musculoskeletal system. On exam, HEENT: unremarkable. Neck muscles are taut, particularly on the left side. The left shoulder demonstrates full passive motion, with normal strength testing. No deformity is observable. Pt. states there is some tenderness over the trapezial area. The reflexes are brisk and symmetric. X-rays of her chest 2 views and C spine AP/LAT are relatively benign, as are complete x-rays of the shoulder.

A: Contusion of upper arm and shoulder

P: 1. Order MRI to rule out torn ligament
    2. Rx Naprosyn
    3. Referral to PT
    4. Referral to orthopedist

James I. Cipher, MD
JIC/mg D: 9/16/08 09:50:16 T: 9/18/08 12:55:01

Let's begin by identifying the key words relating to the diagnosis or diagnoses: the reason *why* Sierra White came to see Dr. Cipher on September 16. Let's go through the notes and pull out the terms.

PATIENT:	WHITE, SIERRA
ACCOUNT/EHR #:	WHITSI001
Date:	09/16/08
Attending Physician:	James I. Cipher, MD

S: This new Pt is a 25-year-old female who was involved in a *2 car MVA* while *driving on the job.* She is complaining about some *neck pain.* She has *tingling into her right hand and both feet.* She states that her *arm hurts* when she tries to pull it overhead. She apparently was told, by a friend, that she should likely need to see a spine doctor, but somehow she came to see me first. PMH is remarkable for kidney trouble. Past bronchoscopy, laparoscopy and kidney stone surgery, otherwise noncontributory as per the medical history form completed by the patient and reviewed at this visit.

O: Ht 5′5″ Wt. 179 lb. R 16. Pt presented in a sling. She was told to use it by the same friend. She states if she does not use it her arm does not feel any different, so I had her remove it. She states that she has not had any prior injury to this area, and has no previous problems with her musculoskeletal system. On exam, HEENT: unremarkable. Neck muscles are taut, particularly on the left side. The left shoulder demonstrates full passive motion, with normal strength testing. No deformity is observable. Pt. states there is some *tenderness over the trapezial area.* The reflexes are brisk and symmetric. X-rays of her chest 2 views and C spine AP/LAT are relatively benign, as are complete x-rays of the shoulder.

A: *Contusion of upper arm and shoulder*

P: 1. Order MRI to rule out torn ligament

2. Rx Naprosyn
3. Referral to PT
4. Referral to orthopedist

You can see from the notes that Ms. White was involved in a *car accident* while on the job. This tells us *how* the patient was injured, leading us to the correct E code. The E code gives you the opportunity to report that she was in a motor vehicle collision.

E812.0 Other motor vehicle traffic accident involving collision with motor vehicle, driver of motor vehicle other than motorcycle, driver

Based on the notes, this is all the information you have about the accident. In the real world, you would need to query the patient to get more details about where the accident occurred, so you could determine whether the claim should be sent to the automobile insurance company or workers' compensation.

Key words and terms that identify *why* Ms. White came to see Dr. Cipher include:

Neck pain

Tingling into her right hand and both feet

Arm hurts

Tenderness over the trapezial area

Contusion of upper arm and shoulder

You learned in anatomy and physiology (or from querying the doctor or from a reference book) that the neck pain, tingling, arm hurting, and tenderness are all component, or included, signs and symptoms of the contusion—the physician's diagnosis.

Go to the alphabetic index of the ICD-9-CM book and look up *contusion.* You will find

Contusion

Arm 923.9

Lower (with elbow) 923.10

Upper 923.03

With shoulder or axillary region 923.09

Which of these listings matches the physician's notes? *Contusion, upper arm with shoulder* matches exactly!

You know that you should *never, never, never* code from the alphabetic index, so let's go into the numeric (tabular) portion of the ICD-9-CM book and check the code suggested by the index.

923.09 Contusion of upper limb, shoulder and upper arm, multiple sites

The description "multiple sites" matches our physician's notes because the shoulder and upper arm are both mentioned.

So the two codes we need to identify *why* Sierra White came to see Dr. Cipher today are

923.09

E812.0

CODING TIP »»

E codes are never first-listed codes.

E codes are never permitted to stand alone.

E codes are only reported for the first health care encounter for the injury.

Now, let's go through the notes to determine the correct procedure codes. Read through the notes and choose the key words that identify *what* the physician did for Ms. White, with regard to the diagnosis.

PATIENT: WHITE, SIERRA
ACCOUNT/EHR #: WHITSI001
Date: 09/16/08
Attending Physician: James I. Cipher, MD

S: This *new Pt* is a 25-year-old female who was involved in a 2 car MVA while driving on the job. She is complaining about some neck pain. She has tingling into her right hand and both feet. She states that her arm hurts when she tries to pull it overhead. She apparently was told, by a friend, that she should likely need to see a spine doctor, but somehow she came to see me first. *PMH* is remarkable for kidney trouble. Past bronchoscopy, laparoscopy and kidney stone surgery, otherwise noncontributory as per the *medical history form* completed by the patient and *reviewed at this visit.*

O: Ht 5'5" Wt. 179 lb. R 16. Pt presented in a sling. She was told to use it by the same friend. She states if she does not use it her arm does not feel any different, so I had her remove it. She states that she has not had any prior injury to this area, and has no previous problems with her musculoskeletal system. On exam, *HEENT: unremarkable. Neck* muscles are taut, particularly on the left side. The left *shoulder* demonstrates full passive motion, with normal strength testing. No deformity is observable. Pt. states there is some tenderness over the trapezial area. The reflexes are brisk and symmetric. *X-rays of her chest 2 views* and *C spine AP/LAT* are relatively benign, as are *complete x-rays of the shoulder.*

A: Contusion of upper arm and shoulder

P: 1. Order MRI to rule out torn ligament
   2. *Rx Naprosyn*
   3. Referral to PT
   4. Referral to orthopedist

During the time that Dr. Cipher spent with Ms. White during this *office visit,* he did the following:

- Took a *detailed history* (pertinent past, family, and/or social history directly related to the patient's problem).
- Examined her HEENT (head, eyes, ears, nose, throat), neck, and shoulder.

This information tells us that, during the office visit, Dr. Cipher examined two body areas (head and neck) and three organ systems (eyes; ears, nose, mouth, and throat; and musculoskeletal). As per the guidelines, this is a *detailed examination.*

- Dr. Cipher's medical decision-making was of a *low complexity.* The possible diagnoses are limited, based on his examination; there are not many treatment options from which to choose; and the complications and comorbidities involved are few to none.
- The notes also identify that Ms. White is a *new patient.*

All these key components lead us directly to the E/M code 99203.

In addition to the evaluation of Ms. White's condition, the notes also indicate that x-rays were taken in the office. Each x-ray must be reported so Dr. Cipher and his facility can be reimbursed for these services.

First, we code for "x-rays of her chest 2 views":

71020 Radiologic examination, chest, two views, frontal and lateral

Second, we have "C spine AP/LAT":

72040 Radiologic examination, spine, cervical; two or three views

NOTE: C spine = cervical spine; AP = anterior posterior; Lat = lateral

Third, we code "Complete x-rays of the shoulder":

73030 Radiological examination, shoulder; complete, minimum two views

Therefore, our claim form for Sierra White's visit with Dr. Cipher on September 16 will show:

Diagnosis codes:	923.09
	E812.0
Procedure codes:	99203
	71020
	72040
	73030

Good job!

Case #2. Frances Franklin

Okay, let's look at another case. Let's read through the case of Frances Franklin and identify the key words relating to the diagnosis, or *why* she came to see Dr. Victors on October 17.

COMMUNITY HEALTH CENTER
A Complete Health Care Facility
159 CENTRAL AVENUE • SOMEWHERE, FL 32811 • 407-555-4321

PATIENT: FRANKLIN, FRANCES
ACCOUNT/EHR #:   FRANFR001

Date: 10/17/08

Attending Physician: Valerie R. Victors, MD

S: This 57-year-old female came for her *routine annual physical exam.* Pt does not smoke, drinks alcohol occasionally, and exercises three times per week. Pt states she has no specific health concerns at this time. I last saw her one year ago.

O: Ht 5'3" Wt. 145 lb. R 20. HEENT: unremarkable; Respiratory: unremarkable; Musculoskeletal: age appropriate. No sign of osteoporosis. Bone density appropriate. Discussed the importance of keeping up her exercise regimen. Comprehensive metabolic panel done, awaiting results.

A: Pt is in good health.

P: 1. Follow-up prn
      2. Schedule screening mammogram

Valerie R. Victors, MD
VRV/mg D: 10/18/08 09:50:16 T: 10/23/08 12:55:01

Chapter 1   How to Abstract Notes

The key words are *routine annual physical exam.* There do not seem to be any other statements pointing toward why Ms. Franklin came to the doctor's office.

Generally, the word *examination* would be used to identify a procedure or service, but in this case, it will actually provide the medical reason why this healthy woman saw the physician. You may remember that the ICD-9-CM includes codes for such occasions—when a person without a current illness or injury needs to meet with a health care provider. These codes are V codes (think preventive).

Go to the alphabetic index in the ICD-9-CM and look up:

Examination (general) (routine) (of)(for) V70.9

    Allergy V72.7

    Annual V70.0

The notes state routine exam, for which the index suggests code V70.9. There is also a listing for annual exam, with suggested code V70.0. An *annual exam* is another term used for routine exam. Go to the numeric listing, and read the descriptions for both codes very carefully.

    V70.0 Routine general medical examination at a health care facility

    V70.9 Unspecified general medical examination

Honestly, the first code, V70.0 is a more specific code and accurately reports what was done for Frances Franklin. This one code tells the whole story as to *why* Ms. Franklin came to see Dr. Victors. Good!

Now, let's review the notes for documentation on *what* Dr. Victors did for Ms. Franklin.

PATIENT: FRANKLIN, FRANCES
ACCOUNT/EHR #:   FRANFR001
Date: 10/17/08

Attending Physician: Valerie R. Victors, MD

S: This 57-year-old female came for her *routine annual physical exam.* Pt does not smoke, drinks alcohol occasionally, and exercises three times per week. Pt states she has no specific health concerns at this time. I last saw her one year ago.

O: Ht 5′3″ Wt. 145 lb. R 20. HEENT: unremarkable; Respiratory: unremarkable; Musculoskeletal: age appropriate. No sign of osteoporosis. Bone density appropriate. Discussed the importance of keeping up her exercise regimen. *Comprehensive metabolic panel* done, awaiting results.

A: Pt is in good health.

P: 1. Follow-up prn
      2. Schedule screening mammogram

Interestingly, the same key words that identify the *why* also identify the *what:* routine annual physical exam. It is clear from the notes that this is an office visit; however, as you look through the documentation, you see that there is no description of the three key components required for a typical evaluation and management code. There is no documentation of a patient history being taken, nor is there any indication of medical decision-making. Therefore, you must look elsewhere in the E/M section.

You know that the diagnosis code (V70.0) is the one for preventive medicine. Again, there is a direct connection to the procedure code for this encounter. Look up *preventive medicine services* in the CPT book alphabetic index. The index recommends the range 99381–99397. Just as with ICD-9-CM, you *never, never, never* code from the alphabetic index. So let's turn to the numeric listing (in the E/M code section) and look at the code descriptions.

The first thing you should note is the long introduction to this subsection. Be certain to read it carefully because it contains important information that coders need to properly assign codes.

Next, you see that the codes are divided into two categories, just like other subsections of this portion of the CPT: new patient and established patient.

Is Frances Franklin a new patient or an established patient? The notes state, "I last saw her one year ago." She is an established patient.

What else do you need to know from the notes to find the correct code? It appears that the codes change based on the age of the patient. How old is Frances Franklin? She's 57 years old.

These details all come together to point us toward the most accurate code:

99396 Periodic comprehensive preventive medicine reevaluation and management of an individual; established patient ;40–64 years

Good coding!

But, wait, you are not finished yet. Dr. Victors has her own way of writing her notes. She has indicated that a comprehensive metabolic panel was performed. If it were to be performed elsewhere, this would state that the panel needed to be done or needed to be scheduled (as the screening mammogram is written).

You would all like our physicians to write their notes in the clearest, easiest to understand manner for us to interpret into codes. Some will, and some won't. It is our responsibility to work with the information given to us, and ask for confirmation or additional details. You are never to assume, guess, or suppose. If it is not documented clearly, you must query. This is in the job description of a professional coding specialist.

So you must code the comprehensive metabolic panel. Looking this up will require you to use your education and knowledge. There are two ways you can find the correct code:

1. You will need to know that the comprehensive metabolic panel is a blood test, and look it up that way in the CPT alphabetic index. You will find:

Blood Tests

    Panels

        Metabolic

            Comprehensive 80053

2. You will need to know that the comprehensive metabolic panel is a lab test, and turn to the Pathology and Laboratory section of the CPT book, the codes that begin with 8.

Either way, you should find the correct code for the test:

80053 Comprehensive metabolic panel

This brings us to the three codes that report the entire story of Frances Franklin and her visit to Dr. Victors on October 17:

Diagnosis code: V70.0

Procedure codes: 99396

                            80053

Good work!

CHAPTER SUMMARY

Abstracting physician's notes is a very important part of a professional coding specialist's responsibilities. It is the only way that you can assure yourself, and those you work for, that you are using the codes that most accurately report the diagnoses and procedures relevant to a particular encounter.

As you read through the notes, you must be careful to identify the key words that relate to why the patient came to see the health care provider for the visit. If the patient is injured or has been poisoned, you must also use codes to notify the third-party payer how and where it happened. The information will also be used so you can send the claim form to the correct insurance carrier.

You will then need to pull out the key words regarding the procedures and services provided to the patient. Be certain to use modifiers, when appropriate, to report special circumstances.

Remember that ancillary services such as durable medical equipment and professionally administered medications are coded from the HCPCS Level II book and services of all kinds provided to a patient who had been admitted into the hospital (an inpatient) will be coded from the ICD-9-CM Volume 3 to reimburse the hospital for what was done.

1. The seven steps of coding include all except

    a. Query the health care provider who wrote the notes.

    b. Abstract the notes to identify key words.

    c. Code from the superbill only.

    d. Link every procedure code to at least one diagnosis code.

2. Key words used to indicate the reason why the patient came to see a health care provider for the encounter will lead you to the correct

    a. Diagnosis code.

    b. Procedure code.

    c. Evaluation and management code.

    d. HCPCS Level II code.

3. Medical necessity is the confirmation that the procedures provided were done so within

    a. The physician's office.

    b. Standards of medical care.

    c. Coding guidelines.

    d. The latest technology.

4. HCPCS Level II codes report the provision of all except

    a. Durable medical equipment.

    b. Transportation services.

    c. Health care supplies.

    d. Prescriptions that are self-administered.

5. ICD-9-CM Volume 3 procedure codes are used to report services and procedures provided to

    a. Patients in an ambulatory care center.

    b. Physician's office.

    c. Hospital inpatient.

    d. Clinic.

6. In SOAP notes, you will most likely find the patient's chief complaint in the section marked

    a. Subjective.

    b. Objective.

    c. Assessment.

    d. Plan.

7. The health care provider will document the observations and results of the physical examination and any diagnostic tests in the section marked

    a. Subjective.

    b. Objective.

    c. Assessment.

    d. Plan.

8. Narrative or progress notes are most often used by

    a. Radiologists.

    b. Family physicians.

    c. Specialists.

    d. Pathologists.

9. When abstracting notes, the identification of what the provider did for and to the patient will lead you to the correct

    a. Diagnosis codes.

    b. Procedure codes.

    c. E codes.

    d. V codes.

10. When the patient's signs and symptoms, as stated in the S portion of the notes, lead the physician to identify a specific diagnosis, codes should identify

    a. The signs only.

    b. The symptoms only.

    c. The diagnosis only.

    d. All of the above.

Allergy and Immunology Cases and Patient Records

INTRODUCTION

The following case studies are from an allergy/immunology office. In a physician's office of this type, a professional coding specialist is likely to see many different health situations.

Allergists, also known as immunologists, are physicians who specialize in the diagnosis and treatment of conditions and diseases that involve the immune system. These health care professionals treat individuals with such concerns as asthma; allergies to food, medications, animals, or environmental elements such as pollen; and autoimmune diseases including human immunodeficiency virus (HIV) and lupus erythematosus.

Allergy/immunology specialists may focus on treating a specific type of condition, such as rheumatoid arthritis, or they may specialize in patients of certain age groups, such as pediatric allergists, who only treat children.

Allergists can be board-certified by the Board of Allergy and Immunology, which is recognized by the American Board of Medical Specialties.

You can use the following cases to practice coding diagnoses, E/M, procedures, DME, or other HCPCS Level II items, as applicable; code for the physician or the facility:

1. Code for the physician.

2. Code for the anesthesiologist, when applicable.

3. Code for the hospital, when applicable.

4. Code for the pathology and laboratory, when applicable.

5. Code HCPCS Level II codes, when applicable.

MORRIS, SHALLERT & ASSOCIATES
Allergy & Immunology
975 CENTRAL AVENUE • SOMEWHERE, FL 32811 • 407-555-4321

PATIENT: BAPTISMA, CORRINE
ACCOUNT/EHR #:   BAPTCO001
Date: 09/16/08

Attending Physician: Suzanne R. Shallert, MD

This fifty-five-year-old female was admitted for a high fever and obtundation. She had been treated with oral antibiotics for left ear fullness (clogged up) and decreased hearing for one week. Three days ago, I saw the patient in the office and her left ear spontaneously drained.

On PE, the patient appears confused and febrile. Her left ear continues to drain. Spinal fluid is turbid and showed 6250 WBC, 330 mg% protein, and 21 mg% glucose.

Two blood cultures are positive for arbovirus. She responded to antimicrobial therapy and except for the reduction of hearing on the left, there are no neurologic sequelae. If patient continues to improve, she can be discharged home tomorrow.

DX. Meningitis due to arbovirus, urban; acute suppurative otitis media

Suzanne R. Shallert, MD

SRS/pw   D: 9/16/08 09:50:16   T: 9/18/08 12:55:01

You Code It!

What are the best, most accurate codes?

_____

_____

_____

MORRIS, SHALLERT & ASSOCIATES
Allergy & Immunology
975 CENTRAL AVENUE • SOMEWHERE, FL 32811 • 407-555-4321

PATIENT: WRIGHT, LEA
ACCOUNT/EHR #:   WRIGLE001
Date: 08/11/08

Consulting Physician: Marcus Morris, MD

Attending Physician: Willard B. Reader, MD

Dr. Reader asked me to consult on this patient, due to PMH of HIV positive status.

    Patient was admitted by Dr. Reader into the cardiology unit with a chief complaint of shortness of breath of approximately one-week duration. PMH: HIV positive in March 2000; manifestation of AIDS in August 2003.

    Patient reports that she has lost approximately twelve pounds within the last four weeks.

    T 102.5° Wt 115 lb. Ht 5'7" Red and blue skin lesions are noted in her mouth, specifically the upper palate. Lesions biopsied earlier today are positive for Kaposi's. Explained diagnosis and treatment options with patient and family at bedside. They will call me when a decision is made.

DX. Kaposi's sarcoma of the palate, secondary to AIDS

_____

Marcus Morris, MD

MM/pw   D: 08/11/08 09:50:16   T: 08/13/08 12:55:01

You Code It!

What are the best, most accurate codes?

_____

_____

_____

MORRIS, SHALLERT & ASSOCIATES
Allergy & Immunology
975 CENTRAL AVENUE • SOMEWHERE, FL 32811 • 407-555-4321

PATIENT: BASCINTRASEN, ERNEST
ACCOUNT/EHR #:   BASCER001
Date: 07/23/08

Attending Physician: Suzanne R. Shallert, MD

History: This 47-year-old male has a history of chronic sinusitis with perennial nasal allergy and several attempts at desensitization using allergy injections. He had several sinus surgery procedures for chronic sinusitis and removal of nasal polyps. He is seen today for the first time and volunteered that he has been "sick all his life." He complained of nasal stuffiness, sinus pressure, ear pressure, and constant post-nasal drainage. He had episodes of asthma which were particularly bad in May when boating on a lake. He frequently felt short of breath with wheezing and had sinus headaches through the frontal and maxillary areas. He had the diagnosis of celiac disease made through a blood test and avoids wheat and gluten. He had eczema as a child and still has occasional patches on the elbows.

Exam: He had small nasal polyps bilaterally with much lymphoid hyperplasia in the posterior pharynx and post-nasal drainage. The exam was otherwise normal. His previous allergy treatment was at a local hospital and he had been treated with antihistamines and topical nasal steroids as well as Atrovent and albuterol lung inhalers.

Skin testing: He reacted quite strongly to dust and dust mites and to the molds and formalin, but did not react to ragweed mixture, grass mixture, or Midwest tree mixture.

Progress note: The patient will be started on treatment 7/24/08 with sublingual antigens appropriate for the testing results for dust, dust mite, Alternaria, Cladosporium, aspergillus, Penicillium, and four other mold mixtures. (He also reacted to formaldehyde, and this was included in the sublingual antigen.) He is given a prescription for Sporanox capsules to be taken twice weekly for yeast and mold colonization. He should continue the sublingual antigens and will be seen again in four to six weeks.

Suzanne R. Shallert, MD

SRS/pw   D: 7/23/08 09:50:16   T: 7/27/08 12:55:01

You Code It!

What are the best, most accurate codes?

_____

_____

_____

MORRIS, SHALLERT & ASSOCIATES
Allergy & Immunology
975 CENTRAL AVENUE • SOMEWHERE, FL 32811 • 407-555-4321

PATIENT: BASCINTRASEN, ERNEST
ACCOUNT/EHR #:   BASCER001
Date: 09/06/08

Attending Physician: Suzanne R. Shallert, MD

Progress notes: Patient shows a very dramatic response. Treatment was effective in just five weeks. Primary allergic treatment using sublingual antigens and Sporanox to decrease mold and yeast growth rapidly has helped him to do better than he has in years. Sublingual treatment will be continued, and he will be seen every six months until testing of the inhalants is negative or near negative. He will be given antibiotics for any acute respiratory infection and followed with antifungals if needed.

Suzanne R. Shallert, MD

SRS/pw   D: 9/06/08 09:50:16   T: 9/18/08 12:55:01

You Code It!

What are the best, most accurate codes?

_____

_____

_____

MORRIS, SHALLERT & ASSOCIATES
Allergy & Immunology
975 CENTRAL AVENUE • SOMEWHERE, FL 32811 • 407-555-4321

PATIENT: BRANCH, BETHANY
ACCOUNT/EHR #:   BRANBE001
Date: 08/11/08

Attending Physician: Willard B. Reader, MD

This 58-year-old female was admitted with cough of thirteen weeks duration. Pt also complained of headache and nasal discharge.

History—She has a history of urticaria and multiple drug allergies including ampicillin, ibuprofen, diclofenac.
    Previously any drug given to her for pain resulted in skin rashes, pruritus and facial edema. She was administered oral paracetamol (500 mg) on admission at 0930. At about 1110, the patient developed severe itching and rash all over the body along with facial edema and swelling of lips. This was quickly followed by change in voice and tachypnea.

Examination—Her blood pressure was 124/80 mm Hg on admission. Respiratory system examination was unremarkable except for tenderness over frontal sinuses. After intake of paracetamol, she was found to have hypotension and altered sensorium. Diffuse rhonchi was heard on auscultation.

Diagnosis: Anaphylactic shock

Testing—Her blood counts revealed hemoglobin of 12.7 g/dl, total leucocyte count of 9,100/mm³ with 3% eosinophils. Chest x-ray and electrocardiogram were normal. X-ray paranasal sinuses was suggestive of frontal sinusitis.

Treatment—Injection adrenaline 0.5 ml (1:1000) was given intramuscularly and rapid infusion of normal saline along with high flow nasal oxygen was started. Intravenous dopamine in normal saline was also started as blood pressure was not recordable. Nebulized salbutamol was given every 15 minutes till bronchospasm was controlled. Hydrocortisone (200 mg) was given intravenously and patient was kept under close monitoring. Injection adrenaline was repeated after 20 minutes and infusion of normal saline and dopamine continued till systolic blood pressure had risen to above 90 mm Hg.
    Patient recovered fully within two hours.

Willard B. Reader, MD

WBR/pw   D: 08/11/08 09:50:16   T: 08/13/08 12:55:01

You Code It!

What are the best, most accurate codes?

_____

_____

_____

MORRIS, SHALLERT & ASSOCIATES
Allergy & Immunology
975 CENTRAL AVENUE • SOMEWHERE, FL 32811 • 407-555-4321

PATIENT: CARLTON, NELSON
ACCOUNT/EHR #:   CARLNE001
Date: 08/11/08

Attending Physician: Marcus Morris, MD

Patient is a 67-year-old male brought into the Emergency Department by ambulance with increasing dyspnea, productive cough, and progressive weakness.

His condition deteriorated quickly and was sent up immediately to the ICU on the second floor. I was called in on consultation.

The patient was intubated and mechanically ventilated. Broad-spectrum antibiotics were ordered and administered IV for septic shock, respiratory failure and Hemophilus influenza pneumonia.

DX. Septic shock with respiratory failure, pneumonia due to H. influenza

___

Marcus Morris, MD

MM/pw   D: 08/11/08 09:50:16   T: 08/13/08 12:55:01

You Code It!

What are the best, most accurate codes?

___

___

___

MORRIS, SHALLERT & ASSOCIATES
Allergy & Immunology
975 CENTRAL AVENUE • SOMEWHERE, FL 32811 • 407-555-4321

PATIENT: WRIGHT, PAUL
ACCOUNT/EHR #:   WRIGPA001
Date: 09/15/08

Attending Physician: Suzanne R. Shallert, MD

S: This new Pt is a 5-year-old male brought to this office by his father. He has been suffering from fatigue and appears to be experiencing moderate edema. Two weeks ago, the father states that the boy had a sore throat. This was treated with over-the-counter medications.

O: Ht 3'3" Wt. 45 lb. R 23. BP 100/80. UA reveals proteinuria and hematuria. CBC indicates RBC, WBC and mixed cell casts common in urinary sediment. Elevated serum creatinine levels, and low creatinine clearance with impaired glomerular filtration evident. Elevated antistreptolysin-O titers, elevated streptozyme and anti-DNase titers, and low serum complement levels. Throat culture shows group A beta-hemolytic streptococcus. Renal ultrasound is unremarkable.

A: Acute post-streptococcal glomerulonephritis secondary to streptococcal pharyngitis

P: 1. Bed rest, fluids
      2. Diet should be no/low sodium
      3. Rx diuretic; antibiotic 7-10 days
      4. Return in 2 weeks for follow-up

Suzanne R. Shallert, MD

SRS/pw   D: 09/15/08 09:50:16   T: 09/17/08 12:55:01

You Code It!

What are the best, most accurate codes?

_____

_____

_____

MORRIS, SHALLERT & ASSOCIATES
Allergy & Immunology
975 CENTRAL AVENUE • SOMEWHERE, FL 32811 • 407-555-4321

PATIENT: HAYES, LEONARD
ACCOUNT/EHR #:   HAYELE001
Date: 09/15/08

Attending Physician: Suzanne R. Shallert, MD

This 55-year-old male comes in with a complaint of bilateral hearing loss and allergy symptoms. He states that his hearing loss has been going on for several years, but he feels the right ear is worse than the left. He does admit to using Q-tips. He was seen by his primary care physician back in August and was told he had no wax impactions. He has had no otorrhea or tinnitus. He has no history of ear surgery, recent skull trauma, or noise exposure.

    The review of systems, past medical history, family history, and social history are per the new patient history sheet dated September 15th.

PE: BP 100/62. HR: 68 T 98.3. The patient is a well-developed, well-nourished male in no apparent distress. Voice is normal. Face: symmetrical with normal salivary glands, and normal facial strength. Pinnae, external auditory canals, and tympanic membranes were normal with no evidence of middle ear effusion, acute infection, or cerumen impaction. The external nose was normal. Nasal cavity has no polyps or purulent drainage. The septum was essentially straight.

    Oral cavity shows no masses or lesions. Normal mucosa. Lips, teeth, and gums are normal. The true vocal cords were mobile bilaterally with no nodules, polyps, or neoplasms in the larynx or hypopharynx. No lymphadenopathy, masses, or thyromegaly.

Audiogram: This revealed essentially normal hearing throughout the frequencies with 100 percent discrimination on the right and 96 percent on the left. Tympanograms were Type A bilaterally.

Impression: Perception of auditory loss; however, no evidence of significant hearing loss by audiogram. Allergic rhinitis that has responded well to allergy shots in the past.

Suzanne R. Shallert, MD

SRS/pw   D: 09/15/08 09:50:16   T: 09/17/08 12:55:01

You Code It!

What are the best, most accurate codes?

_____

_____

_____

MORRIS, SHALLERT & ASSOCIATES
Allergy & Immunology
975 CENTRAL AVENUE • SOMEWHERE, FL 32811 • 407-555-4321

PATIENT: RAYTHES, DEAN

ACCOUNT/EHR #: RAYTDE001

Date: 09/15/08

Attending Physician: Marcus Morris, MD

This 15-year-old male came to the Emergency Room with complaints of fever, headache, malaise, and generalized myalgias. He stated the symptoms have lasted several days. The day of admission, he acutely developed painful swelling of his right wrist.

On examination of his extremities, a lesion was noted on his left shin just below the knee. He had several other lesions on his right arm near the elbow.

Diagnosis: Disseminated gonorrhea (arthritis dermatitis syndrome)

Treatment: Anti-inflammatory drug therapy, plus passive range-of-motion exercises including stretching, active range of motion and muscle strengthening should be done at least twice daily.

Marcus Morris, MD

MM/pw   D: 09/15/08 09:50:16   T: 09/17/08 12:55:01

You Code It!

What are the best, most accurate codes?

_____

_____

_____

MORRIS, SHALLERT & ASSOCIATES
Allergy & Immunology
975 CENTRAL AVENUE • SOMEWHERE, FL 32811 • 407-555-4321

PATIENT: Chesdrake, Sarah
ACCOUNT/EHR #:   CHESSA001
Date: 08/11/08

Attending Physician: Willard B. Reader, MD

Patient is a 23-month-old female seen in our emergency facility. She was brought in by ambulance, accompanied by her father, Roger. Father states that the patient was complaining of pain in her abdomen. He also noted that she was having a bad case of diarrhea. When her stool turned to bright red bloody, he called 911. In addition, he said he also has been having abdominal cramps and a bit of diarrhea himself. Last weekend, he said, Sarah was watching an old Popeye cartoon when she came into the kitchen. He was eating a fresh spinach salad, and she wanted to try it. She ate several mouthfuls.

Pt is listless and showing signs of dehydration. T102, BP 80/65 Immunoassay antigen detection for E. coli, multi-step method ordered. Stool culture confirms the presence of E. coli bacteria.

DX: Hemolytic uremic syndrome due to E. coli bacteria

Admit to PCCU.

Willard B. Reader, MD

DRC/pw   D: 08/11/08 09:50:16   T: 08/13/08 12:55:01

You Code It!

What are the best, most accurate codes?

_____

_____

_____

MORRIS, SHALLERT & ASSOCIATES
Allergy & Immunology
975 CENTRAL AVENUE • SOMEWHERE, FL 32811 • 407-555-4321

PATIENT: GARRISON, JUSTIN
ACCOUNT/EHR #:   GARRJU001
Date: 08/11/08

Attending Physician: Willard B. Reader, MD

This 31-year-old male came in with complaints of clogged sinuses. I have not seen this patient since last year when he was experiencing severe hay fever symptoms. Patient states that he recently started dating a woman who has a pet cat. He noted symptoms the first time he visited her home.

HEENT: His sinuses appear to be congested. Throat and nasal passages are mildly inflamed. Upon visual inspection, the ears appear unremarkable.

Because complete allergy testing had not been done previously, we performed full spectrum, per cutaneous (scratch) testing. Tests confirmed some mild food allergies and a severe allergy to cat dander.

DX: Allergy to animal dander (cat)

Rx: Allegra

PLAN: Patient states he does not want to be dependent on medication for the rest of his life. After discussions of benefits and concerns, he opts to begin weekly desensitization injections.

_____

Willard B. Reader, MD

DRC/pw   D: 08/11/08 09:50:16   T: 08/13/08 12:55:01

You Code It!

What are the best, most accurate codes?

_____

_____

_____

MORRIS, SHALLERT & ASSOCIATES
Allergy & Immunology
975 CENTRAL AVENUE • SOMEWHERE, FL 32811 • 407-555-4321

PATIENT: GARRISON, JUSTIN
ACCOUNT/EHR #:   GARRJU001
Date: 08/30/08

Supervising Physician: Willard B. Reader, MD

Preparation and provision of serum for allergen immunotherapy: single allergen, 6 doses
Single injection of allergenic extract

DX: Allergy to animal dander (cat)

_____

Jonelle Harrison, RN

You Code It!

What are the best, most accurate codes?

_____

_____

_____

MORRIS, SHALLERT & ASSOCIATES
Allergy & Immunology
975 CENTRAL AVENUE • SOMEWHERE, FL 32811 • 407-555-4321

PATIENT: TRUMAINE, BARRY
ACCOUNT/EHR #:   TRUMBA001
Date: 09/09/08

Attending Physician: Suzanne R. Shallert, MD

S: The patient comes in today for follow-up. He has had allergic rhinitis, along with a rash that was difficult to go away. After doing significant exploration, he finally determined that it was Entex that was causing him to get the rash repeatedly. He apparently has taken Sudafed since then, without substantial rash. He states he still continues to smoke. He needs a refill on his Zyrtec. He would like to, perhaps, try Zyrtec D, if that is not going to cause him rash. I warned him against using guaifenesin, as that is likely his allergic component.

O: Blood pressure 102/70, pulse 86, respirations 18, weight 149 pounds. Tympanic membranes clear bilaterally. Nares congested with clear rhinorrhea. Pharynx clear. Neck supple with full range of motion. No adenopathy. No thyromegaly. Lungs clear to auscultation bilaterally. Heart regular rate and rhythm.

A: Allergic rhinitis

P: The patient will be given Zyrtec D, 1 tablet twice a day (#10 samples given). The patient will follow-up as necessary. Should he develop a rash or reaction to medication, he is to stop immediately and use Benadryl. The patient will otherwise follow-up as directed. Should he experience any problems, will follow accordingly.

Suzanne R. Shallert, MD

SRS/pw   D: 9/09/08 09:50:16   T: 9/15/08 12:55:01

You Code It!

What are the best, most accurate codes?

_____

_____

_____

Chapter 2   Allergy and Immunology Cases and Patient Records

Cardiology and Cardiovascular Cases and Patient Records

INTRODUCTION

Cardiologists are physicians who specialize in identifying and treating diseases or conditions of the heart and blood vessels, including conditions such as chest pain (angina), irregular heart rhythms, high blood pressure, congenital cardiac problems, and myocardial infarctions (heart attacks).

These health care professionals run diagnostic procedures that identify the functionality of a person's heart. Therapeutic procedures performed by cardiologists include cardiac catheterizations and angioplasties. Cardiac subspecialties include interventional cardiology, which uses mechanical treatments, such as angioplasty and electrophysiology, in which treatments involve the heart's electrical system.

Cardiovascular surgeons are the specialists who perform surgery on the heart and blood vessels. Most often, these operations are done to open a blockage in the blood vessels leading to the heart, such as in coronary artery disease, or problems with heart valves, such as mitral insufficiency or aortic stenosis.

Cardiologists can be board-certified through the Board of Internal Medicine, and cardiovascular surgeons can be board-certified by the Board of Surgery in general surgery or vascular surgery. The American Board of Medical Specialties recognizes both of these certifications.

You can use the following cases to practice coding diagnoses, E/M, procedures, DME, or other HCPCS Level II items, as applicable; code for the physician or the facility; code inpatient and outpatient services, as applicable:

1. Code for the physician.
2. Code for the anesthesiologist, when applicable.
3. Code for the hospital, when applicable.
4. Code for the pathology and laboratory, when applicable.
5. Code HCPCS Level II codes, when applicable.

WINTER HILLS CARDIOLOGY
420 VENTURA BYPASS • CENTRAL, FL 32811 • 407-555-4798

PATIENT: CAPOZZI, VINCENT
ACCOUNT/EHR #:   CAPOVI001
Date: 08/11/08

Attending Physician: Willard B. Reader, MD

Patient is a 62-year-old male previously seen by Dr. David Bush 18 months ago. The patient has a history of coronary artery disease and hyperlipidemia. He underwent coronary bypass surgery in 1973, by Dr. Howard that involved a left internal mammary artery to left anterior descending. In 1989, he underwent a re-do operation consisting of a right internal mammary artery to left anterior descending, saphenous vein graft to circumflex, and saphenous vein graft to right coronary artery.

He did well until yesterday afternoon when he developed an episode of moderate retrosternal chest pressure radiating to the right shoulder, which was prolonged and lasted until 3:00 a.m., at which time he presented to the ED. He apparently was given one nitroglycerin sublingual, with resolution of symptoms.

The patient is currently asymptomatic on examination and his review of systems is noncontributory.

PE: He is alert, oriented times three, in no acute distress. HEENT: unremarkable. Lungs: clear. Cardiovascular: Regular rate and rhythm. No murmurs and no gallops. Abdomen: Benign. Extremities: No edema. EKG: Normal sinus rhythm with myocardial changes. Lipid Panel: all unremarkable except for a cholesterol of 255. CBC: within normal limits. PT and PTT within normal limits. Cardiac enzymes times one: negative. Chest x-ray: unremarkable.

Admitting DX: Prolonged chest pain with negative electrocardiogram and negative enzymes times one.

Admit for observation to Telemetry. In view of the atypical nature of prolonged chest pain, we will proceed with a screening Cardiolite stress test later today. Nitroglycerin paste was applied on admission; however, it will be held until the stress test is completed. One aspirin a day was started. Further recommendation and interventions will depend on the results from the stress test.

Discharge DX: Coronary atherosclerosis of native coronary artery

Willard B. Reader, MD

DRC/pw   D: 08/11/08 09:50:16   T: 08/13/08 12:55:01

You Code It!

What are the best, most accurate codes?

_____

_____

_____

WINTER HILLS CARDIOLOGY
420 VENTURA BYPASS • CENTRAL, FL 32811 • 407-555-4798

PATIENT: KLACKSON, KEVIN
MRN: KLACKE01
Date: 15 September 2008

Diagnosis: Primary cardiomyopathy with chest pain
Procedure: Arterial catheterization

Physician: Frank Vincent, MD
Anesthesia: Local

PROCEDURE: The patient was placed on the table in supine position. Local anesthesia was administered. Once we were assured that the patient had achieved no nervous stimuli, the incision was made and the catheter was introduced percutaneously. The incision was sutured with a simple repair. The patient tolerated the procedure well and was transferred to the recovery room.

_____

Frank Vincent, MD

FV/mg   D: 9/15/08 09:50:16   T: 9/15/08 12:55:01

You Code It!

What are the best, most accurate codes?

_____

_____

_____

WINTER HILLS CARDIOLOGY
420 VENTURA BYPASS • CENTRAL, FL 32811 • 407-555-4798

PATIENT:	CRAINE, JACOB
ACCOUNT/EHR #:	CRAJA001
Date:	10/15/08

Consulting Physician: Taylor Duggan, MD

Attending Physician: Faron Macavoy, MD

HISTORY OF PRESENT ILLNESS: The patient is a 57-year-old white male with a longstanding history of hypertension, coronary artery disease, chronic obstructive pulmonary disease who was admitted for chest pain. The patient has recurrent pain episodes and is followed by South City Cardiology. The patient has had a stress test prior to admission, which did not reveal any ischemia. The patient is ruled out for myocardial infarction and was stable over two nights in the hospital. He also had a CT scan negative for dissection. The patient was discharged to home in good condition without any further pain. He is to follow up with his primary care physician, Dr. Lorrenez, in one-to-two weeks after discharge and Dr. Macavoy, his cardiologist, two weeks after discharge. He is to resume his home medications.

Taylor Duggan, MD

TD/bje   10/13/08 11:47:39

You Code It!

What are the best, most accurate codes?

_____

_____

_____

WINTER HILLS CARDIOLOGY
420 VENTURA BYPASS • CENTRAL, FL 32811 • 407-555-4798

PATIENT: FELIZ, MARIA
ACCOUNT/EHR #:   FELMA001
Date: 10/15/08

Attending Physician: Taylor Duggan, MD
Chief Complaint: Chest pain

HISTORY OF PRESENT ILLNESS: The patient is a 43-year-old Hispanic female with numerous visits to the emergency room and hospital for chest pain and rule out MI. The patient also has a longstanding history of drug-seeking behavior. She has a history of coronary artery disease, status post PTCAx5, the last episode per her occurred three months ago. The patient was seen in her cardiologist's office today for a Persantine thallium test and the patient was experiencing chest discomfort. She reported shortness of breath, some nausea, no vomiting, some diaphoresis with the pain; the pain was substernal and not pleuritic in nature. She denied any fever or chills. She denied any cough. She denied any lower extremity swelling. The patient is a nonsmoker and has a longstanding history of asthma and COPD. She is on multiple medications for her asthma and COPD. The patient states that she is currently pain-free.

PAST MEDICAL HISTORY: Hypertension, elevated cholesterol, coronary artery disease, status post stenting x5, COPD, anxiety, chronic pain syndrome.

ALLERGIES: Talwin, Keflex

MEDICATIONS: Lasix, Singulair, Zoloft, Theo-Dur, Colace, OxyContin, Baclofen, Levaquin, Norvasc, aspirin, Xanax, Neurontin, Deltasone, Pravachol MDI, Zanaflex, Zantac

SOCIAL HISTORY: The patient does not smoke or drink or use illegal drugs

FAMILY HISTORY: Noncontributory

REVIEW OF SYSTEMS:

PHYSICAL EXAMINATION

VITAL SIGNS: T 97.3; P 115, R 28, BP 154/106. Repeat value of 133/86. O2 saturation 96% on two liters.

GENERAL APPEARANCE: In general, the patient is slightly obese, in no acute distress currently.

HEENT: Normocephalic, atraumatic. Pupils are equal, round, and reactive to light and accommodation, extraocular movements are intact.

NECK: Supple; no JVD or lymphadenopathy

HEART: Regular rate and rhythm, without bruits

CHEST: Coarse, with fine bronchial rales throughout

ABDOMEN: Soft, non-tender, no distention, positive bowel sounds

PELVIC/RECTAL:

EXTREMITIES: No clubbing, cyanosis or edema. 2+ distal pulses.

LABORATORY VALUES: Chest x-ray shows bilateral pulmonary scarring and an elevated right hemidiaphragm, otherwise, no acute pulmonary process. Electrocardiogram shows sinus tachycardia at 111 beats per minute with no acute ST-T wave changes. BMP is normal except for a sodium of 130. CBC reveals a white blood cell count of 14,800; hemoglobin of 14.4 and platelet count of 501,000. D-dimer is greater than 0.5, less than 1. Troponin is pending.

Continued

IMPRESSION:
1. Acute chest pain syndrome in a patient with known coronary heart disease
2. History of coronary artery disease, status post PTCA (percutaneous transluminal coronary angioplasty) x5, the last was three months ago
3. History of COPD and asthma
4. Hypertension
5. History of drug-seeking behavior and chronic pain syndrome
6. Anxiety
7. Elevated cholesterol
8. Leukemoid reaction probably secondary to steroids

RECOMMENDATIONS:
1. This patient has a longstanding history of multiple admissions and visits to the emergency room for chest pain. She has a longstanding history of drug-seeking behavior and noncompliance, however the patient does not have known coronary disease and had a stress test performed at the office of Grosspoint Cardiology on the morning of admission. For this reason, we will admit her for 23-hour observation and rule her out for a myocardial infarction.
2. Will consult Grosspoint Cardiology. The patient is known to them and they may review the results of the stress test from today with her.
3. Will continue her home medications including aspirin and MDI. The patient is not on a beta-blocker secondary to her COPD and asthma. Nitroglycerin will be used p.r.n.
4. CT scan of the chest is pending, as performed by the emergency room staff to rule out PE and dissection.

Taylor Duggan, MD

TD/bje   10/13/08 11:47:39

You Code It!

What are the best, most accurate codes?

_____

_____

_____

WINTER HILLS CARDIOLOGY
420 VENTURA BYPASS • CENTRAL, FL 32811 • 407-555-4798

PATIENT: WALLACE, LEO
ACCOUNT/EHR #:   WALLE001
Date: 10/15/08

Primary Care Physician: Quentin David, MD

Attending Physician: Faron Macavoy, MD
Presenting Complaint/Chief Complaint: Right Leg DVT

HISTORY OF PRESENT ILLNESS: The patient is a 59-year-old male patient, presented to my office today with a four-day history of right leg discomfort and swelling. Patient also complaining of hematuria and smelly urine with no fever or chills, nor dysuria. Patient was sent to have an urgent venous Doppler as he was found on clinical exam to have varicose veins with right calf tenderness and right leg edema. The urgent venous Doppler results were called to me, which is positive for acute right leg DVT. Patient's urinalysis is also positive for blood and urinary tract infection.

PAST MEDICAL HISTORY: Parkinson's disease. Patient stated he had DVT ten years ago in the left leg for which he was treated only with aspirin. He denies any past medical history of urinary tract infection or renal stones.

ALLERGIES: None.

MEDICATIONS: Sinemet, dose unknown, which he is taking three times a day. He is also on Eldepryl 5mg p.o. daily.

SOCIAL HISTORY: Lives alone. He is a widower for six years. Does not smoke.

FAMILY HISTORY:

REVIEW OF SYSTEMS: Denies any fever. No flank pain, no suprapubic pain, no vomiting, no headache, no shortness of breath, no palpitations.

PHYSICAL EXAMINATION

GENERAL APPEARANCE: He is comfortable

VITAL SIGNS: His vitals are stable. He is afebrile. Pulse is 80 beats per minute, BP 122/90

HEENT: Unremarkable

NECK: Supple. No goiter. No carotid bruits

LUNGS: Clear bilaterally

ABDOMEN: Soft. No suprapubic or costovertebral angle tenderness

EXTREMITIES: Examination of his lower extremities reveals bilateral varicose veins. Right calf tenderness is present, as well as right leg edema.

NEUROLOGICAL: Neurological exam reveals Parkinsonian tremors with increased rigidity.

PELVIC/RECTAL:

LABORATORY DATA: Urinalysis, which was done in the office, is positive for blood, Nitrate, and also leukocytes. Venous Doppler, as I mentioned above, is positive for acute DVT, right leg.

ASSESSMENT:
1. Acute DVT (deep venous thrombosis), right leg
2. Urinary tract infection
3. Parkinson's disease

Continued

PLAN:
Patient is admitted to the Mason Hospital for anticoagulation therapy. We will also get routine blood tests, including CBC, chest x-ray, ECG, INR/prothrombin time. Patient will be started on Coumadin. He is also started on Levaquin. We will get sonogram of his kidneys and bladder to rule out any underlying renal pathology for current urinary tract infection. Patient will be managed by Winter Hills Cardiology.

Faron Macavoy, MD

FM/bje   10/13/08 11:47:39

You Code It!

What are the best, most accurate codes?

_____

_____

_____

WINTER HILLS CARDIOLOGY
420 VENTURA BYPASS • CENTRAL, FL 32811 • 407-555-4798

PATIENT: FINNEGAN, IAN
ACCOUNT/EHR #:   FINIA001
Date: 10/15/08

Consulting Physician: Taylor Duggan, MD

Attending Physician: Faron Macavoy, MD

REASON FOR VISIT: Patient is here for preoperative clearance. Dr. Macavoy is the surgeon to repair an aneurysm behind his left knee. He denies any cardiac discomfort or SOB at present.

HISTORY OF PRESENT ILLNESS: Routine clinic follow-up for this 61-year-old male. The patient is scheduled for popliteal aneurysm surgery per Dr. Macavoy. The patient has a history of thoracoabdominal aneurysm operated on by Dr. Macavoy approximately one year ago. Catheterization at that time revealed the right coronary artery to be a dominant vessel diffuse plaquing with two areas of eccentric stenosis of approximately 60-70% in the mid-portion. The circumflex was a small and non-dominant vessel. Ejection fraction was approximately 6%. Medical management was recommended.

    At the present time, there are no symptoms of angina, heart failure or arrhythmias. The patient remains compliant with his diet and medication.

MEDICATIONS: Dynabac 250 mg qd; Rhinocort 4 sp qhs, Darvocet p.r.n.

ALLERGIES: ASA

PHYSICAL EXAMINATION

VITAL SIGNS: BP 148/78; P 80; R 18; Ht 5'5"; Wt 199

NECK: Neck veins are flat. Carotid upstrokes are 2+ and symmetrical and without bruits

CHEST: Clear to auscultation and percussion

HEART: Regular rate and rhythm

ABDOMEN: Benign

EXTR: Palpable aneurysms in both popliteal areas. There is no edema.

CLINICAL IMPRESSION/PLAN:
This information reviewed at length with the patient. Clinically, he remains asymptomatic. In view of his upcoming surgery, I have recommended that he undergo a Persantine Cardiolite stress test. Coronary intervention would only be recommended if a significant amount of reversible ischemia is demonstrated.

Taylor Duggan, MD

TD/bje   10/13/08 11:47:39

You Code It!

What are the best, most accurate codes?

_____

_____

_____

WINTER HILLS CARDIOLOGY
420 VENTURA BYPASS • CENTRAL, FL 32811 • 407-555-4798

PATIENT:	HAYMAN, ALANA
ACCOUNT/EHR #:	HAYAL001
Date:	10/15/08
Attending Physician:	Taylor Duggan, MD
Chief Complaint:	Uncontrolled palpitations with dyspnea

HISTORY OF PRESENT ILLNESS: The patient is a pleasant and elderly 78-year-old Caucasian female, with atherosclerotic peripheral vascular disease, is admitted to the hospital today with new onset uncontrolled atrial fibrillation. She presents with symptomatic palpitations and shortness of breath, and generalized weakness with exertional dizziness. She denies exertional angina pectoris, although her exertional dyspnea is now quite limiting with her palpitations. No dependent edema.

She reports a several month history of worsening left leg claudication. A previous arterial ultrasound has documented a stenosis in her proximal left leg arterial system.

PAST MEDICAL HISTORY: The patient is allergic to PENICILLIN and PREVACID. Environmental allergies to feathers and trees. Gastric intolerance to Mevacor. Historical hypercholesterolemia and peptic ulcer disease. Recorded illnesses are hiatal hernia, gastroesophageal reflux disorder, osteopenia with lumbar compression fracture, and controlled but recurrent supraventricular tachycardia (SVT). Status post hysterectomy and bilateral oophorectomy, and right segmental mastectomy.

FAMILY HISTORY: Both the patient's mother and brother are deceased secondary to colon carcinoma.

SOCIAL HISTORY: Patient is a widow, currently living alone. She is a retired biostatistician. No recent tobacco usage.

REVIEW OF SYSTEMS: This is significant with reported left leg sciatica, recurrent esophageal pyrosis, anxiety, right knee osteoarthritis, and recurrent sinus posterior drainage due to perennial rhinitis.

PHYSICAL EXAMINATION

GENERAL: This reveals a 78-year-old white female complaining of dyspnea and unrestrained palpitations.

VITAL SIGNS: Respiratory rate increased at 20 per minute, BP 100/64 with an irregular pulse

HEENT/NECK: Normocephalic with some erythema of her nasal turbinates. No jugular venous distention or carotid bruits. Cervical kyphosis.

LUNGS: The lungs are clear to auscultation.

HEART: A soft and systolic murmur present. Heart tones are irregular without a gallop.

ABDOMEN: Soft and non-tender to palpitations

EXTREMITIES: No dependent edema. The distal left pedal pulses are reduced.

NEUROLOGIC: Neurologic reflexes symmetric bilaterally.

ADMITTING LAB DATA BASE: The admitting EKG confirms atrial fibrillation.

Continued

IMPRESSION:
1. Paroxysmal and uncontrolled atrial fibrillation
2. Atherosclerotic peripheral vascular disease with left leg claudication
3. Lumbar compression fracture with osteopenia
4. Treated hypercholesterolemia
5. Treated and controlled supraventricular tachycardia
6. Gastroesophageal reflux disorder with hiatal hernia
7. Historical peptic ulcer disease
8. Status post hysterectomy with bilateral oophorectomy
9. Status post right segmental mastectomy
10. Allergic perennial rhinitis
11. Aortic valvular murmur
12. Gastric intolerance to oral Mevacor
13. Environmental allergies to feathers and trees
14. Drug allergies to PENICILLIN and PREVACID

PLAN: Patient has been admitted to GASTRON MEDICAL CENTER today for control and treatment of her rapid atrial fibrillation. Also, her atherosclerotic peripheral vascular disease and progressive claudication will have to be addressed clinically.

Taylor Duggan, MD

TD/bje   10/13/08 11:47:39

You Code It!

What are the best, most accurate codes?

_____

_____

_____

WINTER HILLS CARDIOLOGY
420 VENTURA BYPASS • CENTRAL, FL 32811 • 407-555-4798

PATIENT: LONDON, JOSEPH

ACCOUNT/EHR #: LONJO001

Date: 10/15/08

Surgeon: Taylor Duggan, MD

Asst. Surgeon: Maureen O'Connell, MD

Preop DX: Severe coronary artery disease with unstable angina

Postop DX: Same

Operative Procedure: Cardiac Bypass Grafting

Anesthesiologist: Randolph Sullivan, MD

Anesthesia: General

INDICATIONS: This is a 55-year-old male who underwent evaluation for severe coronary disease. Catheterization demonstrated severe triple vessel coronary disease with a subtotal right coronary artery and significant disease involving the left anterior descending, diagonal and circumflex. We thought the patient could have four bypasses. The left anterior descending disease appeared diffused. Ventricular function was preserved.

PROCEDURE: With the patient in the supine position under general anesthesia, the chest, abdomen, groins, and legs were prepped and draped in standard fashion. Saphenous vein was taken from the right leg and this wound was closed in routine fashion. Simultaneously, the chest was opened through a median sternotomy and the left internal mammary was prepared. The mammary was densely adherent to the back of the sternum at the top and we ended up dividing it at this point. The proximal end was oversewn with 3-0 Prolene and then with #2 silk and the mammary was prepared as a free graft.

We then opened the pericardium and heparinized and cannulated the aorta and right atrium. We went on bypass and cooled down. The aorta was cross-clamped and cardioplegia was infused in the root. We then bypassed the right coronary artery just beyond the acute angle of the heart. It was about 2.0 mm. We then bypassed a marginal, which was in about mid-position, and this was about 2.5 mm vessel.

We then bypassed a diagonal, which was also 2.5 mm. The left internal mammary, used as a free graft, was then used to bypass a 2.0 mm left anterior descending. The aortic cross-clamp was removed and three vein anastomoses were made to the ascending aorta. We then sutured the left internal mammary to the hood of the diagonal vein graft. With flow established in all four grafts, we weaned from bypass with good hemodynamics. The heart was decannulated, protamine was administered and Hemostasis was obtained. Atrial and ventricular pacing wires were attached and chest tubes were inserted. The mediastinum was copiously irrigated out and we closed in layers. The patient tolerated this well and left the operating room for intensive care in stable condition.

Taylor Duggan, MD

TD/bje   10/13/08 11:47:39

You Code It!

What are the best, most accurate codes?

_____

_____

_____

WINTER HILLS CARDIOLOGY
420 VENTURA BYPASS • CENTRAL, FL 32811 • 407-555-4798

PATIENT:	DEL FINNIO, MARTA
ACCOUNT/EHR #:	DELMA001
Date:	10/15/08
Surgeon:	Taylor Duggan, MD
Asst. Surgeon:	Maureen O'Connell, MD
Preop DX:	1. Coronary artery disease
	2. Unstable angina pectoris
	3. Left carotid artery disease
Postop DX:	Same
Operative Procedure:	Cardiac Bypass Grafting
Anesthesiologist:	Randolph Sullivan, MD
Anesthesia:	General

INDICATIONS: This is a 61-year-old female who was admitted at another hospital with unstable angina. At that time, the patient underwent cardiac catheterization. There was some anterior apical hypokinesis. The left anterior descending had an 85 percent proximal narrowing. The right coronary artery had proximal 75 percent narrowing. Carotid ultrasound, arteriogram revealed very significant, severe disease in the carotids.

INTRAOPERATIVE FINDINGS: Cardiac-wise there were no intrapericardial adhesions. They were normal without palpable plaque. The ventricular function was quite preserved. The left anterior descending measured 2.2 mm in diameter and had excellent brisk flow through the left internal mammary artery. The right coronary artery measured 2.4 mm in diameter and the right internal mammary artery had excellent brisk flow.

OPERATION: With satisfactory insertion of monitoring line, induction of anesthesia, standard prepping and draping, for the chest operation, a median sternotomy was performed. We dissected both internal mammary arteries and their pedicles, opened the pericardium, heparinized and cannulated routinely. Cardiopulmonary bypass was initiated. Temperature dropped to 32 degrees. Myocardium was immediately arrested with aortic cross-clamping and infusion of aortic root blood cardioplegia initially, supplemented by retrograde cardioplegia through the coronary sinus. We performed two end-to-side distal anastomoses, using the mammary artery. The left internal mammary artery was passed toward the left anterior descending through a vent made on the left side of the pericardium. As we did with the right internal mammary artery passing through a vent on the right side of the pericardium. Both distal anastomoses were done with continuous running suture of 7-0 Prolene. Rewarming was in progress. Cross clamp released. Myocardial activity resumed spontaneously. Temporary atrial and ventricular wires were placed and pleural and mediastinal cavities drained appropriately with chest tubes. There was satisfactory Hemostasis. Decannulation followed. Heparinization reversed with protamine sulfate. Sternotomy approximated with interrupted #6 wires. The linea alba, fascia, subcutaneous tissue and skin were closed in the usual manner with continuous and interrupted sutures. The patient was transported to the ICU in satisfactory condition.

Taylor Duggan, MD

TD/bje   10/13/08 11:47:39

You Code It!

What are the best, most accurate codes?

_____

_____

WINTER HILLS CARDIOLOGY
420 VENTURA BYPASS • CENTRAL, FL 32811 • 407-555-4798

PATIENT: SUSNOW, FRANK
ACCOUNT/EHR #:   SUSFR001
Date: 10/15/08

Surgeon: Taylor Duggan, MD

Asst. Surgeon: Ethan Harrison, MD
Preop DX: Status post-coronary artery bypass grafting, remote, with closed bypasses.
Postop DX: Same
Operative Procedure: 1. Re-do median sternotomy and open-heart 2. Cardiac Bypass Grafting

Anesthesiologist: Randolph Sullivan, MD
Anesthesia: General

INDICATIONS: This is a 49-year-old male patient who underwent previous coronary artery bypass at the VA Hospital with closure of all the grafts and most recently very unstable angina pectoris. At the time of surgery, which was approached through a re-do median sternotomy due to poor peripheral pulses, we elected to cannulate again the ascending aorta. The left internal mammary artery was a good vessel, which was anastomosed to the junction of the diagonal and the upper left anterior descending. This was a good vessel. We elected to do distal anastomosis to the distal left anterior descending, as well as bypass the circumflex on the right. The operation was accomplished through a re-do median sternotomy.

OPERATION: Following placement of Swan-Ganz catheter and induction of anesthesia, the chest was carefully re-entered. Adhesions were lysed. The patient was heparinized, and we cannulated the ascending aorta. It is worth mentioning the fact that the patient was markedly ischemia with PA pressures in the mid-50s. We instituted cardiopulmonary bypass and hypothermia. The aorta was cross-clamped. Cardioplegia solution was given through the aortic root. Following dissection of the mammary, individual segments of saphenous vein were anastomosed to the circumflex, distal left anterior descending and anastomosed to the circumflex, distal left anterior descending and right coronary artery, which were good vessels. The left internal mammary artery was anastomosed to the upper left anterior descending diagonal junction. The two proximal anastomoses for the right coronary artery and the left anterior descending were performed with aortic cross-clamp in the anterior portion of the ascending aorta. Cross-clamp time was 40 minutes. We released the aortic cross-clamp, following which we performed the proximal anastomoses of the graft to the circumflex to the side of the graft to the left anterior descending. We rewarmed and experienced no difficulty in weaning the patient from cardiopulmonary bypass. Routine decannulation and closure was performed. The patient was taken to the cardiac surgical intensive care unit in satisfactory condition.

Taylor Duggan, MD

TD/bje   10/13/08 11:47:39

You Code It!

What are the best, most accurate codes?

_____

_____

_____

WINTER HILLS CARDIOLOGY
420 VENTURA BYPASS • CENTRAL, FL 32811 • 407-555-4798

PATIENT: CALLMAN, DELMAR
ACCOUNT/EHR #:   CALDE001
Date: 10/15/08

Referring Cardiologist: Simon R. Blackman, MD

Primary Physician: Curtis Le Fran, MD
Office Consultation

CHIEF COMPLAINT: Referral from Dr. Blackman for evaluation for aortic valve replacement due to aortic insufficiency.

HISTORY OF PRESENT ILLNESS: Patient is a 39-year-old black male who relates a history of increasing fatigue as well as occasional palpitations. He denies chest pain, orthopnea, PND, pedal edema, syncope, or pre-syncope. The patient has a three-month history of a known cardiac murmur. This has been evaluated through Dr. Blackman's office. Transesophageal echocardiogram was performed on June 8 at Gaston Medical Center by Dr. Blackman, which showed PA 36/25, mean wedge 19. There is no significant gradient across the aortic value. The left main coronary artery is free of stenosis. The LAD is free of stenosis. The circumflex is free of stenosis. The right coronary artery is free of stenosis. There are no anomalous coronaries noted. Ejection fraction was noted to be 40%. The LV was markedly dilated. The aortic root injection demonstrated severe aortic regurgitation. Because of these findings, the patient is referred for evaluation for aortic valve replacement.

PAST HISTORY:

PAST MEDICAL HISTORY: History of fractured ankles, secondary

ALLERGIES: No known drug allergies

MEDICATIONS: Zestril 20 mg p.o. qd; Alprazolam p.r.n. dose unknown

FAMILY HISTORY: Father has an unknown heart problem. Older brother has had a stroke. Mother has a history of high blood pressure.

SOCIAL HISTORY: The patient has a 30-pack/year history of cigarette smoking. He continues to smoke. He relates daily vodka intake of 2-3 oz. He also relates marijuana use. He works as a delivery driver.

REVIEW OF SYSTEMS: Hematopoietic: The patient denies chronic anemia, easy bruising or previous blood transfusion reaction. HEET: He denies chronic headaches or sinus problems or dental problems. RESPIRATORY: The patient denies chronic cough, wheeze, sputum production, hemoptysis, TB, or pneumonia. CARDIAC: See HPI. He denies varicose veins or claudication. GASTROINTESTINAL: He denies nausea, vomiting, hematemesis, or melena. GENITOURINARY: He denies dysuria, urgency, frequency, hematuria. MUSCULOSKELETAL: The patient denies acutely swollen, painful, or warm joints or history of DVT. ENDOCRINE: The patient denies diabetes mellitus or thyroid disease. NEUROLOGIC: The patient denies stoke, TIA, amaurosis fugax, and syncope.

PHYSICAL EXAMINATION: Well-developed, well-nourished male in no apparent distress. Ht 5'7", wt 157 lb., BP 150/60, P 60 and regular, R 18 and unlabored, T 98.3.

HEENT: Normocephalic, atraumatic. Pupils equal, round, and reactive to light and accommodation bilaterally. Sclerae nonicteric, conjunctivae pink. Oral mucosa is well hydrated, and pink.

NECK: The trachea is midline. There is no jugular venous distension. Carotid pulses are 3+ bilaterally without bruit. There is no thyromegaly noted.

CHEST: The lungs are clear to auscultation and percussion. Excursion is satisfactory. Chest wall is nontender.

HEART: Regular rate and rhythm. Grade III/VI systolic murmur heard at the base. Grade III/VI diastolic murmur heard at the apex and at the base.

Continued

ABDOMEN: Positive bowel sounds, nontender, no organomegaly detected. Abdominal aorta is non-enlarged. There is no abdominal bruit heard.

EXTREMITIES: Radial pulses are 3+ bilaterally. Femoral pulses are 3+ with water hammer pulse. Pedal pulses are intact, 3+. There is no peripheral edema, clubbing, or cyanosis noted.

NEUROLOGIC: The patient is alert and oriented x3. The affect is appropriate. No motor deficits are seen.

IMPRESSION: Severe aortic insufficiency

DISCUSSION AND PLAN: The patient was seen and evaluated by me. Records were reviewed. However, the echocardiogram did not accompany the patient nor did the cardiac catheterization. This will be reviewed at a later date. Aortic valve replacement, device options, autologous blood donation, alternatives, risks, and imponderables were discussed in detail with the patient and his wife. They seem to understand and wish us to proceed. We will consult Dr. Blackman peri-operatively for medical evaluation and treatment of medical management problems.

Taylor Duggan, MD

TD/bje   10/13/08 11:47:39

You Code It!

What are the best, most accurate codes?

_____

_____

_____

WINTER HILLS CARDIOLOGY
420 VENTURA BYPASS • CENTRAL, FL 32811 • 407-555-4798

PATIENT:	HASSAN, SUNIL
ACCOUNT/EHR #:	HASSU001
Date:	10/15/08
Surgeon:	Taylor Duggan, MD
Asst. Surgeon:	Carole Franks, PA and Wayne Hanson, RN
Preop DX:	Severe aortic valve incompetence with class II congestive heart failure and moderately severe left ventricular dysfunction
Postop DX:	Same
Operative Procedure:	Aortic valve replacement with St. Jude model #25A-101, serial #88073284; transesophageal echocardiography; temporary cardiopulmonary bypass with moderate hypothermia; sanguinous cardioplegia with topical hypothermia and warm blood cardioplegic reperfusion.
Anesthesiologist:	Randolph Sullivan, MD
Anesthesia:	General

INDICATIONS: This 43-year-old male was found to have severe aortic valve incompetence with moderately severe left ventricular dysfunction and early onset of symptoms. Operation is undertaken for relief of symptoms, preservation of ventricular function and prolongation of life.

OPERATIVE FINDINGS: The left ventricle was enlarged grade 4/6, and hypertrophied grade 3/6, with reduced LV function diffusely. The ascending aorta was normal. The aortic valve was a tricuspid structure with myxomatous degeneration and prolapse, particularly of the non-coronary cusp.

OPERATION: After induction of general endotracheal anesthesia and placement of appropriate monitoring devices, the patient's chest and legs were sterilely prepped and draped. Primary median sternotomy was performed. The pericardium was opened and pericardial stays placed. Pursestrings were placed in the distal ascending aorta and right atrium. The patient was systemically heparinized and adequate anticoagulation was confirmed. He was cannulated and temporary cardiopulmonary bypass instituted at 2.4 l/min/m² at 32 degrees throughout most of the 58-minute bypass time. The patient was core cooled and topically cooled until ventricular fibrillation ensured. The aortic cross-clamp was placed. The left ventricular vent was placed through the right superior pulmonary vein. Right cardioplegia followed by subsequent direct ostial antegrade cardioplegia was administered and repeated at 20-minute intervals throughout the 39-minute cross-clamp time. An oblique aortotomy was performed. The valve was precisely excised after achieving effective cardiac arrest. The annulus comfortably accepted the 25mm prosthesis. Interrupted non-pledgeted 2-0 Tycron sutures were placed circumferentially around the annulus then passed through the sewing ring of the valve. The valve was seated and the sutures tied and cut. The valve seated nicely. The mechanism worked well. The root was irrigated and as we allowed the left heart to fill with blood, the aortotomy was closed with a double row of running 4-0 Prolene suture. With strong suction on the aortic needle vent and the patient in Trendelenburg position after a dose of warm blood cardioplegia followed by warm blood, the aortic cross-clamp was removed with a 34-minute ischemic time. The heart regained spontaneous rhythm but subsequently required DC cardioversion after some air entered the coronary arteries. The rhythm thereafter remained stable. We completed de-airing by TE guidance, rewarmed the patient. Temporary pacing wires were left on the surface of the right atrium and right ventricle. Two mediastinal

Continued

tubes were placed at separate water-seal suction and to the auto-transfusion device. He was weaned from cardiopulmonary bypass without difficulty. Protamine sulfate was administered, the patient decannulated. Hemostasis was achieved with electrocautery and the wounds closed in layers in the usual fashion. Sterile dressings applied. The sponge, needle, lap, and instrument counts were noted as correct. The patient transported directly to the CVRR in satisfactory condition.

Taylor Duggan, MD

TD/bje   10/13/08 11:47:39

You Code It!

What are the best, most accurate codes?

_____

_____

_____

WINTER HILLS CARDIOLOGY
420 VENTURA BYPASS • CENTRAL, FL 32811 • 407-555-4798

PATIENT: GASDEN, ADELE
ACCOUNT/EHR #:   GASAD001
Date: 10/15/08

Physician: Taylor Duggan, MD

Consulting: Garrett Kildare, MD

PROCEDURE: Intraoperative transesophageal echocardiogram
    Intraoperative transesophageal echocardiography was performed and the procedure note is reported sepa-
rately. This is an echocardiographic interpretation.

FINDINGS: Transesophageal and some transgastric views were obtained. The left ventricle is well visualized.
There is mild-to-moderate global left ventricular systolic dysfunction with left ventricular dilation and an ejection
fraction estimated at 45%. The left ventricle is moderately dilated with end-diastolic dimension approximately 6.5
cm by transesophageal. The aortic valve is well-visualized and it is clearly tricuspid. The aortic root is moderately
dilated. The mitral valve appears to have normal structure and motion with no evidence of prolapse or stenosis.
The aortic valve does not appear to have prolapse. There is no stenosis. The tricuspid valve has normal structure
and motion. The pulmonic valve is not visualized. There is no pericardial effusion or abnormal calcifications seen.

DOPPLER: The aortic valve shows moderate-to-severe aortic insufficiency by color Doppler. Measurements of
the aortic valve annulus appear to be 23-24 mm. The right-sided structures appear to be normal, a PA catheter is
identified.

IMPRESSION:
1. Significant left ventricular dilation with moderately depressed left ventricular systolic function. Ejection
    fraction estimated at 40%.
2. Structurally normal aortic valve, which is tricuspid with a dilated aortic root, with associated aortic insuf-
    ficiency. Taken together these are findings of left ventricular volume overload due to significant aortic
    insufficiency.
3. Postoperative a St. Jude's valve has been placed in the aortic position. There is central trace insufficiency,
    which is within the designed parameters of the valve. There is no perivalvular leak or rocking seen. There is
    no pericardial effusion or other pericardial abnormalities identified. The left ventricular systolic function is
    moderately reduced and estimated at 35-40%.
4. Hemodynamically significant aortic insufficiency with dilated cardiomyopathy secondary to volume overload
    on the left ventricle.
5. Status post aortic valve replacement with a St. Jude's prosthesis appears to be stable and functioning nor-
    mally postoperatively.

Taylor Duggan, MD

TD/bje   10/13/08 11:47:39

You Code It!

What are the best, most accurate codes?

_____

_____

_____

WINTER HILLS CARDIOLOGY
420 VENTURA BYPASS • CENTRAL, FL 32811 • 407-555-4798

PATIENT: ROLANE, JACK
MRN: ROLAJA01
Date: 19 September 2008

Diagnosis: Atrial fibrillation
Procedure: Internal cardiac defibrillator

Physician: Frank Vincent, MD
Anesthesia: Moderate sedation

CLINICAL INFORMATION: A 71-year-old male with a history of paroxysmal atrial fibrillation, on antibiotic therapy, continued paroxysms of atrial fibrillation, now for an atrial defibrillator. We discussed the risks and benefits of this procedure, including 1% less risk of bleeding, infection, injury to the cephalic vein, subclavian vein and right atrium and right ventricular structures, cardiac perforation, clot formation and lead resistance and distal embolization to arms, legs, kidneys, stroke, death and lead dislodgement. He understood and agreed to proceed.

The patient was then taken to the EP laboratory and given Versed and fentanyl for sedation. After receiving 1 gram of Vancomycin for antibiotic prophylaxis, the whole anterior thorax was prepped and draped in the sterile fashion. Pre-gelled electrodes were placed in the posterior thorax with access to the anesthesia monitoring machine. Pre-gelled electrode pads were placed in the anterior and posterior and care taken to verify that the heart had been adequately interfaced between the two pads. After this, he was prepped and draped in a sterile fashion. 1% Lidocaine was then used to anesthetize the left prepectoral area. A 7 cm incision was made in the medial to lateral direction with care taken to verify that the deltopectoral groove was within the incision line. Blunt dissection electrocautery was then used to make the ICD pocket and venotomy technique was then used to cut down to the cephalic vein and introduce the leads. Using venotomy technique, a 0.3 G-tipped guide wire was passed to the level of the left cephalic vein to the subclavian vein. This was then used to pass a 9 French safe sheath to the level of the left subclavian vein. Guide wire remained in place and then the guide wire was removed and the second guide wire was put in place and the sheath was then removed. An 11 French safe sheath was then passed over one of the guide wires. The guide wire dilator was removed and the ventricular lead, a Medtronic lead 6942, 65, serial #TCB115488V was then passed to the level of the inferior vena cava. Under fluoroscopic visualization, leads were then placed in the right ventricular apex. The lead was then sutured in the prepectoral muscle using 2-0 Vicryl suture. Over the second guide wire, a 9 French safe sheath was then passed, guide wire and dilator was removed and an atrial lead Medtronic 6940, 65, serial #TCB023468V was then passed to the level of the right atrium. This is an activation lead and was actively fixed. The following pacing thresholds were noted upon implant. A sense P wave of 4.4 mV, sensory R wave of 10.5 mV, with a capture threshold in the atrium and 1.2 volts at 0.5 msec, the ventricle 0.3 volts at 0.5 msec, lead impedance in the atrium is 819 and the ventricle 518. Each lead was sutured in the prepectoral muscle using 2-0 nylon absorbable suture. The lead in the ICD was then placed in the pocket. The ICD was a Medtronic 7258H, dual AF, serial number of PID, 102351R. Under fluoroscopic visualization, the leads were verified to be in stable position and the ICD was sutured to the prepectoral muscle using 2-0 nonabsorbable suture. A total of two inductions of ventricular fibrillation was then

Continued

induced; each time it was quickly detected, and terminated with an 18 joule biphasic shock, designating the RV electrode and cathode. Defibrillation pressure was established at less or equal to 18 joules. Atrial fibrillation was then induced two times, each time was quickly detected and terminated with a 4 joule biphasic shock. The atrial defibrillation threshold established was less or equal to 4 joules. The patient tolerated the procedure well. The wound was then copiously irrigated with a G-U irrigant and closed in layers using 2-0 Vicryl suture for the first fascial layer, 3-0 Vicryl suture for the second fascial layer and 4-0 Vicryl suture for subcuticular layer. Steri-strips and sterile occlusive dressing were then placed for final wound approximation. The patient was then taken to the recovery room for further monitoring.

Frank Vincent, MD

FV/mg   D: 9/19/08 09:50:16   T: 9/15/08 12:55:01

You Code It!

What are the best, most accurate codes?

_____

_____

_____

Dentistry Cases and Patient Records

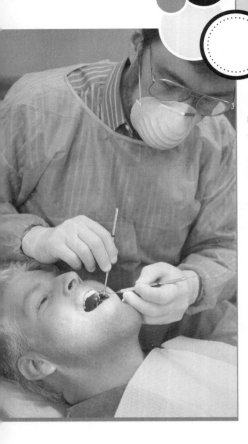

INTRODUCTION

The following case studies are from a dental practice. In a dentist's office, a professional coding specialist is likely to see many different types of health situations, especially preventive health care services.

Dentists are health professionals who specialize in the prevention, diagnosis, and treatment of health problems in the mouth and of the teeth. They will clean out and fill cavities, remove diseased teeth, embed dental implants, and provide cosmetic procedures, such as whitening teeth.

Dentists may specialize, such as:

- Periodontist, who specializes in treating diseases of the gum
- Orthodontist, who straightens crooked teeth
- Endodontist, who specializes in treating nerves of the teeth
- Oral Surgeon, who performs surgical procedures on the mouth and gums
- Prosthodontist, who specializes in tooth restoration

Some dentists may specialize in treating particular age groups, such as pediatric dentists, who only treat children, or those that might only work with those needing dentures.

You can use these cases to practice coding diagnoses, E/M, procedures, DME, or other HCPCS Level II items, as applicable; code for the physician or the facility; code inpatient and outpatient services, as applicable:

1. Code for the physician.
2. Code for the anesthesiologist, when applicable.
3. Code for the hospital, when applicable.
4. Code for the pathology and laboratory, when applicable.
5. Code HCPCS Level II codes, when applicable.

DENTAL ASSOCIATES OF ARRINGTON
9550 ENAMEL BLVD. • MOLAR, FL 32811 • 407-555-4703

PATIENT: PRIESTLY, ERIK
ACCOUNT/EHR #:   PRIER001
Date: 10/15/08

This patient is a 2-year-old boy, brought to the office by his mother, with concerns that he has not been eating normally and has many dark spots on his teeth. He might be having dental pain, but she is not sure. Acetaminophen has been given, and this might be helping to some degree. His mother reports trying to wean him off the bottle. She typically feeds him at night, and he refuses to go to sleep without a bottle of milk or apple juice. She doesn't brush his teeth because he doesn't like it. She has never taken him to a dentist before due to financial reasons. His past medical history and family history are unremarkable.

EXAM: VS T 37.50C. He appears alert and active in no apparent distress. Intraorally, there are opaque brown and grey specks on the enamel surface of several upper primary teeth. The upper central and lateral incisors show extensive decay and are slightly loose. The gingival tissues above the upper right central incisor are slightly swollen. Moderate lesions are visible in the upper canines, upper first molars, and lower first molars. The upper and lower second molars are just emerging through the gingiva. The lower canines and incisors are all intact, with no signs of dental decay.

DIAGNOSIS: Early childhood caries (ECC)

PLAN: His mother is told to wean him off the bottle and to brush his teeth at least twice a day. An appointment is made for her to bring him back for treatment of the ECC.

10/15/08 11:47:39

You Code It!

What are the best, most accurate codes?

_____

_____

_____

DENTAL ASSOCIATES OF ARRINGTON
9550 ENAMEL BLVD. • MOLAR, FL 32811 • 407-555-4703

PATIENT: WOZNIAK, LEONARD
ACCOUNT/EHR #:   WOZLE001
Date: 10/15/08

Leonard is a 41-year-old male with limited finances who is concerned about the appearance of his teeth. He is seeking the best treatment plan for the least amount of money.

Medical History: The patient is alert, normally developed, and is in no distress. Patient takes no medications, denies all organ system disease and allergies.

Dental History: He has received intermittent treatment, and the following teeth were extracted due to caries: #14, 15, 19, 20, 21, 30, 31.

Clinical Findings: Generalized plaque and calculus with staining are evident. There are focal white rough lesions on the mandibular left and right alveolar ridges. These white lesions are asymptomatic and do not rub off.

TREATMENT: A complete series, including bitewings, are taken. Prophylaxis is completed.

PLAN: Patient to return in one week to discuss treatment options for cosmetic measures.

10/15/08 11:47:39

You Code It!

What are the best, most accurate codes?

_____

_____

_____

DENTAL ASSOCIATES OF ARRINGTON
9550 ENAMEL BLVD. • MOLAR, FL 32811 • 407-555-4703

PATIENT: OPPENHEIM, CALLIE
ACCOUNT/EHR #:   OPPCA001
Date: 10/15/08

Patient is a 19-year-old female who has requested a routine examination.

Medical History: No abnormalities are identified.

Dental History: Patient had a congenitally missing permanent tooth and a retained deciduous tooth. The patient's last dental visit was two years ago. The patient has good oral hygiene. She uses a stiff toothbrush and brushes with the left hand.

Clinical Findings: A localized white plaque is present on the attached gingiva buccal to the mandibular right second premolar. The lesion is nontender, slightly thickened, firm, rough and fixed to the surface mucosa and underlying structures. The lesion does not rub off. The patient was unaware of the lesion.

TREATMENT: Complete x-ray series including bitewings. Adjunctive pre-diagnostic exam for mucosal abnormality identification. Patient to return to discuss lab results.

10/15/08 11:47:39

You Code It!

What are the best, most accurate codes?

_____

_____

_____

DENTAL ASSOCIATES OF ARRINGTON
9550 ENAMEL BLVD. • MOLAR, FL 32811 • 407-555-4703

PATIENT: MITCHELL, BRENT
ACCOUNT/EHR #:   MITBR001
Date: 10/15/08

Patient is a 15-year-old male who comes to this office requesting a routine examination.

MEDICAL HISTORY: Patient reports acne. No other abnormalities are identified.

DENTAL HISTORY: The patient has had intermittent dental care. The last dental visit was four years ago.

CLINICAL FINDINGS: White patches are present diffusely and bilaterally on the hard and soft palate, buccal mucosa, dorsum of the tongue, and some areas of the gingiva. The lesions are nontender, thickened, firm, rough and will not rub off. All the white patches are fixed to the surface mucosa, but they are fixed to underlying structures only on the hard palate and gingiva. The patient reports that the lesions are asymptomatic, have been present as long as the patient can remember, have always been in the same location, and have not changed. Other members of the patient's family have had white patches in their mouths.

TREATMENT: Comprehensive oral evaluation, complete x-ray series including bitewings, and accession of tissue samples, both gross and microscopic, including the assessment of surgical margins for presence of disease, of lesions.

DIAGNOSIS: Vitiligo

10/15/08 11:47:39

You Code It!

What are the best, most accurate codes?

_____

_____

_____

DENTAL ASSOCIATES OF ARRINGTON
9550 ENAMEL BLVD. • MOLAR, FL 32811 • 407-555-4703

PATIENT: ULSTER, AARON
ACCOUNT/EHR #:   ULSAA001
Date: 10/15/08

Patient is a 69-year-old male, new to the area. He was referred by Miriam Sanderson.

CHIEF COMPLAINT: The patient complains of a persistent, progressive, erythematous area of three months duration involving the mandibular left retromolar pad. The area is slightly sore. Topical therapy with Nystatin and Triamcinolone acetonide have had no effect on the lesion.

MEDICAL HISTORY: No abnormalities are identified.

DENTAL HISTORY: The patient has worn complete maxillary and mandibular dentures for seven years. The current dentures are six years old. The patient does not wear the dentures at night.

CLINICAL FINDINGS: The lesion is a localized erythematous area involving the crest and lingual aspect of the mandibular left retromolar pad. The lesion is nonpalpable, mildly tender, and fixed to surface mucosa but not to underlying structures.

TREATMENT: Comprehensive periodontal evaluation, new patient; adjustment to complete denture, maxillary, and mandibular.

PLAN: Patient to return if this adjustment does not solve the problem.

10/15/08 11:47:39

You Code It!

What are the best, most accurate codes?

_____

_____

_____

DENTAL ASSOCIATES OF ARRINGTON
9550 ENAMEL BLVD. • MOLAR, FL 32811 • 407-555-4703

PATIENT: DAVIDS, SARAH
ACCOUNT/EHR #: DAVSA001
Date: 10/15/08

Patient is a sixteen-year-old female whom I have not seen in six months.

CHIEF COMPLAINT: The patient has had a sore mouth associated with a white lesion for three weeks. Drinking orange juice makes the discomfort worse. The lesion has been in the same location during the three weeks. The patient has not recently burned the roof of her mouth.

MEDICAL HISTORY: The patient is taking Erythromycin, 250 mg, twice a day for acne.

DENTAL HISTORY: No abnormalities are identified.

CLINICAL FINDINGS: Soft, white plaques, which rub off, are diffusely present on the hard palate. The mucosa underlying the plaques is tender and erythematous.

TREATMENT: Limited oral evaluation – problem-focused; microorganisms collected for culture and sensitivity tests.

DX: Leukoplakia or oral mucosa

10/15/08 11:47:39

You Code It!

What are the best, most accurate codes?

_____

_____

_____

DENTAL ASSOCIATES OF ARRINGTON
9550 ENAMEL BLVD. • MOLAR, FL 32811 • 407-555-4703

PATIENT: GLOUSTINE, MONICA
ACCOUNT/EHR #:   GLOMO001
Date: 10/15/08

Patient is a thirteen-year-old female who requests a routine examination.

MEDICAL HISTORY: The patient recently completed a regimen of penicillin for strep throat.

DENTAL HISTORY: The patient's last dental appointment was eight months ago.

CLINICAL FINDINGS: A sharply delineated, erythematous area is located at the midline of the posterior dorsum of the tongue. The erythematous area is nonthickened, nontender and does not bleed. Several compressible, tender submandibular lymph nodes are palpable bilaterally. The patient was unaware of the lesion.

TREATMENT: Periodic oral examination; bitewings (2); adjunctive pre-diagnostic tests to determine status of lesion.

DIAGNOSIS: Plicated tongue

PLAN: No caries identified. Unremarkable dental examination. Patient to return in two weeks, once results of tests have returned from lab.

10/15/08 11:47:39

You Code It!

What are the best, most accurate codes?

_____

_____

_____

DENTAL ASSOCIATES OF ARRINGTON
9550 ENAMEL BLVD. • MOLAR, FL 32811 • 407-555-4703

PATIENT: VAN HOUSEN, PAUL
ACCOUNT/EHR #:   VANPA001
Date: 10/15/08

Patient is a 48-year-old male.

CHIEF COMPLAINT: The patient is concerned about mucosal lesions of the palate and gingiva covering the mandibular third molars. The palatal lesion is nonpainful. The patient has been aware of it for three weeks, during which time it has increased in size. It has not been treated. The gingival lesions cover the mandibular third molars. Purple patches are present on the skin of the temples bilaterally.

MEDICAL HISTORY: The patient reports hypotension. He states that he was hospitalized for hepatitis-B six years ago. He reports purple skin lesions on the temples and anterior neck of two weeks duration.

DENTAL HISTORY: The patient seeks routine dental treatment every two to three years. He had a dental evaluation of the gingival swelling covering the mandibular third molars approximately two months ago.

CLINICAL FINDINGS: A 3 x 2 cm, purple, surface lesion is present on the hard palate. Purple surface lesions are present around the mandibular third molars, on the temples bilaterally, and on the neck. The skin lesions and the oral mucosal lesions are thickened but flat. All the thickened lesions are compressible, nontender, fixed to surface mucosa and underlying structures, and blanch upon pressure. Ecchymotic areas present at the junction of the hard and soft palate are not thickened. Anterior and posterior cervical lymph nodes and posterior auricular lymph nodes are enlarged, firm, and nontender. The posterior auricular nodes are fixed to surrounding structures.

DIAGNOSIS: Spontaneous ecchymoses

PLAN: Referral to dermatologist

10/15/08 11:47:39

You Code It!

What are the best, most accurate codes?

_____

_____

_____

DENTAL ASSOCIATES OF ARRINGTON
9550 ENAMEL BLVD. • MOLAR, FL 32811 • 407-555-4703

PATIENT: MAC KAY, TRENT
ACCOUNT/EHR #:   MACTR001
Date: 10/15/08

Patient is a four-year-old male.

CHIEF COMPLAINT: The patient's parents are concerned about a pigmented area on the lower lip. The pigmentation has been present for six weeks, is asymptomatic, but is becoming progressively darker. The parents state that the child spends a lot of time in the sun.

MEDICAL HISTORY: No abnormalities are identified.

DENTAL HISTORY: No abnormalities are identified.

CLINICAL FINDINGS: A localized area of pigmentation about 3 mm in diameter is present on the midline of the lower lip. The lesion is nonthickened, nontender and does not blanch.

DIAGNOSIS: Purpura annularis telangiectodes

10/15/08 11:47:39

You Code It!

What are the best, most accurate codes?

_____

_____

_____

DENTAL ASSOCIATES OF ARRINGTON
9550 ENAMEL BLVD. • MOLAR, FL 32811 • 407-555-4703

PATIENT: ASSRHAM, RANDIWAH
ACCOUNT/EHR #:   ASSRA001
Date: 10/15/08

Patient is a 41-year-old female.

CHIEF COMPLAINT: Patient requests a routine examination.

MEDICAL HISTORY: No abnormalities identified.

DENTAL HISTORY: No abnormalities identified. The patient does not wear dentures.

CLINICAL FINDINGS: Multiple, blue-to-black areas with irregular borders are located on the right maxillary tuberosity, hard palate, and soft palate. The pigmented lesions are nontender and smooth to palpation. They do not blanch and do not rub off. Some of the lesions are flat and nonthickened, while other areas are thickened and firm to palpation. All the pigmented areas are fixed to the surface mucosa, but only the thickened areas are fixed to the underlying structures. No radiographic abnormalities are identified. The patient was unaware of the lesions. There are no palpable lymph nodes or other palpable masses. No skin lesions are identified.

TREATMENT: Complete series x-rays, including bitewings; periodic oral examination

DIAGNOSIS: Dyschromia

10/15/08 11:47:39

You Code It!

What are the best, most accurate codes?

_____

_____

_____

DENTAL ASSOCIATES OF ARRINGTON
9550 ENAMEL BLVD. • MOLAR, FL 32811 • 407-555-4703

PATIENT: CARR, ROSEMARY
ACCOUNT/EHR #: CARRO001
Date: 10/15/08

Patient is a 27-year-old female.

CHIEF COMPLAINT: Patient complains of painful oral ulcers of five days duration. The patient has not noticed blisters. The lesions have occurred five times previously, always in the same location. The lesions resolved in two weeks for each episode.

MEDICAL HISTORY: No abnormalities identified.

DENTAL HISTORY: An amalgam restoration was placed in a maxillary right tooth one week ago.

CLINICAL FINDINGS: Multiple ulcers are present on the right hard palate in the first molar region. The lesions are tender when palpated and are not thickened.

DIAGNOSIS: Ulcerative stomatitis

RX: Steroidal cream

10/15/08 11:47:39

You Code It!

What are the best, most accurate codes?

_____

_____

_____

DENTAL ASSOCIATES OF ARRINGTON
9550 ENAMEL BLVD. • MOLAR, FL 32811 • 407-555-4703

PATIENT: DIAZ, LANCE
ACCOUNT/EHR #:   DIALA001
Date: 10/15/08

Patient is a 25-year-old male.

CHIEF COMPLAINT: Patient requests a routine examination.

MEDICAL HISTORY: No abnormalities are identified.

DENTAL HISTORY: No abnormalities are identified.

CLINICAL FINDINGS: Tooth #32 is unerupted and displaced by a well-circumscribed radiolucent lesion associated with the crown of the tooth.

TREATMENT: Comprehensive periodontal evaluation, new patient; complete series x-rays w/bitewings

DIAGNOSIS: Displaced tooth #32; radicular cyst.

10/15/08 11:47:39

You Code It!

What are the best, most accurate codes?

_____

_____

_____

DENTAL ASSOCIATES OF ARRINGTON
9550 ENAMEL BLVD. • MOLAR, FL 32811 • 407-555-4703

PATIENT: MILTON, SILVESTER

ACCOUNT/EHR #:   MILSI001

Date: 10/15/08

Patient is a 58-year-old male.

CHIEF COMPLAINT: The patient reports swelling in the left mandible of 3 months duration. The swelling is not painful.

MEDICAL HISTORY: No abnormalities are identified.

DENTAL HISTORY: No abnormalities are identified.

CLINICAL FINDINGS: Nontender bony expansion is palpated in the left body of the mandible. Radiographic examination reveals a radiolucent lesion with well-defined, corticated borders. No other abnormalities are identified.

DIAGNOSIS: Torus mandibularis

10/15/08 11:47:39

You Code It!

What are the best, most accurate codes?

_____

_____

_____

DENTAL ASSOCIATES OF ARRINGTON
9550 ENAMEL BLVD. • MOLAR, FL 32811 • 407-555-4703

PATIENT: INGRAM, MARK
ACCOUNT/EHR #:   INGMA001
Date: 10/15/08

Patient is a 37-year-old male.

CHIEF COMPLAINT: Patient requests a routine examination.

MEDICAL HISTORY: No abnormalities are identified.

DENTAL HISTORY: No abnormalities are identified.

CLINICAL FINDINGS: During routine radiographic examination (complete series), a radiolucent lesion with sharply defined, corticated borders is noted in the mandibular right body of the mandible. The lesion demonstrates radiopaque areas within the radiolucent region.

DIAGNOSIS: Latent bone cyst of the jaw

10/15/08 11:47:39

You Code It!

What are the best, most accurate codes?

_____

_____

_____

DENTAL ASSOCIATES OF ARRINGTON
9550 ENAMEL BLVD. • MOLAR, FL 32811 • 407-555-4703

PATIENT: MC PHERSON, SALLY
ACCOUNT/EHR #:   MCPSA001
Date: 10/15/08

Patient is a one-year-old female.

CHIEF COMPLAINT: Patient referred for evaluation of mobile teeth and gingival swelling.

MEDICAL HISTORY: Alert, ill-appearing girl. The patient has a history of intermittent malaise, fever and irritability during the past two months. The patient has recently been evaluated by the University Hospital. Examination there revealed axillary lymphadenopathy and marked hepatosplenomegaly. Radiographic examination of the skull revealed numerous, well-demarcated radiolucent lesions of the cranium. Bone marrow biopsy did not reveal abnormal cellular infiltrates. No other abnormalities are identified.

DENTAL HISTORY: No abnormalities are identified.

CLINICAL FINDINGS: The gingival surrounding the erupting deciduous first molars is enlarged, erythematous, nontender and spongy to palpation. The erupting teeth exhibit marked mobility. Panoramic radiograph reveals diffuse horizontal alveolar bone loss.

DIAGNOSIS: Alveolar mandibular hypoplasia

10/15/08 11:47:39

You Code It!

What are the best, most accurate codes?

_____

_____

_____

DENTAL ASSOCIATES OF ARRINGTON
9550 ENAMEL BLVD. • MOLAR, FL 32811 • 407-555-4703

PATIENT: ALLINGTON, CHAD
ACCOUNT/EHR #:   ALLCH001
Date: 10/15/08

Patient is a 68-year-old male.

CHIEF COMPLAINT: Patient requests routine dental care.

MEDICAL HISTORY: Alert, normally developed, in no distress. Carcinoma of prostate treated by surgical excision two years ago. Previous history of cystitis and urinary incontinence subsequent to prostate surgery. No symptoms or abnormalities in past year. Denies cardiovascular, pulmonary, gastrointestinal, allergic disease or abnormality.

DENTAL HISTORY: Multiple tooth extractions secondary to dental caries. No extractions in past six years. Maxillary partial denture constructed ten years ago. Patient does not wear partial at night. Has never had mandibular prosthetic appliance.

CLINICAL FINDINGS: Periodontitis type II, missing teeth, calculus. Complete x-ray series w/bitewings show circumscribed radiolucent area in the left mandibular edentulous second and third molar region. No other abnormalities identified.

10/15/08 11:47:39

You Code It!

What are the best, most accurate codes?

_____

_____

_____

DERMATOLOGY ASSOCIATES OF CAULDWELL
469 EPIDURAL LANE • SUBQUE, FL 32711 • 407-555-7539

PATIENT: BERN, BEBE
MRN: BERBE01
Date: 9 October 2008

Physician: Collin L. Jonston, MD

This new patient is a 19-year-old female who comes in with a complaint of blisters all over her hands. She works in the mailroom of a large International corporation, and is very concerned that this may be a reaction to anthrax exposure.

VITALS: T 98.8, R 16, P regular. Visual inspection of skin disruption reveals no inflammation. Skin scraping is negative for anthrax or other poisons under microscopic investigation.

DX: Pimples

Collin L. Jonston, MD

10/13/08 11:47:39

You Code It!

What are the best, most accurate codes?

_____

_____

_____

DERMATOLOGY ASSOCIATES OF CAULDWELL
469 EPIDURAL LANE • SUBQUE, FL 32711 • 407-555-7539

PATIENT: HEINZ, HARRISON
MRN: HEIHA01
Date: 9 October 2008

Physician: Collin L. Jonston, MD

This 27-year-old male was brought to the Emergency Room via ambulance after sustaining severe chemical burns to his face, neck, arms, and both hands while working at the chemical plant.

Examination reveals 3rd degree burns on his face and both hands, and 2nd degree burns on his neck and arms. Patient is wrapped in sterile gauze and transferred to the Burn Unit.

10/13/08 11:47:39

You Code It!

What are the best, most accurate codes?

_____

_____

_____

DERMATOLOGY ASSOCIATES OF CAULDWELL
469 EPIDURAL LANE • SUBQUE, FL 32711 • 407-555-7539

PATIENT: VAN DYKE, ROBERTA

MRN: VANRO01

Date: 9 October 2008

History & Physical Exam: A 20-year-old African-American female presented to the emergency room with complaints of malaise, myalgia, chills, sore throat, fever, photophobia, diarrhea, neck stiffness, headache, chest pain and "bruise on leg." The patient was in her usual state of health until the day prior to presentation.

On exam, the patient was lethargic, complaining of chest pain with a blood pressure of 89/36. She had a faint, purpuric rash and scattered petechiae on the lower extremities.

Labs: WBC: 27K PLT: 223 PT: 31 INR: 1.23 PTT: 31

Skin biopsy was performed.

Diagnosis: Meningococcemia

_____

Suzanna A. Maconi, MD

SAM/ghh 10/9/08 11:47:39

You Code It!

What are the best, most accurate codes?

_____

_____

_____

DERMATOLOGY ASSOCIATES OF CAULDWELL
469 EPIDURAL LANE • SUBQUE, FL 32711 • 407-555-7539

PATIENT: FORRESTER, MATHIAS
MRN: FORMA01
Date: 9 October 2008

History of Present Illness: This is a 57-year-old African-American male with history of acute lymphocytic lymphoma (ALL) status post bone marrow transplant. He has a history of graft versus host disease. He was recently hospitalized for sepsis. A consult to dermatology was ordered to evaluate a scaly rash of his scalp and feet that has been present for one year. Patient denies pain or pruritus of this eruption. He had been treated with topical triamcinolone with no improvement.

PMH: ALL, GVHD, CMV, bacterial sepsis, DVT

Meds: Prograf, prednisone, acyclovir, bactrim, MS Contin, vancomycin, Cipro, Lexapro

Physical Examination: Diffuse, hyperkeratotic, crusted plaques of the face, scalp, chest, arms, legs and feet (Figs 1-3). Thickened dystrophic nails.

Diagnosis: Crusted (Norwegian) Scabies

Plan: RX Permethrin 5% cream
      Follow-up in office one week.

Suzanna A. Maconi, MD

SAM/ghh 10/9/08 11:47:39

You Code It!

What are the best, most accurate codes?

_____

_____

_____

DERMATOLOGY ASSOCIATES OF CAULDWELL
469 EPIDURAL LANE • SUBQUE, FL 32711 • 407-555-7539

PATIENT: DUFFY, DENNIS
MRN: DUFDE01
Date: 9 October 2008

HISTORY OF PRESENT ILLNESS: Patient is a 58-year-old white male with a history of colon cancer diagnosed in 1999 that was treated with resection and chemotherapy. Three months after surgery, he began to notice the growth of abnormal facial hair. This hair growth progressively worsened, and he presented to the VA Dermatology Clinic in March 2004. At the time of presentation, there was no evidence of recurrence of the primary malignancy; however, the patient was being followed for a one and one-half year history of hoarseness and unexplained mediastinal lymphadenopathy.

PHYSICAL EXAM: Excess growth of fine, lightly pigmented hairs on cheeks, eyelids, nose, and ears.

DIAGNOSIS: Hypertrichosis Lanuginosa Acquisita (Malignant Down)

PLAN: Topical therapy with Epi-Stop and Vaniqa

Suzanna A. Maconi, MD

SAM/ghh 10/9/08 11:47:39

You Code It!

What are the best, most accurate codes?

_____

_____

_____

DERMATOLOGY ASSOCIATES OF CAULDWELL
469 EPIDURAL LANE • SUBQUE, FL 32711 • 407-555-7539

PATIENT: REINGOLD, MELISSA
MRN: REIME01
Date: 9 October 2008

HISTORY OF PRESENT ILLNESS: This 51-year-old Caucasian woman presented to the Dermatology outpatient clinic for a skin examination, and was noted to have a red papule on her left breast. The lesion had been present for one year and was asymptomatic. The patient has a past medical history notable for papillary carcinoma of the same breast two years prior, which was treated with breast conservation surgery and radiation.

PHYSICAL EXAMINATION: The lesion appeared as a firm and non-tender erythematous papule, 4mm. There was no clinical evidence of ulceration. A punch excision of the lesion was performed in clinic.

DIAGNOSIS: Atypical Vascular Proliferation

PROCEDURE: Simple excision is performed.

Suzanna A. Maconi, MD

SAM/ghh 10/9/08 11:47:39

You Code It!

What are the best, most accurate codes?

_____

_____

_____

DERMATOLOGY ASSOCIATES OF CAULDWELL
469 EPIDURAL LANE • SUBQUE, FL 32711 • 407-555-7539

PATIENT: PARKS, CLIFTON
MRN: PARCL01
Date: 9 October 2008

HISTORY OF PRESENT ILLNESS: Patient is a 70-year-old African-American male who presented to the Dermatology Clinic complaining of a painless, slowly enlarging growth on the left side of his nose. The patient noted that the lesion has been present for at least 15 years.

PHYSICAL EXAMINATION: A 2 cm x 1 cm soft skin colored pedunculated nodule was present on the inferior edge of the left nasal ala.

DIAGNOSIS: Polypoid Sebaceous Hamartoma with connective tissue and organoid features

PROCEDURE: Simple excision is performed.

Suzanna A. Maconi, MD

SAM/ghh 10/9/08 11:47:39

You Code It!

What are the best, most accurate codes?

_____

_____

_____

DERMATOLOGY ASSOCIATES OF CAULDWELL
469 EPIDURAL LANE • SUBQUE, FL 32711 • 407-555-7539

PATIENT: EVERSON, REGINA
MRN: EVERE01
Date: 9 October 2008

HISTORY OF PRESENT ILLNESS: This 24-year-old black female developed fevers one week after Cesarean section for twins. She presented to her primary gynecologist who prescribed Keflex for a post-operative wound infection. The patient's fever persisted and she presented to her local hospital. During the patient's hospitalization, she developed an episode of transient visual loss and confusion that was diagnosed as hysterical blindness. She also developed generalized pustules and worsening mental status. She was transferred to the Hospital Medical ICU. I was then called in for this dermatologic consultation.

PHYSICAL EXAM: The patient had fever (41°C), confusion, and a faint systolic ejection murmur heard best at the apex. Her initial dermatologic exam was significant for diffuse pustules on the face, trunk, and extremities. Her recent surgical scar was erythematous with purulent discharge.

TESTING: The patient developed splinter hemorrhages, Roth spots, Janeway lesions, and Osler's nodes over the next few days. The patient's pustules, blood, and CSF were sent for gram stain and culture. She was empirically started on Vancomycin for extended gram-positive coverage. All body fluids sent grew oxacillin-resistant Staphylococcus aureus.

DIAGNOSIS: ORSA (oxacillin-resistant Staphylococcus aureus) endocarditis with septic emboli to skin.

PLAN: IV antibiotics

Suzanna A. Maconi, MD

SAM/ghh 10/9/08 11:47:39

You Code It!

What are the best, most accurate codes?

_____

_____

_____

DERMATOLOGY ASSOCIATES OF CAULDWELL
469 EPIDURAL LANE • SUBQUE, FL 32711 • 407-555-7539

PATIENT: DONNELLSON, CARLA
MRN: DONCA01
Date: 9 October 2008

HISTORY OF PRESENT ILLNESS: A 51-year-old Caucasian female presented to our dermatology clinic with a painful, itchy rash present for one year. Her past medical history is significant for an extensive hot water burn 13 years prior requiring skin grafting. Her review of systems was significant for dull muscle aches, primarily affecting her back and lower legs.

PHYSICAL EXAMINATION: Cutaneous examination revealed multiple violaceous papules and plaques along the edges of graft sites. The upper extremities, lower extremities, and torso were primarily affected with sparing of the head and neck.

A skin biopsy was performed.

DIAGNOSIS: Cutaneous Sarcoidosis

PLAN: Multiple short-term courses of prednisone for temporary relief of her rash and myalgias.

Suzanna A. Maconi, MD

SAM/ghh 10/9/08 11:47:39

You Code It!

What are the best, most accurate codes?

_____

_____

_____

DERMATOLOGY ASSOCIATES OF CAULDWELL
469 EPIDURAL LANE • SUBQUE, FL 32711 • 407-555-7539

PATIENT: CRAWFORD, VELMA
MRN: CRAVE01
Date: 9 October 2008

HISTORY OF PRESENT ILLNESS: The patient is a 43-year-old woman with a history of acute myelogenous leukemia, in remission six weeks after allogeneic bone marrow transplantation, who presented with an eruption of asymptomatic pink papules on her trunk that has appeared over the previous two weeks.

PHYSICAL EXAM: On her lower back and abdomen were scores of firm, pink papules, 4-10 mm in size.

DIAGNOSIS: Leukemia Cutis

PLAN: Referral for chemotherapy

Suzanna A. Maconi, MD

SAM/ghh 10/9/08 11:47:39

You Code It!

What are the best, most accurate codes?

_____

_____

_____

DERMATOLOGY ASSOCIATES OF CAULDWELL
469 EPIDURAL LANE • SUBQUE, FL 32711 • 407-555-7539

PATIENT: WORTHINGTON, WILMA
MRN: WORWI01
Date: 9 October 2008

HISTORY OF PRESENT ILLNESS: This is a 59-year-old white female who over the past 5 months noticed a progressive thickening and darkening of the skin of her palms, dorsal hands, and ventral wrists. She has also noticed a texture change involving the roof of her mouth.

PHYSICAL EXAM: On full-body skin exam she had rugose thickening of the palms with dermatoglyphic accentuation and a velvety appearance. On the soft palate was a velvety-appearing plaque. There were fine vellus hair growth on the forehead, nose, and cheeks. She has otherwise been feeling well without weight loss, fatigue, or other systemic complaints. She is on no medications.

CBC, comprehensive metabolic panel, and liver function tests, chest x-ray, mammogram, and colonoscopy all report negative.

DIAGNOSIS: Tripe Palms and Florid Mucosal Acanthosis

PLAN: With the high association of her skin findings with internal cancer, further work-up is indicated.

Suzanna A. Maconi, MD

SAM/ghh 10/9/08 11:47:39

You Code It!

What are the best, most accurate codes?

_____

_____

_____

DERMATOLOGY ASSOCIATES OF CAULDWELL
469 EPIDURAL LANE • SUBQUE, FL 32711 • 407-555-7539

PATIENT: KOLOZVARY, ADAM

MRN: KOLAD01

Date: 9 October 2008

HISTORY OF PRESENT ILLNESS: The patient is a 30-year-old graduate student who presented after vacationing for the summer in Ecuador. He had developed an itchy rash on both feet and right thigh that started prior to his return to the United States. The lesions continue to spread.

PHYSICAL EXAMINATION: The dorsum of his feet showed several erythematous, papular and vesicular, serpiginous lesions. Minimal crusting was present over several toes.

DIAGNOSIS: Cutaneous Larva Migrans (creeping eruption)

RX: Thiabendazole, 500 mg tabs x3, p.o. bid for 2 successive days

Suzanna A. Maconi, MD

SAM/ghh 10/9/08 11:47:39

You Code It!

What are the best, most accurate codes?

_____

_____

_____

DERMATOLOGY ASSOCIATES OF CAULDWELL
469 EPIDURAL LANE • SUBQUE, FL 32711 • 407-555-7539

PATIENT: BECK, JOSEPH
MRN: BECJO01
Date: 9 October 2008

HISTORY OF PRESENT ILLNESS: This patient is an 80-year-old white male with no significant past medical history who was referred to the dermatology clinic because of several pink "bumps" on his face and trunk. The patient reports that these lesions developed over a period of several months prior to presentation. They are asymptomatic, and are not rapidly growing in size. The patient denies a history of skin cancer or other skin disease.

PHYSICAL EXAMINATION: The patient has several 0.4 to 0.6 cm pink, pearly, telangiectatic papules scattered on the face, chest, and upper arms.

LABORATORY EVALUATION: A complete blood count showed mild thrombocytopenia with platelet count of 60,000. Peripheral blood smear showed mild monocytosis and rare immature myeloid cells.

DIAGNOSIS: Multiple xanthogranulomas, associated with chronic myelomonocytic leukemia.

PLAN: Due to the unusual diagnosis of adult xanthogranuloma, as well as the abnormal CBC, a full work-up was initiated to evaluate the possibility of an underlying systemic malignancy.

REFERRAL to oncology for bone marrow biopsy

RX: Intralesional corticosteroids

Suzanna A. Maconi, MD

SAM/ghh 10/9/08 11:47:39

You Code It!

What are the best, most accurate codes?

_____

_____

_____

DERMATOLOGY ASSOCIATES OF CAULDWELL
469 EPIDURAL LANE • SUBQUE, FL 32711 • 407-555-7539

PATIENT: SCHUMMER, ANISHA
MRN: SCHAN01
Date: 9 October 2008

HISTORY OF PRESENT ILLNESS: This patient is a 24-year-old woman G2P1 at 34 weeks gestation who presented with a "rash" on her hands evident since the first trimester. She denied pain or pruritus and had a similar eruption during her first pregnancy which resolved after delivery. Her past medical history was significant only for gestational diabetes.

PHYSICAL EXAM: The patient had well demarcated erythematous patches symmetrically over her distal phalanges as well as her thenar and hypothenar eminences. The areas completely blanched with pressure.

DIAGNOSIS: Pregnancy associated Palmar Erythema

PLAN: No treatment. Condition is expected to spontaneously resolve after delivery.

Suzanna A. Maconi, MD

SAM/ghh 10/9/08 11:47:39

You Code It!

What are the best, most accurate codes?

_____

_____

_____

DERMATOLOGY ASSOCIATES OF CAULDWELL
469 EPIDURAL LANE • SUBQUE, FL 32711 • 407-555-7539

PATIENT: LIGHTFOOT, YAMIDRA
MRN: LIGYA01
Date: 9 October 2008

HISTORY OF PRESENT ILLNESS: This is a 21-year-old Caucasian female who was referred to this Dermatology clinic for a history of a pruritic eruption secondary to either natural light or tanning beds. The patient states she discontinued tanning and limited her exposure to sunlight over the past six months because of an increasing sensitivity to light. She stated that she would react within a few minutes to light exposure.

PE: The patient was placed in a UVA light box for 40 seconds. As a result of an absence of response, she was immediately placed in a UVB light box for 50 seconds. No reaction to the light occurred and the patient went to the neighboring SunKiss tanning beds. She returned to our clinic with erythematous plaques after less than one minute in the tanning bed. This rash resolved within 30 minutes. Skin biopsy was performed.

DIAGNOSIS: Solar urticaria

PLAN: RX: Antihistamines and light treatment for hardening

Suzanna A. Maconi, MD

SAM/ghh 10/9/08 11:47:39

You Code It!

What are the best, most accurate codes?

_____

_____

_____

DERMATOLOGY ASSOCIATES OF CAULDWELL
469 EPIDURAL LANE • SUBQUE, FL 32711 • 407-555-7539

PATIENT: MC KENZIE, DANIEL
MRN: MCKDA01
Date: 9 October 2008

HISTORY OF PRESENT ILLNESS: This 20-year-old white man presented to the dermatology clinic for evaluation of draining facial nodules. The patient is a member of the military, and is anticipating imminent deployment to the Middle East. His history is notable for being stationed in southern California several months previously, while in basic training. In addition, his family recently adopted a stray kitten that has been sleeping in the same bed with the patient.

The patient reported that when the eruption first appeared, 4-6 weeks prior to his presentation in our office, the lesions looked like "ringworm," with circular pink scaly patches. His primary care physician, Dr. Alendar, treated him at that time with Lotrisone (clotrimazole/betamethasone dipropionate) twice daily. Because the lesions worsened, becoming more painful and swollen, with purulent drainage, his physician then treated him with a course of cephalexin, followed by a course of azithromycin, and finally a course of Augmentin, all while continuing his Lotrisone. The patient also reported that two large "boils" on his face were drained by Dr. Alendar. The patient reported moderate clinical improvement on Augmentin.

The patient presents today for a second opinion. He was concerned this eruption would interfere with his deployment.

PE: Upon presentation, the patient appears as a healthy male in no distress. He is afebrile and vitals are stable. On examination, he is noted to have erythema and inflammation of his lower face and neck, with draining red nodules along his jawline. In addition, he has two pink scaly plaques on his abdomen, each with central pustules.

Four punch biopsies are performed: two for tissue culture and two for histopathologic examination. In addition, wound cultures from the pustules on his abdomen are obtained. A PPD was placed to rule out tuberculosis, and was found to be non-reactive. A chest x-ray is within normal limits.

LAB RESULTS: Tissue and wound cultures taken from the abdomen and the left face revealed the diagnosis.

DIAGNOSIS: Tinea barbae secondary to Trichophytin mentagrophytes

RX: Sporanox, 150 mg, daily for three weeks + topical antifungal cream and a low-potency topical steroid

Suzanna A. Maconi, MD

SAM/ghh 10/9/08 11:47:39

You Code It!

What are the best, most accurate codes?

_____

_____

_____

DERMATOLOGY ASSOCIATES OF CAULDWELL
469 EPIDURAL LANE • SUBQUE, FL 32711 • 407-555-7539

PATIENT: TROTTIER, MARSHALL
MRN: TROMA01
Date: 9 October 2008

HISTORY OF PRESENT ILLNESS: This premature male was born via C-section at 29 weeks of gestation to a 29-year-old G4P2Ab1 female with a monochorionic triplet pregnancy. Marshall was born with extensive skin defects involving the trunk, scalp and extremities. Triplet B died in utero at 14 weeks of gestation. Triplet C died of hydrops fetalis at delivery.

PHYSICAL EXAMINATION: On the flanks, abdomen, and scalp showed sharply demarcated lesions covered with a glistening membrane, an absence of the epidermis and dermis with prominent vasculature. No syndactyly, limb reduction or cleft palate was present. Corneal opacities and glaucoma were present.

LABORATORY FINDINGS: An MRI of the head revealed cerebral dysmorphism posteriorly with absence of the corpus callosum. Colpocephaly, Schizocephaly, & Lissencephaly were also found. Abdominal film revealed mild left hydronephrosis.

DIAGNOSIS: Aplasia Cutis Congenita

PLAN: A skin flap is performed to repair the defect on the vertex of the scalp with good results. The other areas were covered with AlloDerm and skin grafting will be carried out in the future.

Suzanna A. Maconi, MD

SAM/ghh 10/9/08 11:47:39

You Code It!

What are the best, most accurate codes?

_____

_____

_____

DERMATOLOGY ASSOCIATES OF CAULDWELL
469 EPIDURAL LANE • SUBQUE, FL 32711 • 407-555-7539

PATIENT: STRICKLAND, JADE
MRN: STRJA01
Date: 9 October 2008

HISTORY OF PRESENT ILLNESS: This patient is a 49-year-old African-American female presenting with a one-month history of a diffuse-skin eruption. She reported that the eruption was at first mild and became severe one week prior to presentation. The eruption was pruritic and not painful. She denied eye pain, abdominal pain, dysuria, chest pain, dyspnea, myalgia, or arthralgias. She reported an intermittent fever for 3 weeks and facial edema. Past medical history was significant for a subarachnoid hemorrhage six weeks prior to presentation from a ruptured aneurysm which was treated with cerebral aneurysm clipping. She started Dilantin at this time (six weeks prior to presentation) as seizure prophylaxis. Other medications included atenolol, lisinopril, and aspirin.

PHYSICAL EXAMINATION: Vital signs at presentation were: T 39.4 °C, BP 140/90, heart rate 118, and respiratory rate 18. She has significant facial edema with numerous pustules and yellow crust. Her skin reveals an erythroderma with red papules on her arms and legs some of which were vesiculated. Her lips had yellow crust, but she did not have mucosal involvement of the oropharynx, conjunctiva, or vagina. She has an enlarged right anterior cervical lymph node.

LAB FINDINGS: Electrocardiogram revealed sinus tachycardia. Laboratory analysis revealed a WBC of 4.6 x 103/mcl, hemoglobin of 11.6 g/dL, and platelet count of 33 x 103/mcl. The platelet count normalized without transfusion of platelets suggesting that the initial value was a laboratory error. Her eosinophil count was 1.1 x 103/mcl (24% of the WBC). A complete metabolic panel was significant for a slightly elevated AST and ALT of 63 and 58, respectively.

DIAGNOSIS: Drug reaction with eosinophilia and systemic symptoms (DRESS) formerly referred to as drug hypersensitivity syndrome.

PLAN: RX: Systemic corticosteroids

Suzanna A. Maconi, MD

SAM/ghh 10/9/08 11:47:39

You Code It!

What are the best, most accurate codes?

_____

_____

_____

DERMATOLOGY ASSOCIATES OF CAULDWELL
469 EPIDURAL LANE • SUBQUE, FL 32711 • 407-555-7539

PATIENT: SAFKEN, ANTONIA
MRN: SAFAN01
Date: 9 October 2008

HISTORY OF PRESENT ILLNESS: Patient is a previously healthy 7-year-old girl presenting from an outside hospital for evaluation and treatment of swelling of the head and neck. The patient's mother reports that the patient was sleeping on a rarely used hide-a-bed when she awoke in middle of the night crying and complaining of lip pain. Within hours, the patient's mother noted significant swelling of the left lip and face. The patient was taken to a small local hospital. Despite treatment with antihistamines, epinephrine, and IV steroids at the outside hospital, the patient experienced rapidly progressing facial and neck swelling requiring transfer to Children's Hospital. Shortly after admission, the patient was intubated due to a compromised airway. The patient remained intubated in the pediatric intensive care unit for five days. As the swelling slowly resolved, a necrotic papule became apparent on the left lower lip. A dusky depressed linear plaque in a gravitational pattern also developed along the left chin and mandible.

TEST RESULTS: All laboratory results were within normal limits. Imaging of the head and neck revealed extensive soft tissue swelling. As the edema improved and the area of necrosis became visible, a brown recluse bite was suspected. Upon further interview, the patient's father reported seeing a brown spider in the area of the hide-a-bed. Based on the patient's history, the presence of a brown spider, and a clinically compatible lesion, a diagnosis of probable brown recluse bite was made.

DIAGNOSIS: Life-threatening head and neck edema secondary to probable brown recluse spider bite of the lip

PLAN: Thorough cleansing followed by rest, ice, compression, and elevation (RICE) is indicated for mild localized lesions without systemic involvement. RX: Antibiotics, to prevent secondary infection. Aspirin can be used to counteract platelet aggregation. Parents are warned that heat should be avoided as it potentiates the venom's enzymatic activity.

Suzanna A. Maconi, MD

SAM/ghh 10/9/08 11:47:39

You Code It!

What are the best, most accurate codes?

_____

_____

_____

DERMATOLOGY ASSOCIATES OF CAULDWELL
469 EPIDURAL LANE • SUBQUE, FL 32711 • 407-555-7539

PATIENT: VALENTIN, KERI
MRN: VALKE01
Date: 9 October 2008

HISTORY OF PRESENT ILLNESS: This patient is a 43-year-old Caucasian male who was admitted to the hospital with a two-year history of petechial lesions on the bilateral lower extremities and a two-week history of swelling and pain of the right ankle. He denies any history of trauma, bites, tick exposure, or new medications. Additional findings are significant for submucosal hemorrhage of the oral mucosa and gingival hypertrophy with bleeding gums.

PAST MEDICAL HISTORY: noncontributory.

SOCIAL HISTORY: Significant for heavy alcohol consumption of approximately 12 beers/day.

MEDICATIONS: Patient denies any medications at time of admission and denies using recreational drugs.

LABORATORY DATA: Significant for anemia (hemoglobin -11.6, hematocrit - 34.1) and leucopenia (WBC 2.1). CMP panel was within normal limits.

DIAGNOSIS: Scurvy

PLAN: Supplementation with Vitamin C, 100 mg 3-5x/day until a total of 4g is reached then 100mg qd. Patient is counseled to have a diet rich in fruits and vegetables such as grapefruit, lemons, broccoli, green peppers, tomatoes, and cabbage.

Suzanna A. Maconi, MD

SAM/ghh 10/9/08 11:47:39

You Code It!

What are the best, most accurate codes?

_____

_____

_____

DERMATOLOGY ASSOCIATES OF CAULDWELL
469 EPIDURAL LANE • SUBQUE, FL 32711 • 407-555-7539

PATIENT: CROWE, CASSANDRA

MRN: CROCA01

Date: 9 October 2008

HISTORY OF PRESENT ILLNESS: This is a 54-year-old woman complaining of a painless, nonpruritic, nonhealing ulcer on her left nipple that has been evident for six months. The patient denies any discharge.

PAST MEDICAL HISTORY: Hypertension

FAMILY HISTORY: Positive for breast cancer of unknown type in her sister and aunt. Mammogram and ultrasound showed a hypervascular nipple mass.

PHYSICAL EXAM: On physical exam she has a 1.3 x 1.5 cm palpable mass covering 90% of her nipple. There was no peripheral infiltration, no discharge, and no axillary lymphadenopathy. The left nipple is 2 cm higher than the right nipple. Nipple to midline distance is 12 cm on the left and 11 cm on the right. She has moderate fibrocystic changes throughout both breasts.

DIAGNOSIS: Erosive adenomatosis of the nipple

PLAN: Performed successful local excision, tumorectomy, liquid nitrogen and Mohs.

_____

Suzanna A. Maconi, MD

SAM/ghh 10/9/08 11:47:39

You Code It!

What are the best, most accurate codes?

_____

_____

_____

DERMATOLOGY ASSOCIATES OF CAULDWELL
469 EPIDURAL LANE • SUBQUE, FL 32711 • 407-555-7539

PATIENT: BEGAMMO, SHENIKA
MRN: BEGSH01
Date: 9 October 2008

HISTORY OF PRESENT ILLNESS: This 64-year-old Caucasian female presents to the emergency room with a 10-year history of a progressively enlarging ulcer on the right arm. The lesion had never been biopsied or treated. She has not seen a physician for any complaint for 20 years. The patient has hidden the lesion from her family until it was noticed two days prior to her presentation by her son, who brought her to the hospital. She denies pain or decreased range of motion of the right arm. She denies systemic symptoms.

PAST MEDICAL HISTORY: Patient denied any medical conditions.

MEDICATIONS: None.

PHYSICAL EXAMINATION: A large ulcer is present on the right arm, ulcerated to muscle, with rolled, infiltrated borders. There is a palpable 2 cm right axillary lymphadenopathy. A 2.5 x 1 cm slightly brown, telangiectatic, irregularly shaped plaque is present on the right back.

LABORATORY DATA: CBC: WBC: 6.0 (3.8-9.8); Hgb: 2.9 (12.1-15.1); Hct: 10.6 (36.1-44.3); Plt: 445K (140-440K); MCV 52.7 (74-115) CMP: Sodium: 137 (135-145); Potassium: 3.9 (3.3-4.9); Chloride: 106 (97-110); Bicarbonate: 21 (20-28); Creatinine: 0.8 (0.6-1.4); BUN: 10 (8-25); Glucose: 124 (65-199)

Plasma protein: 7.8 (6.5-8.5); Albumin: 3.1 (3.6-5.0); Bili: 0.4 (0.3-1.1); Alk Phos: 82 (38-126); AST: 13 (11-47); ALT: 25 (7-53); INR: 1.31 (0.8-1.2): PTT: 32.8 (23-35)

RADIOGRAPHY: Chest and right humerus radiographs revealed multiple poorly defined nodules over the right lung field, slightly enlarged right hilar shadow, with normal left lung field and cardiac silhouette, and no effusion. A large soft tissue defect was present over the proximal humerus.

DIAGNOSIS: Basal cell carcinomas, metastatic

PROCEDURE: Surgery to remove carcinoma on humerus to be followed by chemotherapy [Cis-platinum]

Suzanna A. Maconi, MD

SAM/ghh 10/9/08 11:47:39

You Code It!

What are the best, most accurate codes?

_____

_____

_____

DERMATOLOGY ASSOCIATES OF CAULDWELL
469 EPIDURAL LANE • SUBQUE, FL 32711 • 407-555-7539

PATIENT: SLATE, ASHLEY
MRN: SLAAS01
Date: 9 October 2008

HISTORY OF PRESENT ILLNESS: This patient is a 39-year-old African-American male who works as a roofer with significant occupational exposure to pigeon droppings who presented last week to the emergency department with a two-week history of fever, chills, nausea, fatigue, and a twenty-pound weight loss. A chest x-ray revealed hilar lymphadenopathy and presumptive treatment for pneumonia was begun with oral levofloxacin.

He returns today with an additional onset of diffuse lymphadenopathy, decreased visual acuity, a tender effusion of the left wrist, and new skin lesions. It is at this time that he was referred to me.

PHYSICAL EXAMINATION: Skin exam reveals multiple skin-color papules and nodules over the face, ranging in size from 3-15 mm. Some of the lesions have central crusting and ulceration. He additionally has a 5 cm firm left submental mass and diffuse lymphadenopathy over his entire body.

LABORATORY STUDIES: HIV: Negative. Three 4 mm punch biopsies are performed for culture and H&E.

DIAGNOSIS: Disseminated Cryptococcus in an apparently immunocompetent patient

RX: Fluconazole, p.o.

PLAN: Long-term follow up to discover whether he has an occult disease causing immunosuppression

___

Suzanna A. Maconi, MD

SAM/ghh 10/9/08 11:47:39

You Code It!

What are the best, most accurate codes?

___

___

___

DERMATOLOGY ASSOCIATES OF CAULDWELL
469 EPIDURAL LANE • SUBQUE, FL 32711 • 407-555-7539

PATIENT: MARTINEZ-ORTIZ, ALIZA
MRN: MARAL01
Date: 9 October 2008

HISTORY OF PRESENT ILLNESS: This is a 45-year-old Hispanic female, with a past medical history significant only for rectal fissures in the 1980's, presenting for an evaluation of a plaque present for 5-6 years on her right temple. The lesion began as a small pink papule. However, throughout the years, it has noticeably been increasing in size. She denies any pruritus, pain, or other symptoms associated with the lesion. Moreover, she has no personal or family history of diabetes mellitus. She had two biopsies performed on the lesion in the past. She states the first biopsy was consistent with a keratinous cyst, and the second biopsy demonstrated a non-specific dermatitis.

PERTINENT MEDICATIONS: Prempro

PHYSICAL EXAM: Physical exam demonstrates a thin, Hispanic female. On the right temple, there is a 5.3 by 6.3 centimeter plaque, which had a pearly, yellow atrophic center that contains prominent telangiectasias. Surrounding the atrophic center, there is a palpable, red-brown border. There are no other similar plaques located anywhere else on her body.

DIAGNOSIS: Necrobiosis Lipoidica located on the face

RX: Thalidomide was initiated at 50 mg each night. In order to reduce the potential risk of thrombosis associated with the usage of Thalidomide, especially given the concurrent use of Prempro and her history of tobacco use, aspirin 81 mg daily was also prescribed. Smoking cessation was encouraged.

_____

Suzanna A. Maconi, MD

SAM/ghh 10/9/08 11:47:39

You Code It!

What are the best, most accurate codes?

_____

_____

_____

DERMATOLOGY ASSOCIATES OF CAULDWELL
469 EPIDURAL LANE • SUBQUE, FL 32711 • 407-555-7539

PATIENT: PICARD, TERRELL
MRN: PICTE01
Date: 9 October 2008

HISTORY OF PRESENT ILLNESS: This is a 55-year-old white male with a one-year history of worsening rash on his face, back, elbows, hips, knees, and palms. He was referred here for evaluation of pruritus and possible tinea versicolor.

PAST MEDICAL HISTORY: Remarkable for primary biliary cirrhosis (PBC), and he is awaiting a liver transplant. In the meantime, he is being treated with ursodiol (Actigall) for his PBC.

PHYSICAL EXAM: Cachectic WM with diffuse jaundice. Peri-orbital yellow papules and plaques and facial telangiectasias. A large V-shaped yellow plaque on his chest back and upper extremities with a distinct line of demarcation. Red-yellow papules and nodules on bilateral elbows and knees. A well-demarcated yellow plaque on his right hip and yellow discoloration of his palmar surfaces were also noted.

LABORATORY VALUES: Total Cholesterol 678, HDL 14, LDL 607, Triglycerides 190. Alkaline phosphatase 721, Bilirubin 6.7, AST 89, ALT 36

DIAGNOSIS: Xanthomatosis secondary to primary biliary cirrhosis-related hyperlipidemia

IMPRESSION: The hypercholesterolemia in PBC is due to reduction in cholesterol secretion, and the treatment mainstay is liver transplantation. Although responses to systemic medications have been poor, ursodiol (Actigall) has been shown in some studies to increase survival, time to transplant, and reduce cholesterol levels. Other agents that may be helpful include azathioprine and cyclosporine. Unfortunately, none of these treatments have been shown to reliably improve xanthomatosis, and this patient will eventually require liver transplantation for survival.

Suzanna A. Maconi, MD

SAM/ghh 10/9/08 11:47:39

You Code It!

What are the best, most accurate codes?

_____

_____

_____

DERMATOLOGY ASSOCIATES OF CAULDWELL
469 EPIDURAL LANE • SUBQUE, FL 32711 • 407-555-7539

PATIENT: MADERA, RUSSEL
MRN: MADRU01
Date: 9 October 2008

HISTORY OF PRESENT ILLNESS: This patient is a 42-year-old firefighter who suffered a flame burn injury to the skin on the left inner thigh 11 months before presentation. He was treated as an outpatient at one of the burn centers where he received topical anti-microbials and dressing changes. The wound healed by epithelialization and hypertrophic scarring.

     The patient was referred to our clinic because the burn scar had become quite hypertrophic and was unresponsive to compression stocking therapy.

PE: Using a visual analog scale of scar pruritus, the patient scored itch intensity at 6/10 (where 10 = unbearable itching) and itch frequency at 6/10 (where 10 = itching at all times). With time, the scar continued to progressively increase in thickness.

IMPRESSION: Therapy is initiated with Avogel hydrogel with 3% salicylic acid in a cream base applied to the scar each night and left for 8 to 10 hours.

Suzanna A. Maconi, MD

SAM/ghh 10/9/08 11:47:39

You Code It!

What are the best, most accurate codes?

_____

_____

_____

DERMATOLOGY ASSOCIATES OF CAULDWELL
469 EPIDURAL LANE • SUBQUE, FL 32711 • 407-555-7539

PATIENT: LUDWIG, HENRIETTA
MRN: LUDHE01
Date: 9 October 2008

HISTORY OF PRESENT ILLNESS: This patient is a 65-year-old woman who underwent open-heart surgery two years ago. She had applied vitamin E topically to the scar for a short period of time without effect. She complained of pain and tenderness, and the scar was very elevated and erythematous.

PE: The patient's scar is 14 cm long, varying from 4 to 6 mm in width, and is elevated by 3 to 4 mm. Symptomatic relief from pruritus and tenderness occurred within 48 hours of applying 2% salicylic acid and hydrogel.

    At this follow-up, the patient reports that after one week of the new regimen, she noted a marked decrease in symptoms and decreased erythema in this area. Regression in the size of the scar was less impressive, but symptomatic relief was significant.

PLAN: Patient to return for another appointment in sixty days.

Suzanna A. Maconi, MD

SAM/ghh 10/9/08 11:47:39

You Code It!

What are the best, most accurate codes?

_____

_____

_____

DERMATOLOGY ASSOCIATES OF CAULDWELL
469 EPIDURAL LANE • SUBQUE, FL 32711 • 407-555-7539

PATIENT: LUDWIG, HENRY
MRN: LUDHE01
Date: 9 October 2008

HISTORY OF PRESENT ILLNESS: This is a 31-year-old white male who was trapped in a burning apartment building when he decided to jump from a window. Pre-assessment by emergency personnel revealed burns to his extremities, scalp, face, thorax, and back (an estimated 90% total body surface area burn). It also appeared he sustained a tibia/fibula fracture of the left leg and a crush injury of the right ankle. He was brought into the emergency room on a 100% oxygen non-rebreathing mask. In the emergency room he was promptly intubated with an oral 7.5 ETT because of suspected inhalation burns. Appropriate analgesics and IV fluids were administered and the patient was placed on mechanical ventilation. He was immediately taken to the burn unit and tanked. He then went to surgery to repair and stabilize his fractures. The following day his total body surface area burns were reassessed from 90% to 60%.

PATIENT COURSE: He developed pleural effusion on the right and right upper lobe pneumonia. Pseudomonas was cultured from his sputum. Escharotomy was required on all ten fingers. Debridement and skin grafting proceeded without complications. The patient had a tracheotomy during the fourth week and is now on 4-hour trachshield trials throughout the day with mechanical ventilatory support at night.

PHYSICAL EXAM IN ER: HR 110, BP 154/110, RR 24, Chest: coarse, CV: RRR
    Pt is alert. IV Fluids started. Burns: 2nd and 3rd degree.

LABS: WBC 16 .1 mm3, Gluc 122 mg/dl, Na 141 mEq/L, K 4.0 mEq/L, Cl 105 mEq/L, Ca 9.5 mEq/L, PO4 3.6 mEq/L, Mg 1.9 mEq/L, Bun 22 mg/dl, Cr 0.9 mg/d

IMPRESSION: A restrictive defect may occur anywhere on the body, but from a respiratory standpoint, chest and abdomen burns are the most life-threatening. The burned skin will restrict chest or abdomen movement, decrease chest wall compliance, and make it very difficult to ventilate the patient.

Suzanna A. Maconi, MD

SAM/ghh 10/9/08 11:47:39

You Code It!

What are the best, most accurate codes?

_____

_____

_____

Emergency Services Cases and Patient Records

INTRODUCTION

The following case studies are from an emergency clinic. In an emergency department or urgent care clinic, a professional coding specialist is likely to see a wide variety of diagnoses and procedures.

Physicians who specialize in emergency, or urgent, care are called emergency medicine specialists, also known as ER doctors. These health care professionals diagnose and treat multiple health care concerns, often in life-threatening situations where decisions must be made quickly. Unlike many other medical specialists, ER doctors must maintain diagnostic and treatment standards for conditions that affect almost all body and organ systems.

Frequently, emergency medical specialists will diagnose and treat the patient to stabilize them and then call in a physician who specializes in the body or organ system involved for a consultation and continued care.

Some emergency medicine specialists may choose to have a subspecialty, such as infectious disease medicine or orthopedics.

Emergency medicine doctors are board-certified by the Board of Emergency Medicine, which is recognized by the American Board of Medical Specialties.

You can use these cases to practice coding diagnoses, E/M, procedures, DME, or other HCPCS Level II items, as applicable; code for the physician or the facility; code inpatient and outpatient services, as applicable:

1. Code for the physician.
2. Code for the anesthesiologist, when applicable.
3. Code for the hospital, when applicable.
4. Code for the pathology and laboratory, when applicable.
5. Code HCPCS Level II codes, when applicable.

NOTE: Despite the fact that most emergency departments are located in a hospital, these services are considered outpatient services for coding.

TYLER EMERGENCY CLINIC
911 QUICK LANE • ANYTOWN, FL 32711 • 407-555-6248

PATIENT: PARKER, PETER
ACCOUNT/EHR #   PARKPE001
Date: 10/1/08

Attending Physician: Valerie R. Victors, MD

S: This 23-year-old male was brought to the ED by ambulance after he was found unconscious on the living room floor this morning. He regained consciousness within several minutes, however, complained of a severe headache and nausea. Pt states that the last thing he remembers he was on a ladder, changing the bulb in the track lighting. He believes he lost his balance trying to reach too far to take out the next light on the track and fell, hitting his head on the coffee table.

O: Ht 5′10″ Wt. 195 lb. R 16. Head: Scalp laceration on the right posterior parietal bone. Bruise indicates trauma to this area. Eyes: PERL. Neck: Neck muscles are tense; there is minor pain upon rotation of the head. Musculoskeletal: All other aspects of the shoulders, arms, and legs are unremarkable. X-rays of skull 2 views, and soft tissue of the neck are all benign.

A: Concussion

P: 1. MRI brain to rule out subdural hematoma is negative
      2. Repair laceration and bandage

Valerie R. Victors, MD

VRV/mg   D: 10/1/08 09:50:16   T: 10/5/08 12:55:01

You Code It!

What are the best, most accurate codes?

_____

_____

_____

TYLER EMERGENCY CLINIC
911 QUICK LANE • ANYTOWN, FL 32711 • 407-555-6248

PATIENT: BLACK, YVONDA
ACCOUNT/EHR #:   BLACYV001
Date: 08/11/08

Attending Physician: Willard B. Reader, MD

Patient is a 35-year-old female seen in our emergency facility. She was brought in by ambulance, accompanied by her daughter. Daughter states that the patient was found unconscious in her bedroom, a bottle of Nytol found empty on the nightstand. Pt exhibited signs of severe depression over the course of the last 3–4 days after being served with divorce papers.

Pt is listless and unresponsive. Respiration labored, BP 80/65, P slow and erratic. Skin pale and moist. Stomach pumped. Pt responding to treatment.

DX: Poisoning by Nytol due to attempted suicide
    Admit to observation unit.
    Call for psychiatric evaluation.

Willard B. Reader, MD

DRC/pw   D: 08/11/08 09:50:16   T: 08/13/08 12:55:01

You Code It!

What are the best, most accurate codes?

_____

_____

_____

Chapter 6   Emergency Services Cases and Patient Records

TYLER EMERGENCY CLINIC
911 QUICK LANE • ANYTOWN, FL 32711 • 407-555-6248

PATIENT: BENTON, EARL
ACCOUNT/EHR #:   BENTEA001
Date: 12/01/08

Attending Physician: Willard B. Reader, MD

S: Pt is a 44-year-old male who comes in with severe pain in the lower right quadrant of his abdomen. He states that the pain is sharp and shoots across his belly from right to left. Patient also states that he has been somewhat nauseated over the last two days.

O: Ht 5′9″ Wt. 177 lb. R 21. T 101.6. BP 130/95. Abdomen appears to be tender upon manual examination. Comprehensive metabolic blood test, general health panel blood work-up, and an MRA, abdomen, angiography are taken. Results of all tests confirm diagnosis of appendicitis.

A: Acute appendicitis, w/o peritonitis

P: Pt to go to hospital immediately to be admitted for appendectomy

Willard B. Reader, MD

WBR/pw   D: 12/01/08 09:50:16   T: 12/01/08 12:55:01

You Code It!

What are the best, most accurate codes?

_____

_____

_____

TYLER EMERGENCY CLINIC
911 QUICK LANE • ANYTOWN, FL 32711 • 407-555-6248

PATIENT: FAWZI, BENITA
ACCOUNT/EHR #:   FAWZBE001
Date: 12/17/08

Attending Physician: Willard B. Reader, MD

S: Pt is a 31-year-old female who comes in with a sharp pain in the center of her torso. She states that the pain, which began approximately one week ago, comes and goes, is more severe at night, and shoots through to her back. The pain is lessened when she drinks a lot of water, and worse after meals.

O: Ht 5′4″ Wt. 125 lb. R 20. T 98.6. BP 110/80. HEENT: unremarkable. Chest sounds normal. Abdominal, B-scan, ultrasound indicates impacted gallstone without obstruction. Surgery is recommended.

A: Gallstone, impacted, no obstruction

P: Pt to call for appointment for surgery

Willard B. Reader, MD

WBR/pw   D: 12/17/08 09:50:16   T: 12/17/08 12:55:01

You Code It!

What are the best, most accurate codes?

_____

_____

_____

TYLER EMERGENCY CLINIC
911 QUICK LANE • ANYTOWN, FL 32711 • 407-555-6248

PATIENT: GEORGES, EDWARD
ACCOUNT/EHR #:   GEORED001
Date: 08/11/08

Attending Physician: Willard B. Reader, MD

S: Pt is a 33-year-old male, who was helping his girlfriend move two days ago. He was lifting a box of books when he felt a sharp pain, "like something ripped" in his lower right abdomen. He states that he has had a sharp, steady pain in his groin. He has vomited several times since the incident.

O: Ht 6'1" Wt. 199 lb. R 18. T 98.6. BP 110/85. Examination reveals an obvious swelling in the inguinal area, just above the right groin. Palpation of the area, while the patient is doing the Valsalva's maneuver confirms inguinal hernia. Digital exam confirms hernia is indirect. Automated differential WBC count is elevated. X-ray of abdomen confirms partial bowel obstruction.

A: Indirect inguinal hernia, unilateral, with partial bowel obstruction

P: 1. Rx Truss
     2. Referral to surgeon

_____

Willard B. Reader, MD

WBR/pw   D: 08/11/08 09:50:16   T: 08/13/08 12:55:01

You Code It!

What are the best, most accurate codes?

_____

_____

_____

TYLER EMERGENCY CLINIC
911 QUICK LANE • ANYTOWN, FL 32711 • 407-555-6248

PATIENT: BENJAMIN, DAVIDA
ACCOUNT/EHR #:   BENJDA001
DATE: 09/16/08

ATTENDING PHYSICIAN: Suzanne R. Taylor, MD

S: Pt is a 49-year-old female complaining of abdominal pain. She states that the pain has been consistent since noon and vomiting since 2 pm. She has been experiencing chills and weakness, as well. No diarrhea. Last BM was a small one at 7 am and again at 2 pm. She was in good health prior to the symptoms at noon. She also has GERD.

Patient had a total hysterectomy three years ago, and a laparoscopic cholecystectomy ten years ago. She quit smoking ten years ago. Current meds: Evista, Prevacid prn.

O: Wt. 140 Ht 5'2" T99 P 90 R 18 BP 128/73. Abdomen distended, tympanic, tender. CT Scan abd/pelvis: Dilated small bowel loop appears to contain semi-solid material in RLQ, compatible with early small bowel obstruction.

EKG: Sinus tachycardia, otherwise normal ECG. Bowel sounds are normal and hypoactive. Breathing pattern is non-labored, breath sounds clear. Heart rhythm: regular. Neck veins: non-distended. Skin: warm, dry, intact.

Peripheral pulses: Normal CBC w/differential: WBC, RBC, HGB, and HCT are high; MCHC is low; all other results unremarkable. Glucose and BUN/Creat are high; anion gap is low, all other chemistry unremarkable. UA: UR is cloudy, glucose high.

A: Small bowel obstruction; pure hypercholesterolemia; diaphragmatic hernia; esophageal reflux

P: Admit to hospital for surgery

Suzanne R. Taylor, MD

SRT/pw   D: 9/16/08 09:50:16   T: 9/18/08 12:55:01

You Code It!

What are the best, most accurate codes?

_____

_____

_____

TYLER EMERGENCY CLINIC
911 QUICK LANE • ANYTOWN, FL 32711 • 407-555-6248

PATIENT: KAHN, ARLENE
ACCOUNT/EHR #:   KAHNAR001
Date: 09/16/08

Attending Physician: Suzanne R. Taylor, MD

The patient is a 7-month-old female infant brought in by paramedics with respiratory distress. During transport, EMT Arthur reports that the patient stopped breathing. Bag mask ventilation with CPR was immediately administered and continued until arrival at the ED. On arrival in the emergency department, the patient is apneic, asystolic, and pulseless. The infant has no IV access. After brief bag mask ventilation, the patient is intubated with a tracheal tube. A colorimetric carbon dioxide capnometer detector device confirms proper tracheal tube placement. Findings now include:

1) Airway/breathing: Breath sounds are equal bilaterally, and there is good chest movement with ventilation.
2) Circulation: No pulse is palpable without chest compressions, and no heart sounds are heard. ECG shows asystole. Oxygen saturation is not obtainable.
3) Vital signs: Heart rate 0, respiratory rate 0, blood pressure unobtainable.
4) Attempts at IV access are unsuccessful.

      Ventilations and chest compressions are continued. Epinephrine 0.5 mg of the 1:1,000 solution is given down the tracheal tube, and an intraosseous line (IO) is inserted into the proximal left tibia. Blood is obtained from the IO needle and is sent for a number of studies including a rapid glucose check. The airway is reassessed, ventilation and chest compressions are continued, and a second dose of epinephrine is given. The patient converts to a sinus bradycardia with a fair blood pressure. After several more minutes of further stabilization, the infant's heart rate is 120 and she is beginning to move and cough against the tracheal tube. The resuscitation is a success.

DX: PCA (pulmocardiac arrest)
     Admit to NICU

_____

Suzanne R. Taylor, MD

SRT/pw   D: 9/16/08 09:50:16   T: 9/18/08 12:55:01

You Code It!

What are the best, most accurate codes?

_____

_____

_____

TYLER EMERGENCY CLINIC
911 QUICK LANE • ANYTOWN, FL 32711 • 407-555-6248

PATIENT: HADDOX, TYLER
ACCOUNT/EHR #:   HADDTY001
Date: 09/16/08

Attending Physician: Suzanne R. Taylor, MD

This patient is a 3-month-old male infant is brought to the emergency department by his father due to continued vomiting and diarrhea. Father states that these symptoms have been ongoing for the last four days. Initial findings in the emergency department include:

Airway: Breath sounds are normal. Airway is patent.

Breathing: Breathing is regular at 45 breaths per minute, unlabored.

Circulation: Proximal pulses are poor, distal pulses are absent, and extremities are cool. Feeling from the 5th toe upwards, the legs are cool up to the knee. Capillary refill is 8 seconds. Heart rate is 209 beats per minute, and blood pressure is 70mm Hg systolic.

ECG: There are narrow QRS complexes with sinus tachycardia on the monitor.

The infant does not recognize his parents, is extremely lethargic, and responds to pain only, with a minimal grimace.

Due to the size of his veins, we are unable to start an IV line. 100% oxygen is started. The mucous membranes of the mouth are pink. An intraosseous (IO) is placed in the left tibia and 20cc/kg of normal saline is infused as rapidly as possible. The infant is then reassessed. Airway and breathing remain stable. The heart rate is now 195. A repeat bolus of 20cc/kg is given and the patient is reassessed. After the 3rd fluid bolus is given, the patient becomes more alert, distal pulses return, and the patient improves throughout resuscitation. The heart rate has come down to 160. However, a rapid bedside glucose analysis reveals a blood sugar of only 32, which is quickly treated.

DX: Compensated hypovolemic shock (and hypoglycemia) secondary to vomiting and diarrhea

_____

Suzanne R. Taylor, MD

SRT/pw   D: 9/16/08 09:50:16   T: 9/18/08 12:55:01

You Code It!

What are the best, most accurate codes?

_____

_____

_____

TYLER EMERGENCY CLINIC
911 QUICK LANE • ANYTOWN, FL 32711 • 407-555-6248

PATIENT: MODAR, SUZANNE
ACCOUNT/EHR #:   MODASU001
Date: 09/16/08

Attending Physician: Suzanne R. Taylor, MD

This patient is a 5-year-old female who was hit by a car when she ran out into the street after her baseball. Paramedics report that when they arrived at the scene, the child was unconscious. Multiple abrasions were on her
face, chest, abdomen and extremities. Her left thigh was noticeably deformed and swollen. Because she demonstrated very shallow respirations, she was immediately intubated with in-line cervical spine immobilization. Two
large bore IV lines where placed and she was then rushed to the trauma center.

    Exam: VS T 37.0, P160, RR ventilated via the tracheal tube at 20, BP 100/80, oxygen saturation 97%. She
is still unresponsive and being ventilated via the tracheal tube. Her pupils are briskly reactive to light. There is
excellent chest wall rise and fall via ventilation through the tracheal tube. There are numerous abrasions over her
face, chest, abdomen and lower extremities. The abdomen is distended with decreased bowel sounds. Her pelvis
is stable, but her left thigh is obviously swollen and tense. Distal perfusion to all four extremities seems adequate.
The remainder of the physical examination is unremarkable.

    A CT scan of her head reveals a small occipital lobe contusion but no cerebral edema or hemorrhage. The
CT scan of her abdomen reveals a small splenic laceration and a mild contusion of the right kidney. Chest and
extremity x-rays reveal a displaced mid-shaft left femur fracture and a small right pulmonary contusion. Her
cervical spine and pelvic x-rays are normal. After appropriate stabilization interventions, she is admitted to the
pediatric intensive care unit. Her intracranial, pulmonary and splenic injuries are managed with supportive care
and her femur fracture is reduced with open reduction and internal fixation.

DX: Displaced mid-shaft femur fracture, pulmonary contusion, splenic laceration, contusion to the kidney, multiple lacerations
    Admit to pediatric unit for observation.

_____

Suzanne R. Taylor, MD

SRT/pw   D: 9/16/08 09:50:16   T: 9/18/08 12:55:01

You Code It!

What are the best, most accurate codes?

_____

_____

_____

TYLER EMERGENCY CLINIC
911 QUICK LANE • ANYTOWN, FL 32711 • 407-555-6248

PATIENT: WERNER, JEFFREY
ACCOUNT/EHR #:   WERNJE001
Date: 09/16/08

Attending Physician: Suzanne R. Taylor, MD

This 7-year-old male is brought into the ED by his father due to his inability "to catch his breath." He states that his son has just recently recovered from a cold, but has continued to cough. The father reports that the child often coughs in fits with post-tussive emesis, will sometimes turn blue in the face, and makes a "gasping-like" noise when he tries to inhale after a coughing episode. Currently, he is complaining about a pain in his chest and shortness of breath. According to the father, the onset of these symptoms began "after one of those coughing fits this morning." There is an ill contact in the house (a grandmother who has been coughing for the last 3 months).

Exam: VS T 37.1, HR 94, RR 28, BP 115/77, Oxygen saturation 93-95% in RA, height is 50-75th %ile, and her weight and head circumference are both in the 10-25th %ile. He is sitting on the exam table, leaning forward, taking quick breaths with some nasal flaring. He has slightly asymmetrical chest movements (the right chest wall moves less than the left) and he has decreased breath sounds with hyper-resonance and decreased tactile fremitus on the right as well. His PMI and trachea are normally positioned, his sensorium is normal, and he has regular and symmetrical radial and femoral pulses. The nurse, Robin Spinner, places the patient on 2 liters/minute of oxygen via nasal cannula.

     After 45 minutes, the patient's vitals are relatively unchanged except that his oxygen saturation is now 100% on the 2 liters/minute of oxygen. He is switched to a non-rebreather mask with a FiO2 of 100% and sent for a PA and lateral CXR. Radiologist confirms diagnosis.

DX: Right, simple, primary spontaneous pneumothorax, about 12% in size

Tx: Admitted to the hospital for observation and continued oxygen therapy.

Suzanne R. Taylor, MD

SRT/pw   D: 9/16/08 09:50:16   T: 9/18/08 12:55:01

You Code It!

What are the best, most accurate codes?

_____

_____

_____

TYLER EMERGENCY CLINIC
911 QUICK LANE • ANYTOWN, FL 32711 • 407-555-6248

PATIENT: CAPPELLI, JILL
ACCOUNT/EHR #:   CAPPJI001
Date: 09/16/08

Attending Physician: Suzanne R. Taylor, MD

This patient is a 25-year-old female brought to the ED by her roommate with vomiting and nausea. The roommate states that the patient had an argument with her boyfriend last night. She woke up early this morning saying that she feels sick. The patient admits that last night she took some pills at 2100. She has vomited 3-4 times at home. The roommate brought in the bottle of pills, which she states was just purchased the day prior. The bottle is marked as having acetaminophen 500mg tablets in a quantity of 30 tablets. There are 8 tablets remaining in the bottle (maximum 11 grams of acetaminophen ingested).

Exam: VS T 37.2, P 88, R 18, BP 110/70, weight 50kg. She is alert, quiet, shaking her head yes/no to questions, with poor eye contact. Her skin is pink with good perfusion. Her oral mucosa is moist. Heart is regular with a normal rhythm and rate. Lungs are clear with good aeration. Her abdomen is soft, with normoactive bowel sounds, minimal epigastric tenderness, no rebound, and no guarding. She is alert, oriented, and walks about the room without difficulty.

   50 grams of activated charcoal with sorbitol is administered PO. She is also given 10 grams of N-acetylcysteine orally. An acetaminophen level, aspirin level, blood and urine toxicology screen and beta-HCG are drawn. The acetaminophen level drawn at 8.5 hours post-ingestion is 150 mcg/mL.

DX: Vomiting and nausea caused by poisoning by acetaminophen, attempted suicide

Tx: She is hospitalized for further treatment as well as a psychiatric evaluation.

_____

Suzanne R. Taylor, MD

SRT/pw   D: 9/16/08 09:50:16   T: 9/18/08 12:55:01

You Code It!

What are the best, most accurate codes?

_____

_____

_____

TYLER EMERGENCY CLINIC
911 QUICK LANE • ANYTOWN, FL 32711 • 407-555-6248

PATIENT: ORTNER, LOUISA
ACCOUNT/EHR #:   ORTNLO001
Date: 09/16/08

Attending Physician: Suzanne R. Taylor, MD

This patient is a 27-year-old female who presents to the clinic in obvious pain. She states that she just returned yesterday from a weekend camping trip and is experiencing pain and redness in the antecubital fossa of her right arm. She does not report any known history of trauma or insect bites. Upon further history, it is learned that she had applied an insect repellent containing 50% DEET to exposed areas of the skin including the neck, arms, and lower extremities. She had used lower concentrations of DEET repellents in the past, with no reported history of adverse skin reactions. On this occasion, the insect repellent was applied approximately 18 hours prior to the onset of symptoms. She reports that she did not wash the treated skin at the end of the day. She does not report applying sunscreen or taking any medications prior to the onset of the rash. No other unusual exposures are reported.

EXAM: There is a well-demarcated area of erythema apparent in the right antecubital fossa. It is warm and tender to palpation. There are no other abnormal findings on physical examination.

DX: Erythematous rash, an adverse skin reaction associated with DEET

PLAN: Patient is told to expect that in about 2 days, hemorrhagic blisters will form in the erythematous area, and that about two days after that, the bullae should spontaneously rupture, leaving a shallow ulceration which will resolve over the course of the following 10 days.

Suzanne R. Taylor, MD

SRT/pw   D: 9/16/08 09:50:16   T: 9/18/08 12:55:01

You Code It!

What are the best, most accurate codes?

_____

_____

_____

TYLER EMERGENCY CLINIC
911 QUICK LANE • ANYTOWN, FL 32711 • 407-555-6248

PATIENT: FRANCO, ILIANA
ACCOUNT/EHR #:   FRANIL001
Date: 03/05/08

Attending Physician: Suzanne R. Taylor, MD

This patient is a 59-year-old female brought in by her daughter. She states she is feeling anxious, hyperventilating, and suffering paresthesia in both hands and feet. She complains of shortness of breath which she states is worse since taking meds for anxiety. She denies any pain. Pt is currently under the care of a psychiatrist, Dr. Kennedy, for two weeks.

PMH: Pt has history of asthma, depression, and hypertension. Pt states that she lost her husband two years ago and she has been having trouble since. She was prescribed Zoloft and felt that she has been more anxious since taking it.

Current Meds: 50 mg bid Zoloft, 1 tab qd lisinopril; 20 mEq qd potassium; 0.5 mg bid lorazepam

Exam: BP: 155/83; P 95; R 26 ECG: normal sinus rhythm, left ventricular hypertrophy with repolarization abnormality; CBC: all within normal levels; Cardiac enzyme: 65; PT: normal; PTT: slightly low; CXR – PA and Lat: Lungs clear. Pt. Calmed down with reassurance and emotional support.

DX: Depressive disorder; anxiety disorder

Plan: Xanax 1 mg PO tid; Pt to follow-up with Dr. Kennedy

Suzanne R. Taylor, MD

SRT/pw   D: 3/05/08 09:50:16   T: 3/07/08 12:55:01

You Code It!

What are the best, most accurate codes?

_____

_____

_____

PATIENT: OSTERMAN, SHEILA
ACCOUNT/EHR #:   OSTESH001
Date: 07/15/08

Attending Physician: Suzanne R. Taylor, MD

History of present illness: A 77-year-old woman is playing Bingo in a large hall when she suddenly slumped forward and hit her head on the table, scattering pieces in every direction. No seizure activity is noted, but she has some loss of bladder control and when she wakes five minutes later she is confused and tired. Onlookers call 911 and EMTs brought her into the ED.

On arrival to the emergency department, the patient is alert and oriented to person, place and time, though somewhat tired. She complains of some dizziness and a mild headache.

Her vital signs on arrival are BP 188/90, P112, R 16, SaO2 98% on room air and an oral temperature of 99 F.

Review of systems prior to episode: No headache or aura, no chest pain, no palpitations, no nausea or vomiting, no fever, no cough. Bowel movements regular, no melena or rectal bleeding. The ROS is essentially negative.

Past Medical History: COPD treated with inhalers. No history of CAD, no neurologic history. She has never had chest pain or angina.

Social History: Former smoker (40 pack year history), quit 15 years ago. No significant alcohol history, widowed with 4 children living in the Providence area.

Medications: Vitamin B12, Aspirin (which she takes for aching knees).

Physical exam:
General: Cachectic appearing elderly female in no acute distress.

HEENT: Mild frontal contusion, no other apparent injury. Pupils equal, round and reactive to light. No signs of hemotympanum or oropharyngeal erythema.

Neck: non-tender.

Chest: Breath sounds clear bilaterally.

Cardiac: Normal S1S2 with a 2/6 high-pitched apical holosystolic murmur radiating to the axilla.

Abdomen: soft, non-tender.

Rectal exam: deferred.

Neuro: Cranial nerve function intact to careful testing, no cerebellar findings, reflexes brisk but symmetric. No sensorimotor deficit.

Labs:
CBC: Hgb 10.7 (MCV 81), WBC 12.7 (80% PMN's), platelets 242 (slight anemia)

Chem 7: Na 140, K 3.7, Cl 104, CO2 26, BUN 13, Cr 0.7 (all within normal limits)

Cardiac Enzymes: CK 63, AST 32, LDH 467; PT: 11.3, INR 1.0, PTT 23

Chest x-ray: no acute infiltrate or cardiopulmonary process, mild cardiomegaly

The dramatic anterior ST elevations are the most striking feature of this patient's presentation. The ECG, coupled with the history of syncope, make it very tempting to initiate thrombolysis to treat an evolving anterior wall myocardial infarction. Given the history of syncope and headache, however, it was decided to obtain a head CT.

Continued

The CT clearly demonstrates a massive subarachnoid hemorrhage. In retrospect, heparinization and thrombolysis do not seem as prudent an option. For starters, the patient's hypertension at presentation is a relative contraindication to thrombolysis—this case provides an argument for taking those contraindications seriously.

As for our concern for a co-existing myocardial infarction, on subsequent review of the ECG one notes that the prominent ST elevations exist in the absence of any reciprocal ST depressions in the inferior leads. Moreover, the ECG remained static over time, further supporting the notion that no acute event was taking place.

An emergency echocardiogram of this patient's heart demonstrated an aneurysm of the anterior myocardial wall, an anatomic finding which we felt could explain her ST elevations.

Suzanne R. Taylor, MD

SRT/pw   D: 7/15/08 09:50:16   T: 7/19/08 12:55:01

You Code It!

What are the best, most accurate codes?

_____

_____

_____

TYLER EMERGENCY CLINIC
911 QUICK LANE • ANYTOWN, FL 32711 • 407-555-6248

PATIENT: CHESSER, EVAN
ACCOUNT/EHR #:   CHESEV001
Date: 09/05/08

Attending Physician: Suzanne R. Taylor, MD

A 31-year-old Hispanic male presents with "the worst headache ever." He states that at 1100 he felt the acute onset of bitemporal as well as occipital headache. The patient admits to accompanying nausea, vomiting, weakness in the upper extremities, and complains "it hurts to move my neck." He denies fevers, chills, change in vision, difficulty speaking or swallowing, chest or abdominal pain, dysuria, or change in bowel habits.

Medications: Phenytoin 300mg daily

Allergies: NKDA

PMH: Seizure d/o for several years, unknown etiology

SH: Denies tobacco, alcohol, drug use; No HIV risks; Immigrant from Dominican Republic

Review of systems: 2-3 day h/o cough with yellow sputum production and fevers, some dyspnea

Physical Examination: In general, he was an alert, oriented male who was holding head in moderate discomfort, moaning.

VS: T 98.0 (t) HR 110 RR 24; BP 148/85; Pox 99% RA

HEENT: PERRLA, EOMI, No icterus, No injected conjunctiva, Fundi are clear, No photophobia.

LUNGS: Decreased BS Right base, +crackles, LL-CTA.

CARDIAC: Tachy, regular, no murmurs

ABDOMEN: Soft, ND, NT. No guarding or rebound.

RECTAL: brown, ob negative

EXT: Good peripheral pulses; no edema; grimaces with bilateral leg raising.

Skin: no rashes

Continued

NEURO: Moves all extremities to command, reflexes symmetric, CNS grossly symmetric, No deficits noted.

Labs: WBC 13.5; Hgb/Hct16/46.2; Plt 305; Na 142; K 4.5; Cl 100; Bicarb 23; Glucose 130; BUN/Cr 25/1.0; Coags: Normal; U/A Normal; Dilantin 7

CXR – normal; MRI

DX: Neurocystocercosis

Plan: Praziquantel. Six month follow-up scheduled.

Suzanne R. Taylor, MD

SRT/pw   D: 9/05/08 09:50:16   T: 9/07/08 12:55:01

You Code It!

What are the best, most accurate codes?

_____

_____

_____

TYLER EMERGENCY CLINIC
911 QUICK LANE • ANYTOWN, FL 32711 • 407-555-6248

PATIENT: GRANNAU, BEN
ACCOUNT/EHR #:   GRANBE001
Date: 09/05/08

Attending Physician: Suzanne R. Taylor, MD

HPI: A 23-year-old male presents to the ED complaining of back pain since the previous night. The back pain is dull and not localized to any particular area. He also complains of nausea (no vomiting), neck pain and headache. He has had similar back pain intermittently for months, but it is worse today. His ROS is positive for photophobia, subjective fevers and generalized weakness. He denies dysuria, frequency, urgency, hematuria, visual changes or focal weakness or numbness.

PMH is negative except for "neck surgery" for cancer, which he had several months ago. He takes some medicines but he doesn't remember what they are, and he didn't bring them along. He is allergic to penicillin ("it makes me swell up").

FH is unremarkable.

SH: He lives with his wife. He does not drink or smoke.

ROS: As in the HPI. He has felt fairly tired with intermittent back pain for months.

Physical Examination: T 101.8 po HR 109 RR 22 BP 88/49

Generally, he is a flushed uncomfortable male appearing moderately ill.

HEENT: Normal, with a normal funduscopic examination. Neck was supple, with a well-healed thyroidectomy scar.

Lungs were clear to auscultation.

Cardiac examination: Regular tachycardic rhythm, without murmurs or gallops.

Abdominal examination: Normal. There was normal rectal tone.

Extremities: Some back pain with straight leg raise on the left, full pulses and no evidence of arthropathy.

Skin: Flushed but there were no rashes.

Neurologic examination: Normal mental state (although s/w agitated), fluent Spanish, intact cranial nerves, and normal motor examination.

CBC: WBC 5.2, Hgb 12.3, Hct 37.1, Plt 198. Diff: 81% segs, 12% lymphs, 5% monos; Chem7: Na 140 Cl 100 BUN 8 glc 86; The patient's calcium level was 4.9.; K 3.5 C02 24 Cr 0.7; PT 12.6 PTT 29

Continued

U/A negative; UCG negative; CXR, CTLS spine series normal

CSF no wbcs, no rbcs, protein 11, glucose 57

DX: Parathyroid insufficiency; Hypocalcemia, secondary to hypoparathyroidism

Suzanne R. Taylor, MD

SRT/pw   D: 9/05/08 09:50:16   T: 9/07/08 12:55:01

You Code It!

What are the best, most accurate codes?

_____

_____

_____

PATIENT: CLAIBORNE, WALTER
ACCOUNT/EHR #:   CLAIWA001
Date: 09/09/08

Attending Physician: Suzanne R. Taylor, MD

28-year-old male with no significant PMH presented to the ED by ambulance complaining of bilateral lower extremity weakness.

He was in stable health until 3 weeks prior, when he noted progressive cramping, pain and weakness in his legs. A week after, he was treated at another hospital for low back pain with hydrocodone and a muscle relaxant. His back pain resolved gradually, but bilateral thigh pain and weakness persisted. On the morning of admission, the patient tried to rise out of bed but immediately fell to the floor with lower extremity paraparesis.

He denied recent injury, fevers, viral symptoms, headache, diplopia, paresthesias, numbness, arm weakness, arthralgias, incontinence, nausea, vomiting, diarrhea, or previous neurologic deficits.

PMH: Motorcycle accident seven years ago without sequelae.

MED: None

ALLERGIES: None

SOC: Single, employed as a truck driver. Intermittently chews tobacco. Occasional alcohol. Denied intravenous drug use.

FH: No history of paraparesis, paraplegias, or neurological diseases.

ROS: Anxious over the last month with occasional insomnia. Eight to twelve pound weight loss over several months without dieting. No history of recent travel. No blood transfusions. No noted tick or insect bites and no insecticide exposure. No recent URI's.

Physical Examination
Vitals: Temp: 96.2 BP: 127/68 P: 107 R: 20

General: Thin young man who appears anxious.

HEENT: PERRL, sclera anicteric, fundi unremarkable, dentition poor. Neck supple, no lymphadenopathy, palpable thyroid.

CV: tachy normal S1/S2, soft 2/6 holosystolic murmur over LSB. CHEST: clear to auscultation.

ABD: normoactive bowel sounds, no organomegaly.

EXT: no clubbing, cyanosis, or edema; hands and feet warm and dry.

NEURO: Alert and oriented; fluent; CN intact; motor nl bulk, decreased tone in lower extremities, power 4/5 in upper extremities B, 2-3/5 in bilat lower extremities, distal weaker than proximal. Reflexes 2+ and brisk diffusely; toes go down to plantar stim; No clonus. Sensation intact to light touch, pin-prick, temperature, proprioception. Coordination intact in UE's (limited by weakness in lower extremities. Gait not tested.

EKG: SR, 97 bpm. Otherwise normal.

Continued

Labs:

Chem7: Na 143 K 1.8 CL 109 CO2 23 BUN 15 CR 0.6 GLU 110

CBC: WBC 5.5 HB 14.7 HCT 42.8 PLT 246 DIFF 73 poly 16 lymph

CSF: normal protein, glucose, cell count and diff.

Etc: ESR 6 Ca 9.8 Mg 1.6 Phos 4.7 CPK 398 U/A normal

LFTs normal.

CXR: Normal; LS Spine Series: Normal

DX: Hypokalemic periodic paralysis, associated with hypothyroidism

---

Suzanne R. Taylor, MD

SRT/pw   D: 9/09/08 09:50:16   T: 9/13/08 12:55:01

You Code It!

What are the best, most accurate codes?

_____

_____

_____

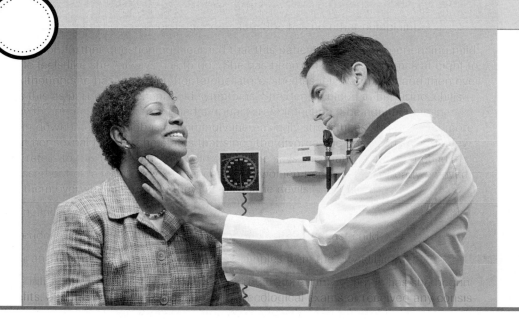

CHAPTER

7

Endocrinology Cases and Patient Records

INTRODUCTION

Endocrinologists are physicians whose specialty involves the diagnosis and treatment of abnormalities of the endocrine system. These common health concerns include diabetes insipidus, hypothyroidism, and diabetes mellitus. Such conditions are usually systemic, meaning that they can affect the entire body and are often chronic.

Endocrinologists can be board-certified through the Board of Internal Medicine, which is recognized by the American Board of Medical Specialties.

You can use these cases to practice coding diagnoses, E/M, procedures, DME, or other HCPCS Level II items, as applicable; code for the physician or the facility; code inpatient and outpatient services, as applicable:

1. Code for the physician.
2. Code for the anesthesiologist, when applicable.
3. Code for the hospital, when applicable.
4. Code for the pathology and laboratory, when applicable.
5. Code HCPCS Level II codes, when applicable.

MEDICAL ASSOCIATES OF ENDOCRINOLOGY
6899 LYMPHATIC PATH • NODINE, FL 32811 • 407-555-4661

PATIENT: ROLLINS, KIM
ACCOUNT/EHR #:   ROLLKI001
Date: 09/16/08

Attending Physician: Suzanne R. Taylor, MD

This 53-year-old female came to see me today with complaints of profuse sweating, tremors, and polyuria. I have not seen her for six months when she came for treatment of her carpal tunnel syndrome. She has IDDM.

Glucose test indicated that her diabetes was out of control. I adjusted her dosage. Patient was given Insulin IM. I spent 40 minutes counseling her on the proper manner of giving herself insulin injections and answering other concerns she had related to her disease.

DX: Diabetes mellitus, insulin-dependent, uncontrolled

___

Suzanne R. Taylor, MD

SRT/pw   D: 9/16/08 09:50:16   T: 9/18/08 12:55:01

You Code It!

What are the best, most accurate codes?

___

___

___

MEDICAL ASSOCIATES OF ENDOCRINOLOGY
6899 LYMPHATIC PATH • NODINE, FL 32811 • 407-555-4661

PATIENT: STANTON, IMOGENE
ACCOUNT/EHR #:   STANIM001
Date: 08/11/08

Attending Physician: Willard B. Reader, MD

S: Pt is a 71-year-old female, visited at home for a regular check of her Type I uncontrolled diabetes mellitus. She has exhibited the initial stages of diabetic gangrene on her left lower leg during her last visit, two weeks ago.

O: BP 130/70; she looks well. Her chest is clear and the cardiac examination is unremarkable. Examination of the leg shows no edema, redness, or heat in the lower extremity. HEENT: unremarkable.

A: Type 1 diabetes uncontrolled; diabetic gangrene

P: 1. Referral to orthopedist, appointment scheduled next week, possible BKA
     2. Continue on meds and treatments prescribed for gangrene
     3. Adjust dosage of insulin to maintain proper glucose levels

Willard B. Reader, MD

WBR/pw   D: 08/11/08 09:50:16   T: 08/13/08 12:55:01

You Code It!

What are the best, most accurate codes?

_____

_____

_____

MEDICAL ASSOCIATES OF ENDOCRINOLOGY
6899 LYMPHATIC PATH • NODINE, FL 32811 • 407-555-4661

PATIENT: PERMANENTE, MORRIS
ACCOUNT/EHR #:   PERMMO001
Date: 09/16/08

Attending Physician: Suzanne R. Taylor, MD

Procedure: Vitrectomy followed by laser panretinal photocoagulation

An ocutome is used to go behind the iris and cut and suction the vitreous mechanically.

    After the vitreous removal, an endolaser is used to treat the remaining retinal disorders in all four retinal quadrants and prevent further retinal hemorrhage.

DX: Juvenile diabetes, insulin-dependent; severe retinal hemorrhage; microaneurysmal diabetic retinopathy

Suzanne R. Taylor, MD

SRT/pw   D: 9/16/08 09:50:16   T: 9/18/08 12:55:01

You Code It!

What are the best, most accurate codes?

_____

_____

_____

MEDICAL ASSOCIATES OF ENDOCRINOLOGY
6899 LYMPHATIC PATH • NODINE, FL 32811 • 407-555-4661

PATIENT: SHEPARD, CHARLES
ACCOUNT/EHR #:   SHEPCH001
Date: 08/11/08

Attending Physician: Willard B. Reader, MD

S: Pt is a 31-year-old male complaining of an unhealed sore on his left foot. He states the sore is of three weeks duration with no evidence of healing despite multiple home remedies and over-the-counter treatments. Pt is a type II diabetic for six years.

O: Wt 195, Ht 5'7" T 99, BP 150/90; HEENT: unremarkable. Left extremity shows a diabetes-related ulcer directly above the third phalange. Ulcer is debrided (skin and subcutaneous tissue), ointment applied, and a bandage placed. Patient is given wound care instructions.

A: Type 2 diabetes; ulcer of midfoot

P: Pt to return in 2 weeks for follow-up

_____

Willard B. Reader, MD

WBR/pw   D: 08/11/08 09:50:16   T: 08/13/08 12:55:01

You Code It!

What are the best, most accurate codes?

_____

_____

_____

MEDICAL ASSOCIATES OF ENDOCRINOLOGY
6899 LYMPHATIC PATH • NODINE, FL 32811 • 407-555-4661

PATIENT:	KELLOGG, COLE
ACCOUNT/EHR #:	KELLCO001
Date:	08/11/08

Attending Physician: Willard B. Reader, MD

Surgeon: Colleen Infanti, MD

Patient is a 28-year-old male with insulin-dependent (type I) diabetic nephropathy and chronic renal failure. He presents today for an arteriovenous shunt for dialysis.

    A Cimino-type direct arteriovenous anastomosis is performed by incising the skin of the left antecubital fossa. Vessel clamps are placed on the vein and adjacent artery. The vein is dissected free and the downstream portion of the vein is sutured to an opening in the artery using an end-to-side technique. The skin incision is closed in layers.

_____

Colleen Infanti, MD

CI/pw   D: 08/11/08 09:50:16   T: 08/13/08 12:55:01

You Code It!

What are the best, most accurate codes?

_____

_____

_____

MEDICAL ASSOCIATES OF ENDOCRINOLOGY
6899 LYMPHATIC PATH • NODINE, FL 32811 • 407-555-4661

PATIENT: JIMENEZ, ANNA
ACCOUNT/EHR #:   JIMEAN001
Date: 07/26/08

Attending Physician: Suzanne R. Taylor, MD

S: This Pt is a 23-year-old female who was diagnosed with juvenile diabetes three years ago. She presents today with complaints of problems with her hands and feet, getting numb on occasion. In addition, she has experienced bouts of pain in her extremities.

O: Ht 5'3" Wt. 219 lb. R 23. BP 150/100. Casual plasma glucose values shown to be 220 mg/dl (normal <199). Feet and hands are cool to the touch indicating poor circulation. Slight edema noticed in left metatarsal and all periphery.

A: Juvenile diabetes mellitus, uncontrolled; Peripheral angiopathy

P: 1. CT of lower extremities
    2. Full blood work up
    3. Adjust insulin dosage
    4. Return in 10 days for follow-up

Suzanne R. Taylor, MD

SRT/pw   D: 07/26/08 09:50:16   T: 07/29/08 12:55:01

You Code It!

What are the best, most accurate codes?

_____

_____

_____

MEDICAL ASSOCIATES OF ENDOCRINOLOGY
6899 LYMPHATIC PATH • NODINE, FL 32811 • 407-555-4661

PATIENT: MOGDONAVICH, MAGDALENA

ACCOUNT/EHR #:   MOGMA001

Date: 10/15/08

HISTORY: Magdalena is a 27-year-old female referred to me by Dr. Jonas with depression, insomnia, increased facial fullness, and a recent increase in facial hair. She has also had an episode of depression and acute psychosis following uncomplicated delivery of normal baby boy nine months previously. Her menses have been irregular since their resumption after the birth (she is not breast-feeding).

PHYSICAL EXAM: Heart rate: 90 beats per min, BP 146/110. Her face is puffy with an increase in facial hair and ruddy complexion. There is no truncal obesity, peripheral wasting, or striae.

LABS: Serum electrolytes, white cell count, and hemoglobin and hematocrit are all within normal limits.

DX: Cushing's syndrome

PLAN: Patient to return in one week with her husband to discuss treatment options.

Derrick Alexander, MD

10/15/08 11:47:39

You Code It!

What are the best, most accurate codes?

_____

_____

_____

MEDICAL ASSOCIATES OF ENDOCRINOLOGY
6899 LYMPHATIC PATH • NODINE, FL 32811 • 407-555-4661

PATIENT: HELGSTROM, INGRID
ACCOUNT/EHR #: HELIN001
Date: 10/15/08

HISTORY: This patient is a 40-year-old female who presents with a six-month history of increasing fatigue. For the past three months she has suffered recurrent upper respiratory infections, poor appetite, abdominal cramps and diarrhea. During this time, she lost 25 lb. She has also noted joint pains, muscle weakness, and dizzy spells following exercise, and she has not menstruated for the past 3 months. Patient was referred to this office by her family physician, Dr. Farina.

PHYSICAL EXAM: Ht 5′4″ Wt 102 lb. Heart rate 86; BP 120/65 when supine. After one minute of quiet standing, the heart rate is 120, BP 90/58, and she became dizzy. Her thyroid gland was diffusely enlarged and the bowel sounds were hyperactive.

Initial testing evaluated thyroid, electrolyte, and renal status. Her sodium is significantly low and her potassium is high, consistent with sodium loss and potassium retention by the renal tubules in mineralocorticoid deficiency. TSH is elevated, though not severely so, and is consistent with borderline hypothyroidism. The hemoglobin is also low. The morning cortisol is low and the ACTH is quite high.

DX: Addison's Disease

PLAN: The patient is instructed to carry an identifying bracelet or card indicating a need for increased steroid dosage during stress or injury. She is informed that thyroid replacement therapy may become necessary in the future.

Derrick Alexander, MD

10/15/08 11:47:39

You Code It!

What are the best, most accurate codes?

_____

_____

_____

MEDICAL ASSOCIATES OF ENDOCRINOLOGY
6899 LYMPHATIC PATH • NODINE, FL 32811 • 407-555-4661

PATIENT: GRISSOM, MARIETTA
ACCOUNT/EHR #: GRIMA001
Date: 10/15/08

HISTORY: Patient is a 48-year-old female, referred by her psychiatrist, Dr. Knutzon, with a past history of mental illness and a new onset of bizarre psychotic behavior. She has been well for the past two years.

PAST MEDICAL HISTORY: No history of bone pain, recent fractures, or kidney stones. The patient denies use of diuretics (e.g., thiazides, which can raise calcium). Her most recent breast exam, mammography, and chest x-ray, taken two months ago, did not suggest malignancy. Stool analysis for occult blood was negative.

PHYSICAL EXAM: Ht 5'5" tall Wt 138 lb. Heart rate 80; BP 130/75. The physical exam is otherwise normal except that she is confused as to the current location, date, and year.
   Routine hematology and chemistry tests were normal. A blood sample was sent for parathyroid hormone (PTH) analysis. In the meantime, the patient and her family are questioned further.
   Intact parathyroid hormone is mildly elevated in a setting of markedly elevated calcium and depressed phosphate.

DX: Primary hyperparathyroidism

CLINICAL COURSE: Treatment options are discussed with the patient. She agrees to surgery. Exploratory surgery of neck is scheduled for next week.

___

Derrick Alexander, MD

10/15/08 11:47:39

You Code It!

What are the best, most accurate codes?

___

___

___

MEDICAL ASSOCIATES OF ENDOCRINOLOGY
6899 LYMPHATIC PATH • NODINE, FL 32811 • 407-555-4661

PATIENT: PETAKKI, WARREN
ACCOUNT/EHR #:   PETWA001
Date: 10/15/08

HISTORY: This 35-year-old male has been referred to me by Dr. Waterman with an elevated blood pressure (188/112, seated) at his yearly physical exam. Previous exams noted blood pressures of 160/94 and 158/92. On questioning, patient admits episodes about twice a month of apprehension, severe headache, perspiration, rapid heartbeat, and facial pallor. These episodes had an abrupt onset and lasted 10-15 minutes each.

PHYSICAL EXAM: Thirty minutes after the initial blood pressure measurement, the seated blood pressure is 178/110 with a heart rate of 90. The blood pressure after 3 min of standing is 152/94 with a heart rate of 112. The optic fundi showed moderately narrowed arterioles with no hemorrhages or exudates.

LABS: Routine hematology and chemistry studies are within the reference ranges and a chest film and EKG are essentially normal. A 24-hour urine specimen is collected for analysis of catecholamines and catecholamine metabolites. Plasma catecholamines are also assayed. Urinary catecholamines and catecholamine metabolites are all elevated. Plasma norepinephrine is markedly elevated, but epinephrine is within the normal range. A CT scan of the adrenals revealed an 8 cm mass on the left side.

DX: Pheochromocytoma

CLINICAL COURSE: Treatment options are discussed with the patient. The patient is treated with alpha and beta-blockers (catecholamine receptor blocking agents) for several weeks. Abdominal surgery for removal of the pheochromocytoma will be scheduled once patient's BP is down.

Derrick Alexander, MD

10/15/08 11:47:39

You Code It!

What are the best, most accurate codes?

_____

_____

_____

MEDICAL ASSOCIATES OF ENDOCRINOLOGY
6899 LYMPHATIC PATH • NODINE, FL 32811 • 407-555-4661

PATIENT: FEATHERLITE, CARLITA

ACCOUNT/EHR #:   FEACA001

Date: 10/15/08

HISTORY OF PRESENT ILLNESS: Referred by her obstetrician, Dr. Laurence, this 26 year-old Caucasian female states that she has been having heart palpitations. She states that the palpitations have been constant over the past two weeks but seem worse at nighttime. When asked to describe them, she states that they are regular and it feels as if her heart is going to jump out of her chest. She denies chest pain, shortness of breath or lightheadedness. She has felt a bit warm of late but denies any frank diaphoresis. It is of note that she recently delivered a normal baby boy during an uncomplicated delivery 5 1/2 weeks before this visit. She says she has loose stools occurring approximately 4 times/day. She complains of feeling tired but unable to get a good night sleep. She states that she feels as if her mind is racing. She denies any nausea, vomiting or abdominal pain. She also denies myalgias, arthralgias, fevers or chills. She denied heat or cold intolerance.

PAST MEDICAL HISTORY: Post partum status and the abnormal thyroid function tests. The patient had a radio-active iodine uptake scan which was normal and subsequently had thyroid auto-antibodies determined positive for anti-thyroglobulin and anti-microsomal antibodies. A thyroid biopsy was also performed and revealed diffuse, lymphocytic infiltration, a characteristic histologic picture of post partum thyroiditis.

PHYSICAL EXAMINATION: Patient is a thin, white female in no apparent distress. BP 146/90, pulse 96 and regular, temp 37 C degrees taken orally. Her review of systems revealed clear lungs, normal heart rhythm, normal abdomen and a normal neurological response although she showed a fine tremor of the hands. Her neck is supple with no lymphadenopathy and her thyroid is approximately 1.5 times normal in size, symmetrically enlarged, firm, non-tender with carotids palpable bilaterally without bruits.

LAB RESULTS: CBC (WBC 14.2, Hct, 38.6, MCV normal, platelet count normal, differential 56% neutrophiles, 7% bands, 34% lymphocytes and 3% monocytes) and a chemistry screen that included electrolytes (NA 142, K 3.6, Cl 101, CO2 22), glucose 86, BUN 26, creatinine 1. Thyroid panel includes thyroxine 16.2 (NL 4-13), T3 resin uptake 34% (NL 25 - 35%) and a TSH of <0.05 (NL 0.3 5.0).

DIAGNOSIS: Post-partum auto-immune thyroid syndrome

PLAN: Rx for beta-blockers to reduce the heart palpitations.

Derrick Alexander, MD

10/15/08 11:47:39

You Code It!

What are the best, most accurate codes?

_____

_____

_____

MEDICAL ASSOCIATES OF ENDOCRINOLOGY
6899 LYMPHATIC PATH • NODINE, FL 32811 • 407-555-4661

PATIENT: ELLISON, TIFFANY
ACCOUNT/EHR #:   ELLTI001
Date: 10/15/08

This 11-year-old Caucasian female was referred by her family doctor, Dr Frieda, with complaints of excessive facial hair and a deepening of her voice.

PAST MEDICAL HISTORY: At the age of 8 it was noted that she had a rather early appearance of pubic hair growth, showed evidence of acne on her forehead, had increased amounts of apocrine sweat gland activity and yet had little evidence of breast development or signs of menarche. As part of her mildly presenting symptoms of androgen excess, she had a DHEA-S blood level drawn at the time that was 600 ng/ml. She was in the 90th percentile for height and weight. The diagnostic impression at this time was precocious adrenarche. This was based on a mildly elevated DHEA-S level, normal serum estradiol and a bone age of 10 1/2 years. Over the next three years, this young girl experienced progression of her facial acne and began to show increasing evidence of facial hair growth. Her acne manifestation prompted a dermatologic consultation that resulted in treatment with Retin-A and tetracycline. She also started to experience significant weight loss that reached 15 pounds by the time she was 11. This was partially attributed to an intense ballet program and her desire to lose weight at the suggestion of her ballet teacher. Her family physician however became concerned with her overt manifestations of virilism and referred her to me.

PHYSICAL EXAMINATION: Patient is a thin, white female with virilizing features including excessive facial hair, a deep voice and considerable cystic acne. Her evaluation included an MRI of the adrenals and ovaries and an ACTH stimulation test. A diagnosis of delayed onset congenital adrenal hyperplasia was considered but hormone analysis revealed a normal baseline cortisol, 17 hydroxyprogesterone and 11 deoxycortisol levels. The cortisol level however did not stimulate beyond the baseline level following Cortrosyn stimulation. She also has markedly elevated levels of DHEA-S for her age at 3,000 ng/ml, and an elevated testosterone level at 218 ng/dl. Her bone age is 13 with a chronological age of 11. An MRI scan revealed a right adrenal mass with a normal left adrenal suggesting a right adrenal tumor.

DIAGNOSIS: Virilizing tumors of the adrenal gland

PLAN: Treatment options are discussed with the patient and her parents. She will be scheduled for surgery to excise the right adrenal mass. It is expected that a successful outcome of the surgery will show her elevated androgen levels to return to normal for her age and pubertal status.

Derrick Alexander, MD

10/15/08 11:47:39

You Code It!

What are the best, most accurate codes?

_____

_____

_____

MEDICAL ASSOCIATES OF ENDOCRINOLOGY
6899 LYMPHATIC PATH • NODINE, FL 32811 • 407-555-4661

PATIENT: CRAIG, THEODORE
ACCOUNT/EHR #: CRATH001
Date: 10/15/08

HISTORY OF PRESENT ILLNESS: This 50-year-old African-American male presents today because he has become quite cantankerous with his co-workers and family. He states these symptoms have been noted for approximately the past year or so. He states he has pain in his back, legs, and hands but has no clinical evidence of inflammatory arthritis, such as heat and redness.

PHYSICAL EXAMINATION: Middle-aged gentleman with erratic behavior, tenderness on his right index finger, as well as RT and LT hands. Augmented peristalsis.

LAB TEST RESULTS:
Hemoglobin 14.7 g
Hematocrit 48%
WBC 7430 nl diff.
Serum calcium 13 mg/dL (Nl 10.5)
PTH elevated to 3 SI units (Nl =1)
Urine Nl.
Alkaline Phosphatase 7 (nl 1-4 B units)

IMAGING STUDIES:
Thyroid scan, Normal
X-ray, HAND, RT, shows bony resorption of distal phalange of index finger

DX: Parathyroid adenoma

PLAN: Discussed surgical options with patient. Patient agrees and procedure is scheduled for two weeks.

_____

Derrick Alexander, MD

10/15/08 11:47:39

You Code It!

What are the best, most accurate codes?

_____

_____

_____

Family Practice Cases and Patient Records

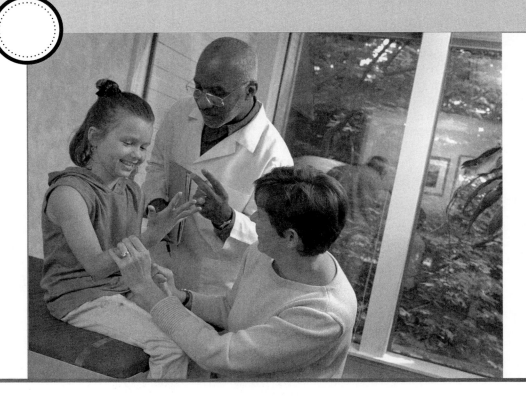

INTRODUCTION

The following case studies are from a family health practice. In a family health practice, a professional coding specialist is likely to handle many different kinds of health situations, especially preventive health care services.

Family medicine practices are health care facilities that specialize in the total health care of the individual and the family. These physicians diagnose and treat a variety of health conditions and diseases in patients of all ages and both sexes. In addition, they are primarily responsible for providing preventive health care advice and procedures, such as vaccinations, annual physical examinations, and age-appropriate screenings.

Family health care specialists may be board-certified by the American Board of Family Medicine, which is recognized by the American Board of Medical Specialties.

You can use these cases to practice coding diagnoses, E/M, procedures, DME, or other HCPCS Level II items, as applicable; code for the physician or the facility; code inpatient and outpatient services, as applicable:

1. Code for the physician.
2. Code for the anesthesiologist, when applicable.
3. Code for the hospital, when applicable.
4. Code for the pathology and laboratory, when applicable.
5. Code HCPCS Level II codes, when applicable.

Note: It is not unusual for family physicians to treat heart disease (cardiology), diabetes (endocrinology), infants (neonatology), children (pediatrics), etc. You can use the other chapters in this book to practice coding those conditions.

FAMILY DOCTORS ASSOCIATES
123 MAIN STREET • ANYTOWN, FL 32711 • 407-555-1234

PATIENT: KRAMDEN, RONALD
ACCOUNT/EHR #:   KRARO001
Date: 11/23/08

Attending Physician: James Healer, MD

This 35 year-old male was last seen by me in August. He presents today for a pre-employment health examination. Patient denies any symptoms or health-related concerns; states he quit smoking in September; drinks on occasion (socially).

Wt. 193 lb. B/P: 120/85, P 25, R reg. T 98.6 HEENT: unremarkable; Cardiopulmonary sounds within normal standards. Abdomen: unremarkable. UA, dipstick, non-automated w/o microscopy and Gen Health panel normal. Circulation good at extremities.

Screening form completed and signed.

_____

James Healer, MD

JHW/mg   D: 011/23/08 09:50:16   T: 011/25/08 12:55:01

You Code It!

What are the best, most accurate codes?

_____

_____

_____

FAMILY DOCTORS ASSOCIATES
123 MAIN STREET • ANYTOWN, FL 32711 • 407-555-1234

PATIENT: FRANKLIN, FRANCES
ACCOUNT/EHR #:   FRAFR001
Date: 10/18/08

Attending Physician: Valerie R. Victors, MD

S: This 57-year-old female came for her routine physical exam. Pt does not smoke, drinks alcohol occasionally, and exercises three times per week. Pt states she has no specific health concerns at this time.

O: Ht 5'3" Wt. 145 lb. R 20. HEENT: unremarkable; Respiratory: unremarkable; Musculoskeletal: age appropriate. No sign of osteoporosis. Bone density appropriate, as per test results. Discussed the importance of keeping up her exercise regimen.

A: Pt is in good health.

P: 1. Follow-up prn
    2. Comprehensive metabolic panel, awaiting results
    3. Schedule screening mammogram
    4. Schedule screening colonoscopy

Valerie R. Victors, MD

VRV/mg   D: 10/18/08 09:50:16   T: 10/23/08 12:55:01

You Code It!

What are the best, most accurate codes?

_____

_____

_____

FAMILY DOCTORS ASSOCIATES
123 MAIN STREET • ANYTOWN, FL 32711 • 407-555-1234

PATIENT: KELLER, ANDRIENNE
ACCOUNT/EHR #:   KELAN001
Date: 12/21/08

Attending Physician: James I. Cipher, MD

S: This Pt is a 35-year-old female who was here six months ago for her annual physical. Today, she presents with a cut in the palm of her right hand. Pt states that she was hanging ornaments on her tree and a glass ball broke in her hand. She is otherwise healthy and has no other stated health concerns.

O: Pt laid back on the examination table and her right hand was draped in a sterile fashion. A topical antiseptic is applied and the superficial laceration, measuring 2.0 cm in length was checked for residual glass shards. None were found and the wound was cleansed and a simple repair was accomplished with a tissue adhesive.

A: Superficial laceration of the right hand, 2.0 cm

P: Follow-up in ten days.

_____

James I. Cipher, MD

JIC/mg   D: 12/21/08 09:50:16   T: 12/22/08 12:55:01

You Code It!

What are the best, most accurate codes?

_____

_____

_____

FAMILY DOCTORS ASSOCIATES
123 MAIN STREET • ANYTOWN, FL 32711 • 407-555-1234

PATIENT: BURNHAM, KERRY
ACCOUNT/EHR #:   BURKE001
Date: 12/21/08

Attending Physician: Donald J. Peters, MD

S: This Pt is a 27-year-old female who was here two years ago. Today, she presents for a prophylactic vaccination required by her new job, working as a laboratory technician. She is otherwise healthy and has no other stated health concerns.

O: Vaccine was administered. I gave the patient a brochure with information about the vaccine and possible side effects to watch for reactions.

A: Inoculation against smallpox, IM

P: Follow-up prn

_____

Donald J. Peters, MD

DJP/mg   D: 12/21/08 09:50:16   T: 12/22/08 12:55:01

You Code It!

What are the best, most accurate codes?

_____

_____

_____

FAMILY DOCTORS ASSOCIATES
123 MAIN STREET • ANYTOWN, FL 32711 • 407-555-1234

PATIENT: DAUPHINE, DOLORES
ACCOUNT/EHR #:   DAUDO001
Date: 2/05/08

Attending Physician: James Healer, MD

S: Pt is a 15-year-old female seen in our office for a physical exam as a requirement for her admission to the Marlberry School for Girls.

O: BP 130/95 P normal R normal Ht 5′0″ Wt 165 lb. HEENT: unremarkable. Heart and lung sounds unremarkable. Pt is clinically obese. Elevated blood pressure noted. Extensive discussion with pt regarding her weight, the health risks associated with obesity, and the options available to her.

A: Obesity, benign essential hypertension

P: 1. Complete school admission form
      2. Referral to nutritionist for diet and exercise regime
      3. Return for check-up in 6 months

James Healer, MD

JH/mg   D: 02/05/08 09:50:16   T: 02/08/08 12:55:01

You Code It!

What are the best, most accurate codes?

_____

_____

_____

FAMILY DOCTORS ASSOCIATES
123 MAIN STREET • ANYTOWN, FL 32711 • 407-555-1234

PATIENT: TRENTON, BASIL
ACCOUNT/EHR #:   TREBA001
Date: 2/05/08

S: Pt is a 43-year-old male who comes to the office today, accompanied by his wife, for a follow-up visit for his hypertension. After addressing the issues related to his hypertension, the patient says, "By the way doc, I am so tired. I've been having trouble sleeping. Are sleeping pills all right to take?" His wife states. "You need to do something about his sleeping. He snores so loud it is ridiculous. He keeps me up all night with that noise. When I finally get to sleep, he sometimes kicks me and wakes me up as he gasps for air."

PAST MEDICAL HISTORY: Significant only for obesity and hypertension.

FAMILY HISTORY: Noncontributory. Patient denies psychiatry history.

SOCIAL HISTORY: The patient denies any alcohol use or abuse, caffeine use, stimulants, or street drug abuse or history of it.

MEDICATIONS: Patient only takes thiazide diuretic for control of hypertension and denies nocturia.

Patient denies palpitations, diaphoresis, tremor, or any other signs of thyroid disease. When asked if he sleeps alone, pt states "I never sleep alone and my partner never has any complaints." ROS: Pt denies arthritis, burning sensation when eating foods, and abdominal pain associated with meals, or angina. Pt denies leg weakness and pain when performing activities or at rest.

PHYSICAL EXAMINATION

VITAL SIGNS: Temp 38.1; blood pressure 150/80; pulse 80; respiration 16; weight 250 lb; height 5'3".

GENERAL: Obese male, generally awake/alert/oriented. Speech understandable and comprehensible, without slurring or hesitation. No infection identified; uvula, palate are midline, noninflamed, and normal in size. There are no masses palpable in the thyroid. Chest wall absent for deformities, breathing is deep with regular rate, good air exchange without wheezes or egophony. Heart exam within normal limits. Abdominal exam within normal limits. Neurological exam is grossly intact.

TEST RESULTS: Labs come back with elevated hemoglobin & hematocrit, normal WBCs, normal renal function, normal thyroid panel. Polysomnogram is ordered.

A: Obstructive sleep apnea

P: 1. Rx: Continuous positive airway pressure (CPAP) equipment
      2. Recommend weight loss. Offer of referral to nutritionist.

James Healer, MD

JHW/mg   D: 02/05/08 09:50:16   T: 02/08/08 12:55:01

You Code It!

What are the best, most accurate codes?

_____

_____

_____

FAMILY DOCTORS ASSOCIATES
123 MAIN STREET • ANYTOWN, FL 32711 • 407-555-1234

PATIENT: WITZKE, REBECCA
ACCOUNT/EHR #:   WITRE001
Date: 2/05/08

This patient is a 34-year-old Caucasian woman who presents complaining of headaches.

History of Present Illness: She describes her current headaches as happening every day in mid-afternoon for the past month. The pain is steady, non-pulsatile, and starts in the occipital region with bilateral radiation to the frontal area. There is no associated aura or photophobia. She is not awakened from sleep with the headaches and she does not wake up in the morning with a headache. Tylenol lessens the discomfort "sometimes."

When asked if there were any other complaints Mrs. Witzke wishes to discuss, she mentions significant stress at home regarding her 11-year-old son. Her concern centers on continued problems with discipline. "He just won't listen to me anymore—he's always beating up on his little brother and getting into fights at school. His grades have really dropped and he might even be held back this year. I just don't know what to do." In reviewing Mrs. Witzke's chart I note she has been in to our office seven times over the past year.

SOCIAL HISTORY: Patient is a college graduate who works part-time as a nursery school teacher. She and her husband, an accountant, have two sons, ages eleven and six. Further discussion reveals that Mrs. Witzke's husband has become increasingly controlling over the past few years. In fact, he often calls home up to ten times per day, making sure Mrs. Witzke comes home right after work or appointments and stays at home until he returns from work. Mrs. Witzke then discloses that he grabbed her around the neck once. "But it was only once . . . and that was a few weeks ago. It was probably my fault, because dinner wasn't ready when he got home, and he becomes kind of hypoglycemic."

The patient also states her husband shoved her a few months ago in the kitchen during a dispute over how she has been handling their son. The following day she went to the ED after work. X-rays of her lower extremities showed no fractures, but significant swelling persisted in her knees for a few weeks. Mrs. Witzke reassured me that she feels safe going back to her home, and that she in fact does not want to leave.

PERSONAL MEDICAL HISTORY: Hypothyroidism and headaches

MEDICATIONS: Synthroid l25mcg each day, Tylenol 650mg two or three times a day

VITAL SIGNS: Temp 98.1; BP 135/85; pulse 80; respiration 20; weight 145 lb; height 5'3".

GENERAL: Her physical exam is unremarkable with normal vital signs and neurological exam.

LABS: TSH from 6 months ago = 0.l5mcg/mL and cholesterol two years ago = 172mg/dL.

A: Stress headaches

Continued

P: I supplied the patient with the phone number for the National Domestic Violence Hotline (1-800-799-SAFE). I explained that they are available at all times and can give her the location of the nearest shelter. I called in a report to the Hotline at 3:42 p.m.

James Healer, MD

JHW/mg   D: 02/05/08 03:50:16   T: 02/08/08 12:55:01

You Code It!

What are the best, most accurate codes?

_____

_____

_____

FAMILY DOCTORS ASSOCIATES
123 MAIN STREET • ANYTOWN, FL 32711 • 407-555-1234

PATIENT: PRICE, JANICE
ACCOUNT/EHR #:   PRIJA001
Date: 2/05/08

S: This new patient is a 56-year-old white female with a four-month history of increasing fatigue and frequent urination. She denies fever, chills, back pain, or hematuria. She denies any recent viral illnesses. Appetite is normal. Fatigue is chronic over the past few months, which has made it difficult for her to carry out her duties as a cashier at a local grocery store.

PAST MEDICAL HISTORY: Hypertension - well controlled; Menopause age 53

PAST SURGICAL HISTORY: Tonsillectomy age 6, Cholecystectomy age 51

FAMILY HISTORY:
- Father deceased, age 68 of myocardial infarction. History included HTN & AODM.
- Mother deceased, age 74 of ruptured aortic aneurysm. History included osteoarthritis and HTN.
- Brother alive age 61 - AODM, HTN, BPH.
- Maternal grandmother deceased, age 54 of breast cancer
- Maternal grandfather deceased, age 31 of industrial accident
- Paternal grandmother deceased, age 70 of a stroke. History included HTN, AODM, obesity.
- Paternal grandfather deceased, age 45 of myocardial infarction.

SOCIAL HISTORY: Married, rare alcohol intake and has never smoked. Employed as a cashier in a local grocery store. Three grown children. Good relationship with her husband. Completed high school education.

MEDICATIONS: Hydrochlorothiazide 12.5mg daily; Conjugated estrogen 0.625mg daily, Medroxyprogesterone acetate 2.5mg daily

O: Height 5'1" and weight is stable at 190 lb. B/P 146/88 Pulse 82 Resp. 16

OPTHALMOLOGIC EXAM - PERRLA, EOMI
FUNDUSCOPIC EXAM - disc sharp, macula appears normal, vessels without nicking, no abnormalities noted

CARDIAC EXAM - regular rate and rhythm, without murmur, rub, gallop PMI normal

PULSES - femoral, popliteal, dorsalis pedis, posterior tibial normal. No bruits noted.

FOOT EXAM - skin and nails free from breaks in the skin/ulcers, 6mm callous plantar surface of L foot, monofilament testing reveals normal sensation. Proprioception intact R & L. Gait reveals pronation during walking.

THYROID - smooth, not enlarged, no nodules palpated

SKIN EXAM - multiple nevi (normal appearing), few seborrheic keratoses on back, no skin lesions or ulcers noted.

NEUROLOGIC EXAM - grossly intact

DENTAL EXAM – anodontia, upper and lower dentures removed - no ulcers or lesions noted. Well fitted dentures.

Continued

A: Diabetes mellitus (type 2), hypertension, and obesity.

P: Rx: Lisinopril 10 mg daily for her blood pressure; atorvastatin (Lipitor) 10 mg each evening for her hypercholesterolemia, and aspirin 81 mg daily. Referral to a dietician and diabetes educator for diet and exercise guidance. Rx home blood glucose monitor, blood pressure monitor

James Healer, MD

JHW/mg   D: 02/05/08 03:50:16   T: 02/08/08 12:55:01

You Code It!

What are the best, most accurate codes?

_____

_____

_____

FAMILY DOCTORS ASSOCIATES
123 MAIN STREET • ANYTOWN, FL 32711 • 407-555-1234

PATIENT: ESTRADA, DAWN
ACCOUNT/EHR #:   ESTDA001

Date: 2/05/08

S: This new patient is a 35-year-old African-American female complaining of pain when she urinates. She is a divorced mother of three children ages 3, 5, and 9. She admits to having multiple sexual partners. She has not used any form of birth control since undergoing tubal ligation after the birth of her last child. She is not sure when her last menstrual period was because her menses have always been irregular. She thinks it was 6 weeks ago. Other than a recent URI, she states that she has been in good health. She has no other complaints.

HISTORY OF PRESENT ILLNESS: Upon further questioning I learned that this patient has been experiencing mild pelvic pain. She also says that she feels like she "always has to go." She has been waking up 4-5 times at night to urinate for the last two nights. Although she has not taken her temperature, she has felt warm now and then over the past week but she dismisses this as part of her recent cold symptoms. She denies blood in her urine, chills, or an increased sense of urgency to urinate. She has never had a urinary tract infection. She admits that she has been feeling fatigued and run down lately. Her job is becomingly increasingly stressful as she takes on more responsibility. When asked about her sexual history, she states that since the divorce she has been seeing a few guys she met in local clubs. She refers to this as "sowing her wild oats." She says she married and had children at such a young age that she missed out on a lot of the experiences other women her age have already enjoyed. She loves her children but finds them overwhelming when they "act like little devils."

PAST MEDICAL HISTORY: Asthma, allergic rhinitis

PAST SURGICAL HISTORY: Appendectomy age 13; Tubal ligation after the birth of her last child

MEDICATIONS: Albuterol inhaler and Claritin, as often as she can get samples from the city clinic

SOCIAL HISTORY: Patient works full-time as an assistant manager in a retail store. Only recently has she begun receiving health insurance benefits. She has not had regular annual gynecological exams or received any consistent health care. She drinks 2-3 beers per day, usually more on the weekends to help her deal with the stress of her children. She denies tobacco or illicit drug use.

FAMILY HISTORY: Mother - diabetes type 2, hypertension. Father died last year of an MI at age 60.

PHYSICAL EXAMINATION

VITALS: Temp 99.0, Pulse 82, BP 127/84, Resp 16/min

HEENT: Head normocephalic. PERRL. EOMI. Oropharynx and TMs clear.

NECK: Some nodal enlargement in the anterior cervical chain. Non-tender.

CV: S1, S2, RRR. No murmurs, rubs, or gallops appreciated.

CHEST: Good air exchange. Slight expiratory wheezes over upper lung fields. No crackles. No CVA tenderness.

ABDOMEN: +BS. soft, ND. Diffuse lower quadrant tenderness. Marked suprapubic tenderness. No rebound or guarding.

EXTREMITIES: Peripheral pulses strong and equal bilaterally. DTRs 2+ upper and lower extremities.

RECTAL: not performed

GYNECOLOGICAL: Normal external genitalia without lesions. Cervix and vaginal wall appeared normal. No bacteria or fungus were seen on KOH prep and wet mount. GC and chlamydia cultures sent. Bimanual exam shows normal size uterus, no cervical motion tenderness, and no adnexal masses or tenderness.

Continued

Chapter 8   Family Practice Cases and Patient Records

TEST RESULTS: UA dipstick positive for UTI

DX: Urinary Tract Infection, pathogenic strains of E. coli

RX; Septra, p.o. 1 TAB b.i.d. x3

James Healer, MD

JHW/mg   D: 02/05/08 03:50:16   T: 02/08/08 12:55:01

You Code It!

What are the best, most accurate codes?

_____

_____

_____

FAMILY DOCTORS ASSOCIATES
123 MAIN STREET • ANYTOWN, FL 32711 • 407-555-1234

PATIENT: LYND, GORDON
ACCOUNT/EHR #:   LYNGO001
Date: 2/05/08

S: This patient is a 46-year-old, middle-aged, well-appearing male, slightly overweight, who comes to see me in the office for a physical exam before taking up a new exercise program he heard about on TV. I have not seen this patient in two years. He has no significant past medical history and is generally in good health. He works as a busy executive at an amusement park, and his wife thinks that he could stand to lose a few pounds.

FAMILY HISTORY: Both parents still living, although his father just had a triple bypass operation a year ago at age 72. He knows of no other history of heart disease or hypertension.

SOCIAL HISTORY: The patient explains that he currently has not been making the time for exercise in his busy schedule. He is interested in trying to walk at lunchtime 3-4 days a week for about a half hour. He drinks 2 cups of coffee in the morning at work every day. He does not smoke, and he drinks a glass of wine 2 nights a week with dinner.

PAST MEDICAL HISTORY: His past BPs have been running in the 130s-140s over 80s-90s.

MEDICATIONS: Multivitamin.

O: VITAL SIGNS: Ht 6 ft O in. Wt 210 lb. BP 156/94 P 82 R 12 T 98.3

ROS reveals no shortness of breath, no palpitations, no headache or sweats, no orthopnea, paroxysmal nocturnal dyspnea, or lower extremity edema.

MENTAL STATUS: Alert and oriented x 3.

CRANIAL NERVES: II - XII intact

FUNDI: No retinopathy, no AV nicking, no papilledema. No exophthalmos.

NECK: No thyromegaly, no carotid bruits, no JVD

HEART: PMI in the MCL, non-displaced, non-enlarged. No sternal heave. S1 S2 present, regular, no S3 or S4, no murmurs, no rubs.

LUNGS: Chest is symmetric with equal breath sounds. No changes to percussion.

ABDOMEN: BS present, normoactive, no renal or aortic bruits. Soft, nondistended, nontender, no striae. No hepatosplenomegaly.

EXTREMITIES: Upper: radial pulses 2+ bilateral. Lower: No edema, erythema. DP and femoral pulses 2+ bilateral.

Continued

LAB RESULTS: U/A, CBC, electrolytes, renals, glucose, cholesterol, and ECG are within normal limits.

A: Essential hypertension

P: Patient is told to come back in 6 weeks for a BP re-check.
Rx: Hydrochlorothiazide, 25 mg

James Healer, MD

JHW/mg   D: 02/05/08 03:50:16   T: 02/08/08 12:55:01

You Code It!

What are the best, most accurate codes?

_____

_____

_____

FAMILY DOCTORS ASSOCIATES
123 MAIN STREET • ANYTOWN, FL 32711 • 407-555-1234

PATIENT: LAFONE, MICHELLE
ACCOUNT/EHR #:   LAFMI001
Date: 2/05/08

This patient is a 56-year-old African-American woman who is well-known to me. Eight years ago I diagnosed her with type II diabetes mellitus, and she is here today for a regular check-up (including her feet) and to go over her most recent lab results.

PAST MEDICAL HISTORY: She is currently taking medications to control her blood sugars. She checks herself about once a day, sometimes forgetting, and usually runs around 130s to 160s. She is post-menopausal, over-weight and her blood pressure has been around 142/90 the past several visits. She has no other significant past medical history. She last visited her ophthalmologist 6 months ago and has not had any retinopathic changes yet.

SOCIAL HISTORY: She does not smoke or drink alcohol.

FAMILY HISTORY: Her father died at age 70 from renal failure from diabetes, but her mother is alive and well, having just had triple heart bypass surgery last year.

MEDICATIONS: Metformin, Rosiglitazone

LAB RESULTS: Her HbA1c is 8.1%, and she has some microalbuminuria (60 mg/d). A BUN and Cr are 35 and 1.3 respectively. A fasting lipid profile revealed: Total cholesterol 262, LDL 174, HDL 50, Triglycerides 162.

A: Diabetes mellitus, type 2, essential hypertension

Rx: Captopril, 25 mg, t.i.d.

I explained to the patient the benefits this medication will have for her, emphasizing its importance in decreasing the progression of renal impairment. I also reiterated to her the importance of controlling her blood glucose levels. She seems to comprehend my advice and agrees to begin taking the Captopril as well as to pay closer attention to her glucose checks.

James Healer, MD

JHW/mg   D: 02/05/08 03:50:16   T: 02/08/08 12:55:01

You Code It!

What are the best, most accurate codes?

_____

_____

_____

FAMILY DOCTORS ASSOCIATES
123 MAIN STREET • ANYTOWN, FL 32711 • 407-555-1234

PATIENT: PICKARD, BARNEY
ACCOUNT/EHR #: PICBA001
Date: 2/05/08

This patient is a 74-year-old patient of mine for the past 20 years. He is a retired construction worker who now lives at home alone after his wife's recent death. He has COPD from years of smoking, but quit 12 years ago. I asked the patient how he is doing with the diuretic I had prescribed and he good-naturedly responded that he hasn't been able to keep track of it real well now that his wife isn't there nagging him all the time. I explain to him that it is important for him to take his medication. He states, "Hey, doc, come on, I'm 74 already and haven't had any health problems! What's the big deal anyways?" I patiently stress further to Mr. Pickard the importance of this medication. He agrees to try harder to stay on schedule with his HCTZ. "It'll be just like punchin' the clock, doc; no problem."

PAST MEDICAL HISTORY: He had an appendectomy as a child and three inguinal hernia repairs during his working life. He has long-standing HTN and that has never been well-controlled. We tried him on clonidine, methyldopa, and prazosin back when those were the choice drugs. I recently switched him to hydrochlorothiazide (25 mg) from clonidine to see if it couldn't make an impact on his BP.

FAMILY HISTORY: He can't remember what his parents died from, but thinks it was "old age."

VITAL SIGNS: BP 176/104.

DX: Essential hypertension

Rx: Nifedipine

James Healer, MD

JHW/mg   D: 02/05/08 03:50:16   T: 02/08/08 12:55:01

You Code It!

What are the best, most accurate codes?

_____

_____

_____

FAMILY DOCTORS ASSOCIATES
123 MAIN STREET • ANYTOWN, FL 32711 • 407-555-1234

PATIENT: CHASTEN, LORRAINE
ACCOUNT/EHR #:   CHALO001
Date: 2/05/08

This patient is a 45-year-old white female with complaints of abdominal pain. She sees me yearly for her gyneco-logic exam but does not regularly visit for any other reason. She states that her pain began about 3 weeks prior to her presentation and has gradually worsened. The pain is sharp in nature and located in the middle of her upper abdomen, just below her rib cage. It occurs most often between meals and is relieved with meals only to recur several hours later. She denies any weight loss, anorexia, dysphagia, diarrhea or constipation. Her stools are a bit darker than usual but without any signs of bright red blood. She has never had pain like this in the past, is uncertain as to its cause, and has been using some over-the-counter antacid without relief. Her last menstrual period was 3 weeks prior to her presentation and was of the usual timing (q 28 days) and duration (5 days). Her abdominal pain did not worsen during the time of her menses. She does not consider her periods heavy.

PAST MEDICAL HISTORY: She has three healthy children delivered by cesarean section but no other surgery. She has a history of seasonal allergies for which she takes over-the-counter anti-histamines with good relief.

MEDICATIONS: None. She denies use of aspirin or nonsteroidal products.

ALLERGIES: Meperidine (Demerol) caused her to break out in a rash, her only medication allergy.

SOCIAL HISTORY: She is physically active, running two or three miles every other day. She uses condoms and spermicidal lubricant for birth control. She is sexually active with her boyfriend of the last 6 months, with whom she feels safe and supported; she has no history of domestic violence. She has never contracted a sexually trans-mitted disease. She has smoked one pack of cigarettes a day for 25 years, rarely drinks alcoholic beverages, and uses no other substances. She works as a legal secretary for a large law firm. Her oldest child, a son, is away at college; her two youngest children are at home including a 12-year-old daughter recently diagnosed with a learn-ing disability. She had all of her children by her former husband from whom she's been divorced for three years. She reports some stress related to being a single parent and sharing custody but does not believe that this is the cause of her abdominal pain.

FAMILY HISTORY: Her father is alive and well despite suffering a myocardial infarction at age 62. Her mother died from colon cancer at age 60. She has two sisters who are alive and well, ages 40 and 47.

PHYSICAL EXAMINATION: She is a thin white female, appearing her stated age. Her weight at this visit is 125 pounds. Her blood pressure is 110/67mmHg supine and 105/60mmHg standing. Her heart rate is 68/min supine and 72/min standing. Her conjunctiva are without pallor, mucus membranes are moist. There are no oral lesions. Neck is without bruits or thyromegaly. Lungs are clear to auscultation and percussion. Heart is regular without murmurs rubs or gallops. Abdomen is soft, non-distended with normoactive bowel sounds. There is epigastric tenderness to palpation without rebound or guarding. Murphy's sign is positive. Stool is dark brown and tests guaiac negative for occult blood. Deep tendon reflexes are 2+ and equal. Skin is without lesions.

Continued

CARROLTON DIGESTIVE MEDICINE, PA
765 SWOLLOW PATH • PASSING, FL 32811 • 407-555-7985

PATIENT: MILLER, JUDITH
ACCOUNT/EHR #:   MILJU001
Date: 10/15/08

Admitting Diagnosis: Gastrointestinal hemorrhage

HISTORY OF PRESENT ILLNESS: The patient is a 71-year-old white female who presents with maroon stools. The patient noticed several episodes of maroon stools with clot yesterday. She called on the phone, was told to come to the Emergency Room. The patient did not come to the ER and instead came to the office. There, she was noted to have normal vital signs and maroon stools in the rectal vault. The patient is now admitted for further evaluation.

PAST MEDICAL HISTORY: The patient denies any previous history of gastrointestinal bleeding. She does have a history of arthritis and has been on Daypro.

ALLERGIES: Bactrim

SOCIAL HISTORY: Negative for smoking or drinking

FAMILY HISTORY: Noncontributory

REVIEW OF SYSTEMS: Notable for marked anxiety

PHYSICAL EXAMINATION

GENERAL: This is a well-developed, well-nourished, white female who was markedly anxious.

VITAL SIGNS: Pulse 80, BP 130/70

HEENT: Conjunctivae pink. Sclerae anicteric

NECK: Without jugular venous distention

LUNGS: Clear

HEART: Regular rhythm

ABDOMEN: Bowel sounds present, nontender, no rebound or guarding. NO masses or organomegaly.

EXTREMITIES: No cyanosis, clubbing or edema

Continued

RECTAL: Exam revealed maroon stools.

IMPRESSION: 1. Gastrointestinal bleeding, etiology to be determined; 2. Anxiety; 3. Allergy to Bactrim

SUGGESTIONS: 1. Follow vital signs closely; 2. Colonoscopy; 3. Gastroscopy if colonoscopy is negative; 4. Transfuse p.r.n

Harold R. Carrolton, MD

HRC/fa 10/15/08 11:47:39

You Code It!

What are the best, most accurate codes?

_____

_____

_____

CARROLTON DIGESTIVE MEDICINE, PA
765 SWOLLOW PATH • PASSING, FL 32811 • 407-555-7985

PATIENT: MILLER, JUDITH
ACCOUNT/EHR #:   MILJU001
Date: 10/15/08

Procedure: Colonoscopy
Indications for Procedure: Gastrointestinal bleeding

DESCRIPTION OF OPERATION: The patient was placed in the left lateral decubitus position. She was gradually sedated with 10 mg of intravenous Versed and 50 mg of intravenous Demerol. Her perirectal area was inspected and no lesions noted. Digital examination revealed no masses or tenderness. The Olympus single channel colonoscope was introduced into the rectum and directed under visual control through the sigmoid, descending, transverse, and ascending colon to the cecum. Position of the cecum was confirmed by visualization of the ileocecal valve, ballottement and transillumination. The mucosa throughout the colon was intact without evidence of edema, erythema, or friability. The patient had extensive diverticulosis with circular muscle hypertrophy. There were no masses or polyps. There was no bleeding in the lower GI tract.

   The colon was decompressed and the endoscope removed. The patient tolerated the procedure well.

IMPRESSIONS: 1. Uncomplicated diverticulosis
               2. Internal hemorrhoids
               3. No evidence of any bleeding in the colon

Harold R. Carrolton, MD

HRC/fa 10/15/08 11:47:39

You Code It!

What are the best, most accurate codes?

_____

_____

_____

CARROLTON DIGESTIVE MEDICINE, PA
765 SWOLLOW PATH • PASSING, FL 32811 • 407-555-7985

PATIENT: MILLER, JUDITH
ACCOUNT/EHR #:   MILJU001
Date: 10/15/08

Procedure: Gastroscopy and biopsy
Indications for Procedure: Gastrointestinal bleeding and negative colonoscopy

DESCRIPTION OF OPERATION: The patient had received 10 mg of intravenous Versed and 50 mg of intravenous Demerol for sedation. The oropharynx was anesthetized with Cetacaine spray. The Olympus video gastroscope was then passed through the cricopharyngeal muscle into the esophagus, stomach, and duodenum. The esophagus was unremarkable. The stomach was entered. There was evidence of multiple gastric ulcers involving the antrum and prepyloric area. There was some blood adherent to the ulcers along the anterior aspect of the antrum. There was no active bleeding noted. The duodenal bulb and duodenal sweep were unremarkable. The endoscope was returned to the stomach and retroflexed. The cardia was observed and no additional lesions identified. Biopsies were taken of the ulcers for histology. The patient tolerated the procedure well.

IMPRESSIONS: 1. Multiple small gastric ulcers

Harold R. Carrolton, MD

HRC/fa 10/15/08 11:47:39

You Code It!

What are the best, most accurate codes?

_____

_____

_____

CARROLTON DIGESTIVE MEDICINE, PA
765 SWOLLOW PATH • PASSING, FL 32811 • 407-555-7985

PATIENT: PATCHMON, PETER
ACCOUNT/EHR #:   PATPE001
DATE: 10/15/08

Preop Diagnosis: Acute cholecystitis, cholelithiasis
Postop Diagnosis: Acute cholecystitis, cholelithiasis
Procedure: Laparoscopic cholecystectomy

Surgeon: Derick Marks, MD
Assistant: Frank Scottsboro, MD

Anesthesia: General endotracheal
Findings at Surgery: Pericholecystic adhesions, large gallstones

DESCRIPTION OF OPERATION: After the induction of general endotracheal anesthesia, the patient's abdomen was prepped and draped in the usual sterile manner and a small infraumbilical incision was made in the skin and carried down to the linea alba which was grasped with a clamp and incised in a vertical manner. The peritoneum was entered under direct vision. Stay sutures were placed in the fascia. The Hasson introducer was placed. Pneumoperitoneum was established and following this, three additional trocars were placed in the abdomen: One in the left epigastrium and two in the right upper quadrant, all 5 mm. Following this, the gallbladder was grasped with cephalad retraction of the gallbladder fundus and lateralward retraction of the gallbladder infundibulum. The dissector was employed to take down the peritoneum overlying the gallbladder infundibulum and cystic duct junction. When this was well delineated on both the anterior and posterior surfaces of the cystic duct, the 5 mm endoscopic clip applier was inserted and two clips were placed on the patient's side, on the gallbladder side of the cystic duct and it was transected. Further dissection in the triangle of Calot revealed the cystic artery, which was handled in an identical manner. The remainder of the dissection was performed using the Bovie spatula cautery and the liver bed was dry. A 10 to 15 mm camera change-out was performed and the camera was inserted into the left epigastric port. A toothed clamp was passed through the umbilicus to grasp the gallbladder, which was then removed through the umbilicus in a standard manner. Following this, the operative field was copiously irrigated with saline and the return was clear. All three upper abdominal ports were seen to exit the abdomen under direct vision and with the Hasson introducer removed, the fascial incision was closed with a 2-0 Vicryl figure-of-eight suture. The skin at the umbilicus was closed with a 4-0 Maxon subcuticular suture. Steri-strips were applied at all sites. The patient tolerated the procedure well.

ADDENDUM: There were three cystic artery branches; each was doubly clipped and transected.

Derick Marks, MD

DM/fa 10/15/08 11:47:39

You Code It!

What are the best, most accurate codes?

_____

_____

_____

CARROLTON DIGESTIVE MEDICINE, PA
765 SWOLLOW PATH • PASSING, FL 32811 • 407-555-7985

PATIENT: HART, LOUIS
ACCOUNT/EHR #:   HARLO001
DATE: 9/15/08

Admission Diagnosis:
1. Abdominal pain with symptomatic cholelithiasis
2. History of depression
3. History of degenerative joint disease

Final Diagnosis:
1. Abdominal pain secondary to cholelithiasis, status post laparoscopic cholecystectomy
2. History of depression
3. History of degenerative joint disease

DISCHARGE INSTRUCTIONS: Medications – Keflex 500 mg one tablet four times a day for one week, Percocet one tablet four times a day p.r.n for pain, Vicodin one or two tablets p.o q4h p.r.n for pain. Recommended follow-up in my office in about two weeks' time, and also recommended to follow with the surgeon in about seven-to-ten days' time.

HOSPITAL COURSE: Patient is a pleasant 39-year-old Caucasian male with a past medical history of degenerative joint disease and a history of depression. He presented to my office with a chief complaint of right upper quadrant pain. The patient had been evaluated by the Emergency Room on August 31, 2007 with a sonogram, which revealed multiple echogenic foci, consistent with stones. As the patient was not getting any better and he was symptomatic, he was admitted electively for possible cholelithiasis and evaluation of his abdominal pain for possible cholecystectomy.

    The patient was admitted to the surgical floor. We obtained a surgical consultation from Dr. Carter's group. Following the surgical evaluation, the patient underwent laparoscopic cholecystectomy. The patient's postoperative course was unremarkable. He was tolerating the pain better on pain medication. Once the patient was advanced on his diet and clinically improved and he was afebrile, he was discharged with the above discharge instructions, to be followed up on an outpatient basis.

Harold R. Carrolton, MD

HRC/fa 9/15/08 11:47:39

You Code It!

What are the best, most accurate codes?

_____

_____

_____

CARROLTON DIGESTIVE MEDICINE, PA
765 SWOLLOW PATH • PASSING, FL 32811 • 407-555-7985

PATIENT:	KINCAIDE, WENDY
ACCOUNT/EHR #:	KINWE001
Date:	9/15/08

HISTORY OF PRESENT ILLNESS: The patient, age 59, had been admitted to this medical center because of abdominal pain. She complained of lower abdominal pain starting on September 1st. Since that time, she has had loose stools and complained of marked fatigue. Her appetite has been poor and she has been aware of a low-grade fever.

The patient complained of similar symptoms about six months ago. At that time, studies included an upper GI series, barium enema and colonoscopy, which were reported as normal. She has continued to have some lower abdominal discomfort.

Prior to this admission, CT scan of the abdomen, revealed thickening of the cecal wall and proximal ascending colon. A ruptured appendix with perforation and abscess formation was suspected.

PAST MEDICAL HISTORY: Revealed known hypertension. She has a history of seizure disorder, her last seizure being 27 years ago. She stated she had tumors removed from her left inguinal area approximately 25-30 years ago, the nature of which she is not certain. She has been treated for hypertension for the past three or four years.

ALLERGIES: Dilantin

PHYSICIAL EXAMINATION

VITAL SIGNS: BP 122/70, Wt 128, T 100.2

GENERAL: The patient appeared to be in moderate pain on admission.

SKIN/MUCOUS MEMBRANES: There was no cyanosis or venous distention.

HEART: Heart sounds were regular and normal.

LUNGS: Clear

BREASTS: Revealed no masses

ABDOMEN: Soft with tenderness in the lower abdomen to palpation. There were no masses or organomegaly detected. The tenderness was noted especially in the right lower quadrant.

RECTAL: Normal and stool negative for occult blood

PELVIC: Unremarkable

EXTREMITIES: There was no dependent edema. Weak pedal pulses were present bilaterally.

LABORATORY STUDIES: Hemoglobin 11.4, hematocrit 33, WBC 11.6. Comprehensive metabolic profile – normal. Urinalysis – normal. Chest x-ray revealed no evidence of cardiopulmonary disease. DEXA: The bones were noted to be osteopenic. EKG revealed normal sinus rhythm and nonspecific T wave changes.

SUMMARY: On September 15th, Dr. Larry Garrett performed exploratory laparotomy, appendectomy and right salpingo-oophorectomy. Patient had an uneventful postoperative course. She was discharged on September 18, 2008.

DISCHARGE DIAGNOSIS: 1. Acute and chronic appendicitis with perforation and abscess formation
2. Hypertension
3. Seizure disorder
4. Allergy to DILANTIN

Continued

DISCHARGE MEDICATIONS: 1. Ziac 5mg daily
2. Mysoline 250 mg three times per day
3. Tylenol #3 one or two 3-4h, p.r.n for pain
4. Cefaclor 250 mg q8h for one week

DISCHARGE INSTRUCTIONS: Patient was instructed to restrict her activities and to contact myself and Dr. Garrett after discharge for follow-up

Harold R. Carrolton, MD

HRC/fa 9/15/08 11:47:39

You Code It!

What are the best, most accurate codes?

CARROLTON DIGESTIVE MEDICINE, PA
765 SWOLLOW PATH • PASSING, FL 32811 • 407-555-7985

PATIENT:	PHARMANE, CATHERINE
ACCOUNT/EHR #:	PHACA001
DATE:	4/17/08
Preop Diagnosis	Chronic appendicitis with abscess
Postop Diagnosis	Same
Surgeon	Alma Beach, MD
Anesthesia	General
Operative Procedure	Laparotomy with appendectomy and right salpingo-oophorectomy

INDICATIONS: The patient is a 51-year-old female, admitted on April 17, 2008, with abdominal pain. The patient complained of lower abdominal pain starting on April 8th. Since that time, she had loose stools and complained of marked fatigue. Her appetite was poor and she had been aware of a low-grade fever. The patient had similar complaints approximately six months ago. At that time, studies included an upper GI series, barium enema and colonoscopy, which were reported as normal. Prior to this admission, a CT scan of the abdomen was performed, which revealed a thickening of the cecal wall and proximal ascending colon. A ruptured appendix with perforation and abscess formation was suspected. Plans were made for surgery.

DESCRIPTION OF OPERATION: The patient was taken to the operating room and placed in the supine position. After general endotracheal anesthesia was administered, a Foley catheter was placed and then her abdomen was prepped and draped in the usual sterile fashion.

A knife was used to make a right paramedian incision and dissection taken down through the subcutaneous tissues. The anterior rectus sheath was divided and blunt dissection accomplished through the rectus muscles. The posterior rectus sheath and peritoneum were then opened sharply, as well. There was a large inflammatory mass noted in the right lower quadrant. There was an abscess cavity entered and this was cultured. The cecum was identified and the tinea were followed to where the appendiceal origin should be. However, there was a great deal of inflammation in this area. The right tube and ovary were involved, as well.

There was a tubular structure heading into the retrocecal area, which appeared to be the remnant of the appendix. This was followed back to the appendix and a straight clamp placed across it. This was then doubly tied with 0-Vicryl ties. The structure was adherent to the tube and ovary, a large inflammatory mass. The tube and ovary were excised by clamping their blood supply and tying these off with 0-Vicryl ties, as well. The specimen was passed off the table.

Continued

The area was irrigated with copious amounts of saline. Hemostasis was good. A 10 mm Blake drain was placed in the abscess cavity and taken out through a lateral stab incision. This was secured in place with a 2.0 nylon suture. Again, the abdomen and pelvis were irrigated and suctioned out. The posterior rectus sheath and peritoneum were closed with a running 0-Vicryl suture and the anterior rectus sheath closed with a running #1 PDS suture. The subcutaneous tissues were irrigated with saline and the skin closed with staples.

The patient tolerated the procedure well and there were no complications. She returned to recovery in stable condition.

Alma Beach, MD

AB/fa 4/17/08 21:47:39

You Code It!

What are the best, most accurate codes?

_____

_____

_____

CARROLTON DIGESTIVE MEDICINE, PA
765 SWOLLOW PATH • PASSING, FL 32811 • 407-555-7985

PATIENT: ANATOLE, RENE
ACCOUNT/EHR #:   ANARE001
Date: 6/19/08

HISTORY OF PRESENT ILLNESS: This patient is a 43-year-old white male who has been having severe epigastric and right upper quadrant pains radiating to his right shoulder since June 13th. This occurred after fatty food. He took Zantac over the counter and Gas-X, but this didn't help him. He had had intermittent episodes that are severe. He remains quite tender in the right upper quadrant. He has been belching quite a bit as well.

He presented to the ER early the morning of June 18 for evaluation of this. Yesterday, he underwent ultrasound of the abdomen, and PIPIDA scan, which showed some delay emptying into the duodenum, but otherwise was normal on the PIPIDA scan and no stones were seen on the ultrasound.

Today, he underwent a biliary tract ejection fraction evaluation and a CT of the abdomen and pelvis. The gallbladder ejection fraction was 17%, which is markedly low, and the CT showed a minimally dilated distal common bile duct without any obvious mass effect, stones, etc., and no other pathology.

He will present to the hospital for purposes of esophagogastroduodenoscopy. He has had a Helicobacter pylori infection in the past, and to rule out any cause such as peptic ulcer disease, reflux esophagitis, etc. for his pain, and then, if all this is negative, then he will undergo laparoscopic cholecystectomy. He was placed on Zantac yesterday, 150 mg bid and was switched to Prilosec today.

PMH: Negative with the exception of the above.

PAST SURGICAL HISTORY: Appendectomy and multiple ear surgeries.

ALLERGIES: None known of.

SOCIAL HISTORY: No tobacco, minimal alcohol.

FAMILY HISTORY: The patient was adopted.

REVIEW OF SYSTEMS: Negative with the exception of the above.

PHYSICAL EXAMINATION

GENERAL: Reveals a well-developed, well-nourished white male in no acute distress

VITAL SIGNS: BP 126/80, T 98.1, P 80, R 16

HEENT: Head is atraumatic, normocephalic

NECK: Supple, trachea midline

CHEST: Clear

HEART: Regular rhythm

ABDOMEN: Tender in the epigastric and right upper quadrant region. There are no masses or organomegaly.

EXTREMITIES: No cyanosis, clubbing or edema

NEUROLOGIC: Grossly intact

IMPRESSION: 1. R/O peptic ulcer disease, reflux esophagitis, etc.
                  2. Biliary dyskinesia

Continued

PLAN: 1. Esophagogastroduodenoscopy
       2. Laparoscopic cholecystectomy if no obvious reason for this patient's discomfort is found

Harold R. Carrolton, MD

HRC/fa 6/19/08 11:47:39

You Code It!

What are the best, most accurate codes?

CARROLTON DIGESTIVE MEDICINE, PA
765 SWOLLOW PATH • PASSING, FL 32811 • 407-555-7985

PATIENT: STEVENS, MARIBELLA
ACCOUNT/EHR #:   STEMA001
Date: 9/15/08

Preop Diagnosis: Severe abdominal pain, R/O peptic ulcer disease, esophagitis, etc.
Postop Diagnosis: Minimal duodenitis
Operation Performed: Esophagogastroduodenoscopy

Surgeon: Lawrence Garrett, MD

Anesthesia: Topical

PROCEDURE IN DETAIL: After an adequate topical anesthetic was achieved using viscous Xylocaine, the Olympus upper GI endoscope was passed per orally and advanced down the esophagus through the GE junction and then in through the stomach, in through the pylorus, into the duodenum.

This study revealed the presence of some minimal friability in the duodenum. Some minimal duodenitis could be seen. The remainder of the examination appeared to be within normal limits, including the remainder of the stomach and esophagus.

The GE junction was at 40 cm; there is no hiatus hernia, there is no evidence of reflux esophagitis, there was no clear-cut gastritis, there were no peptic ulcers, etc. No evidence of neoplasm.

The endoscope was withdrawn, the above findings were reconfirmed. The patient tolerated the procedure well. A biopsy of the antrum was taken for CLO-test.

Lawrence Garrett, MD

LG/fa 9/15/08 11:47:39

You Code It!

What are the best, most accurate codes?

_____

_____

_____

CARROLTON DIGESTIVE MEDICINE, PA
765 SWOLLOW PATH • PASSING, FL 32811 • 407-555-7985

PATIENT: CHAMBERS, DUANE
ACCOUNT/EHR #:   CHADU001
Date: 9/15/08

Preop Diagnosis: COLON CANCER SCREENING
Postop Diagnosis: 1. A 4 mm polyp in the proximal rectum, not biopsied
                           2. Normal sigmoid, descending colon, transverse colon, ascending colon,
                              cecum, and ileum
Procedure: Colonoscopy to the ileum with hot biopsy polypectomy

Physician: Albert Mathews, MD

Anesthesia: Conscious sedation

PROCEDURE IN DETAIL: The patient was identified in the endoscopy room, sedated with 4 mg of Versed and 100 mcg of Fentanyl. The colonoscope was advanced to the ileum. On the way out, the mucosa was examined thoroughly and hot biopsy done in the rectum.

Once the procedure was completed, he was kept in the room for an EGD. Preparation was good.

IMPRESSION: Proximal rectal polyp, about 4 mm

PLAN: EGD now.

Albert Mathews, MD

AM/fa 9/15/08 11:47:39

You Code It!

What are the best, most accurate codes?

_____

_____

_____

CARROLTON DIGESTIVE MEDICINE, PA
765 SWOLLOW PATH • PASSING, FL 32811 • 407-555-7985

PATIENT: WOODS, BETHANY
ACCOUNT/EHR #:   WOOBE001
Date: 9/15/08

CHIEF COMPLAINT: This is a 45-year-old white female, referred by Dr. Hallowing, with complaints of abdominal pain. She states that her pain began about 3 weeks prior to her presentation and has gradually worsened. The pain is sharp in nature and located in the middle of her upper abdomen, just below her rib cage. It occurs most often between meals and is relieved with meals only to recur several hours later. She denies any weight loss, anorexia, dysphagia, diarrhea or constipation. Her stools are a bit darker than usual but without any signs of bright red blood. She has never had pain like this in the past, is uncertain as to its cause, and has been using some over-the-counter antacid without relief. Her last menstrual period was 3 weeks prior to her presentation and was of the usual timing (q 28 days) and duration (5 days). Her abdominal pain did not worsen during the time of her menses. She does not consider her periods heavy. She uses condoms and spermicidal lubricant for birth control. She is sexually active with her boyfriend of the last 6 months, with whom she feels safe and supported; she has no history of domestic violence. She has never contracted a sexually transmitted disease.

PAST MEDICAL HISTORY: She has three healthy children delivered by cesarean section but no other surgery. She has a history of seasonal allergies for which she takes over-the-counter anti-histamine with good relief. She takes no other medications.

ALLERGIES: Meperidine (Demerol) caused her to break out in a rash, her only medication allergy.

FAMILY HISTORY: Her father is alive and well despite suffering a myocardial infarction at age 62. Her mother died from colon cancer at age 60. She has two sisters who are alive and well, ages 40 and 47.

SOCIAL HISTORY: She is physically active, running two or three miles every other day. She has smoked one pack of cigarettes a day for 25 years, rarely drinks alcoholic beverages, and uses no other substances. She uses no aspirin or nonsteroidal products. She works as a legal secretary for a large law firm. Her oldest child, a son, is away at college; her two youngest children are at home including a 12-year-old daughter recently diagnosed with a learning disability. She had all of her children by her former husband from whom she's been divorced for three years. She reports some stress related to being a single parent and sharing custody but does not believe that this is the cause of her abdominal pain.

Physical Examination: She is a well-appearing thin white female, appearing her stated age. Wt 120 pounds, unchanged from her previous visit six months before. BP 110/67mmHg supine and 105/60mmHg standing. Heart rate: 68/min supine and 72/min standing. Respiratory rate is 12. T 98.8°F. Her conjunctiva are pale, sclera are anicteric, mucus membranes are moist. There are no oral lesions. Neck is without bruits or thyromegaly. Lungs are clear to auscultation and percussion. Heart is regular without murmurs, rubs, or gallops. Abdomen is soft, non-distended with normoactive bowel sounds. There is epigastric tenderness to palpation without rebound or

Continued

guarding. Murphy's sign is negative and there is no organomegaly. Stool is dark brown and tests guaiac positive for occult blood. Deep tendon reflexes are 2+ and equal. Skin is without lesions.

DIAGNOSIS: Infection with H pylori.

PLAN: RX: Antibiotics and a proton-pump inhibitor.

Albert Mathews, MD

AM/fa 9/15/08 11:47:39

You Code It!

What are the best, most accurate codes?

_____

_____

_____

CARROLTON DIGESTIVE MEDICINE, PA
765 SWOLLOW PATH • PASSING, FL 32811 • 407-555-7985

PATIENT: MONTANA, JOANNE
ACCOUNT/EHR #: MONJO001
Date: 9/15/08

CHIEF COMPLAINT: Joanne is a 51-year-old female whom I have not seen in two years. She comes in complaining of abdominal pain. This pain is very different from abdominal pain that she suffered one year ago. Now her pain is sharp and stabbing, though still located in the mid-epigastrium. The pain occurs about 45 minutes after eating and lasts less than an hour. The pain occasionally radiates over her right shoulder. She notes the pain is the worst after her favorite meal, pizza.

PHYSICAL EXAMINATION: She is a thin white female, appearing her stated age. Wt 125 pounds. BP 110/67mmHg supine and 105/60mmHg standing. Heart rate: 68/min supine and 72/min standing. Her conjunctiva are without pallor, mucus membranes are moist. There are no oral lesions. Neck is without bruits or thyromegaly. Lungs are clear to auscultation and percussion. Heart is regular without murmurs rubs or gallops. Abdomen is soft, non-distended with normoactive bowel sounds. There is epigastric tenderness to palpation without rebound or guarding. Murphy's sign is positive. Stool is dark brown and tests guaiac negative for occult blood. Deep tendon reflexes are 2+ and equal. Skin is without lesions.

TESTS: Sonogram performed in office reveals presence of gallstones.

DIAGNOSIS: Cholelithiasis

PLAN: Discuss the recommendation for a laparoscopic cholecystectomy. All benefits and risks are reviewed. Patient decides to go ahead with the procedure. Surgery scheduled for two weeks from Friday.

Albert Mathews, MD

AM/fa 9/15/08 11:47:39

You Code It!

What are the best, most accurate codes?

_____

_____

_____

CARROLTON DIGESTIVE MEDICINE, PA
765 SWOLLOW PATH • PASSING, FL 32811 • 407-555-7985

PATIENT: STEVENSON, CHRISTOPHER
ACCOUNT/EHR #:   STECH001
Date: 9/15/08

CHIEF COMPLAINT: This patient is a 41-year-old male, referred by Dr. Sherman, with complaints of abdominal pain. He states that the pain is intermittent and accompanied by bouts of diarrhea. Between bouts of pain with diarrhea (which predominate) he is constipated with small hard stools. He describes the pain as crampy without localization. Patient denies weight gain or loss, but constantly feels bloated. Dairy products and caffeine exacerbate his diarrheal symptoms. His diet includes limited fiber intake. He remains with the same partner. They are considering marriage and this is the source of some friction between him and his youngest child, now a sophomore in high school.

PHYSICAL EXAMINATION: He is mildly anxious but in no acute distress and is non-ill appearing. His weight is 162 pounds, blood pressure is normal, he is not tachycardic, and he is afebrile. His physical examination, including abdominal and rectal examinations, are unremarkable; stool is guaiac negative.

DIAGNOSIS: Irritable bowel syndrome (IBS)

PLAN: Rx psyllium to regulate bowel function and alleviate symptoms. Discuss with patient that the fact that his diarrheal symptoms are aggravated by dairy products suggests that he may have a component of lactose intolerance. We also discuss in detail dietary interventions for IBS such as keeping a food diary to discover any associations of symptoms with specific dietary intake.

Albert Mathews, MD

AM/fa 9/15/08 11:47:39

You Code It!

What are the best, most accurate codes?

_____

_____

_____

CARROLTON DIGESTIVE MEDICINE, PA
765 SWOLLOW PATH • PASSING, FL 32811 • 407-555-7985

PATIENT:	FINSTER, PETER
ACCOUNT/EHR #:	FINSPE001
Date:	04/08/08

Preop Diagnosis:	Malignant polyp in sigmoid colon
Postop Diagnosis:	Malignant polyp in sigmoid colon
Procedure:	Laparotomy, intraoperative colonoscopy for polypectomy site localization, sigmoid colectomy with colorectal anastomosis
Anesthesia:	General endotracheal

INDICATIONS FOR OPERATION: This is a 57-year-old male who was found to have a malignant polyp in the sigmoid colon. The pathology was reviewed and a colectomy was recommended. All risks, benefits, and alternatives were explained and he consented to surgery. He received a full mechanical and antibiotic bowel preparation preoperatively. Deep venous thrombosis prophylaxis was accomplished with the PAS stockings.

DESCRIPTION OF PROCEDURE: The patient was brought to the operating room and after the induction of general endotracheal anesthesia, a Foley catheter was inserted. He was placed in the modified lithotomy position in the Allen stirrups. Rectal irrigation was performed until clear with saline and Betadine. The abdomen was shaved, prepped with Betadine solution, and draped in a sterile fashion. An infraumbilical transverse incision was made and carried down through the anterior rectus sheath. The rectus muscle on the right side was divided with electrocautery. The epigastric arteries were individually clamped, divided, and ligated with #0 Vicryl. The incision was carried down across the midline to the right rectus muscle and this was partially divided. Exposure was then accomplished with the Burke-Walter retractor. Palpation of the liver, gallbladder, and stomach was normal. The small bowel was normal in appearance. The sigmoid colon had diverticulosis, but there was no palpable tumor noted. At this point, I introduced the colonoscope transanally and localized an ulcer consistent with the polypectomy site at the 25 cm level. This site was marked in the serosa with a Vicryl suture. I then rescrubbed and regowned and gloved and proceeded with the operation. The sigmoid colon and descending colon were mobilized and reflected medially, incising along with white line of Toldt. We carried the mobilization until the distal descending colon was quite mobile. The left ureter was identified and kept out of harm's way. We then divided the distal descending colon at its junction with the sigmoid colon with the 75 mm linear stapler. The mesentery at the sigmoid at the point was then divided between clamps, ligating with #0 Vicryl. The superior rectal artery was divided and was suture ligated with #0 Vicryl. This allowed us access into the vasculature plane and we carried this in a caudal direction over the sacral promontory into the presacral space. Once we were below the marked site, we divided the rectal mesentery between clamps, ligating with #0 Vicryl. Once we had achieved a good margin, we came across the superior rectum with a TA-55 mm linear stapler. The specimen was then excised and removed and sent off the field. The specimen was opened to make sure that we had achieved a good margin and that we had the polypectomy site and indeed we have achieved both. The descending colon was then mobilized a little further until the anastomosis could be created to be completely tension free. The end of the descending colon was then prepared by clearing some of the mesentery, thereby exposing the serosa. We quarantined the peritoneal cavity with towels, exposing the descending colon. The staple line was opened and a pursestring of #0 Prolene was created. The detached head of the 29 mm ILS stapler was then secured in place with this pursestring suture. The descending colon was well vascularized. The ILS 29 mm stapler was then introduced transanally and advanced all the way up to the staple line of the rectum. The instrument was opened and the rod came out at the level of the staple line. We then connected the descending colon to the rectum via the stapler, closed the instrument, and fired. Two perfect donuts were retrieved and a circular anastomosis was created. The pelvis was then filled with saline. Air was insufflated transanally descending the descending colon to the anastomosis and there was no air leak noted. We then irrigated the pelvis and the abdominal cavity with saline solution until clear. I changed my gown and gloves at this point and proceeded with draping the omentum over the small intestine. The posterior rectus sheath was closed with a running #1 PDS suture. The rectus muscle was irrigated

Continued

and the anterior rectus sheath was then closed with a running double-stranded #1 PDS suture. The subcutaneous tissue was irrigated. The skin was infiltrated with 20 cc of 0.5% Marcaine. The skin was then closed with a running subcuticular #4-0 Vicryl. This was reinforced with Steri-Strips. A dressing was applied. The patient tolerated the procedure well and left the operating room in stable condition. The final sponge, needle, and instrument counts were correct times two. There were no Intraoperative complications.

Harold R. Carrolton, MD, surgeon
Sander Lawrence, assistant surgeon

HRC/fa 04/08/08 11:47:39

You Code It!

What are the best, most accurate codes?

_____

_____

_____

Gerontology Cases and Patient Records

INTRODUCTION

The following case studies are from a gerontology practice. In a physician's office of this type, a professional coding specialist is likely to see many different kinds of health situations, especially preventive health care services.

Geriatric specialists, also known as geriatricians, are typically family medicine physicians or internists specializing in the diagnosis and treatment of conditions and diseases of older adults. As individuals get older, their health concerns become greater and more serious. For example, a 40-year-old diagnosed with the flu will usually be out of work for a few days; however, for an 80-year-old, a case of the flu can be life-threatening. These health care professionals may care for their patients in their office, in the patient's home, or in a nursing home or assisted living facility.

Geriatric medicine specialists may be board-certified in family medicine, internal medicine, or geriatric medicine by the American Board of Family Practice or the Board of Internal Medicine. Both of these boards are recognized by the American Board of Medical Specialties.

You can use these cases to practice coding diagnoses, E/M, procedures, DME, or other HCPCS Level II items, as applicable; code for the physician or the facility; code inpatient and outpatient services, as applicable:

1. Code for the physician.
2. Code for the anesthesiologist, when applicable.
3. Code for the hospital, when applicable.
4. Code for the pathology and laboratory, when applicable.
5. Code HCPCS Level II codes, when applicable.

ADULT HEALTH ASSOCIATES
720 LONG STREET • ETERNITY, FL 32711 • 407-555-7322

PATIENT: ANDERSON, LAWRENCE
ACCOUNT/EHR #:   ANDELA01
Date: 04/22/08

Attending Physician: James Healer, MD

This 89-year-old male was seen in his room at the Sun City Nursing Home for his regular annual check-up. Pt is stable and doing well on his current regime of medications. PE shows age appropriate condition. HEENT unremarkable. Coordination with resident medical director to review and affirm medical plan of care.

_____

James Healer, MD

JHW/mg   D: 04/22/08 09:50:16   T: 04/25/08 12:55:01

You Code It!

What are the best, most accurate codes?

_____

_____

_____

PATIENT: ALDERS, STEFAN
ACCOUNT/EHR #:   ALDEST01
Date: 04/22/08

Attending Physician: Amanda Christoper, MD

This new patient is a 76-year-old male, referred to me by Dr. Theodore Lee, the family physician. He resides in his own two-story house where he enjoys listening to the radio and the occasional record and tending to his garden. He denies ever marrying and states that he does not have any children. He attended one year of community college, after which he obtained employment as a clerk in a lawyer's office. He kept this job for 40 years and retired when he was 67. He has an older brother, who was killed during World War II, and an older sister (80 years old) who resides in a nearby nursing home and whom he visits occasionally. His native language is French, however, he speaks and understands English very well. He still drives his own car for occasional trips but has expressed concern lately about getting lost when driving outside of his neighborhood.

The patient attends an Adult Day Program affiliated to a Senior Center twice a week. He has had several falls over the last six months and fractured a rib during the last fall incident, four months ago. Currently, he receives nursing service from Home Care once a week to monitor medications. He visits his sister once a week in a nearby nursing home, but the frequency of the visits has lessened over the past few months.

Over the past month or so, day program staff noticed the patient's personal appearance is deteriorating. There are days when he wears soiled clothes, and his hair is not always clean or even combed. Patient showed up at the Center on the wrong day for pre-planned activities, three times in the past two months. It appears that he is forgetting the names of staff and other members of the group, even those whose names he knew. He appears more withdrawn and seems to have trouble following conversations. Maxine Shaw, MSW, the social worker at the adult day program recommended this geriatric assessment to Dr. Lee, who referred the patient to me.

ASSESSEMENT: The patient has a history of being a highly anxious person; he has a history of benzodiazepine use, as well as a history of psychiatric admissions for depression and anxiety. He states he has been experiencing increased anxiety following a diagnosis of skin cancer seven months ago. He has asthma and uses Ventolin for control of symptoms. He states that he frequently calls his family physician, Dr. Theodore Lee, regarding the asthma attacks.

VITAL SIGNS: Temp: Afebrile; Resp: 17 – accessory muscle use unremarkable; BP: 125/85 supine, 128/80 sitting, and 125/85 standing; Weight: 145 lb. relatively stable (according to patient records from Dr. Lee); P normal; Pulse Oximeter O2 sat: 80%

ATTITUDE: Patient is compliant and appears to be slightly resentful of the idea that something is wrong with him. He is slightly slow in some responses.

GAIT: Patient is mildly unstable. Movement is slow, unsteady, and purposeful. At times, it appears that he tries to move and his feet are not quite following.

FOLSTEIN MINI-MENTAL STATUS EXAM (MMSE): Score of 19 indicating possible depression and some cognitive impairment.

INTEGUMENTARY SYSTEM: Skin is slightly pale; some diminished elasticity; slightly dehydrated. No signs of skin cancer, decubitus ulcers, or other ulcerations or wounds. There is some bruising, mostly on extremities, all of which appear to be normal for a patient of this age. No lesions are evident. HEAD: No signs of head trauma; no signs of Paget's disease.

EYES: Screening funduscopic examination is negative for cataracts. Visual fields for glaucoma—mild bilateral cataract developing in left eye; Snellen Eye chart for rapid test of visual acuity is normal.

Continued

EARS: Bilateral hearing aids for SNHL in the left ear and a mixed hearing loss in the right ear as a result of a stapedectomy when he was a child, which caused a conductive hearing loss. Some cerumen impaction, which is normal for patients who wear hearing aids.

NOSE: No nasal obstruction

OROPHARYNX: Patient wears upper and lower dentures that appear to fit correctly. No evidence of leukoplakia, cancers, erosions. Throat examination results show no throat infections or airway obstruction.

NECK: ROM is unremarkable. Lymph nodes show no signs of malignancy. Cervical lymph nodes show no signs of infection, trachea is not deviated from midline, thyroid gland – no nodules indicating malignancy, thyromegaly in negative for hyperthyroidism. Carotid arteries – possible carotid occlusion. Thromboembolic risk is moderate and auscultation for bruits is negative.

LYMPH NODES: Posterior auricular, preauricular, supramandibular, anterior and posterior cervical, supraclavicular, axillary, inguinal lymph nodes are all unremarkable.

SPINAL/BACK: Evidence of moderate kyphosis. There is no spinal tenderness or any associated kyphos. There is some flank tenderness near the area of the previous rib fracture. Back mobility is limited.

CHEST/LUNG: No signs of pulmonary edema, obstructive lung disease, pneumonia, or TB.

HEART: PMI and character of apex beat—unremarkable; parasternal lifts and thrills—unremarkable; no added heart sounds (S3/S4) or murmurs; carotid beat during auscultation (for upstroke for AS)—unremarkable.

PERIPHERAL VASCULAR: Pulses checked: Bilateral temporal—OK, carotid—slow, brachial—OK, radial—OK, femoral—OK, popliteal—OK, dorsalis pedis—OK, posterior tibialis—OK.

ABDOMINAL: Unremarkable

MUSCULOSKELETAL/EXTREMITY: Cyanosis, clubbing, edema, capillary refill appear unremarkable; no deformities; patient's shoes seem to be too large, thereby affecting gait; muscle strength and ROM is limited and not outside of age-appropriateness.

NEUROLOGIC: Gait/fall risk: "get up and go" test (coordination and strength), Tandem Romberg, retropulsion, 360 degree turn—slow, affected. Coordination is within age range; however, strength is a concern. Wasting (local and generalized) and stigmata of stroke and common motor diseases is somewhat apparent. Cerebellar exam: finger to nose, rapid alternating movements, heel-knee to shin, Romberg—all slow but functional.

GENITOURINARY EXAM: Digital rectal examination—unremarkable; patient denies fecal impaction or urinary frequency.

DX: Arteriosclerosis, rule out normal pressure hydrocephalous

PLAN: Screening for arthritidis; Hemoccult test; MRI head; carotid artery angiography—bilateral

---

AMANDA CHRISTOPER, MD

AC/mg   D: 04/22/08 09:50:16   T: 04/25/08 12:55:01

You Code It!

What are the best, most accurate codes?

_____

_____

_____

ADULT HEALTH ASSOCIATES
720 LONG STREET • ETERNITY, FL 32711 • 407-555-7322

PATIENT: WOLLENBERG, LINDSAY

ACCOUNT/EHR #:   WOLLLI01

Date: 04/22/08

Attending Physician: Louis R. Ferguson, MD

This new patient is a 77-year-old female, who has been referred to me by her internal medicine physician, Dr. King. Patient reports a sudden hearing loss following a month of fullness in both ears attributed to altitude changes (recent airplane trip across country) and swimming. She states that she experienced unilateral loss (on the left side), preceded by dizziness and rushing in left ear.

    Tympanometry testing completed in office during this visit.

    Right ear shows normal thresholds, tympanogram results and reflexes.

    Left ear exhibits severe hearing loss (pure tone average (PTA) and speech recognition thresholds (SRT) 70 dB hearing level (HL) - masked right ear) and poor word recognition scores, normal ipsi- and contralateral stapedial reflexes.

DX: Unilateral sensorineural hearing loss, left ear

PLAN: Follow-up with patient in two weeks for further evaluation of continued services.

_____

LOUIS R. FERGUSON, MD

LRF/mg   D: 04/22/08 09:50:16   T: 04/25/08 12:55:01

You Code It!

What are the best, most accurate codes?

_____

_____

_____

PATIENT: MAYOR, ROLLAND
ACCOUNT/EHR #:   MAYORO01
Date: 04/22/08

Attending Physician: James Healer, MD

This patient is a 75-year-old male who lived on his family-owned tree farm outside of the city for most of his adult life. I am seeing him for the first time today due to concerns by his daughter about his recent falls.

PATIENT/SOCIAL: In October, he moved into a townhouse located in the suburb of Geneva, retiring from the farm due to his declining ability to manage the business. His townhouse is a two-story, single-family home. The kitchen, living room, bathroom, laundry, and storage facilities are located downstairs, and the bedroom and main bathroom are on the second floor.

The patient has never learned to drive a car and has relied on public transportation or his children since his wife died six years ago.

He is a member of the Kiwanis Club and the local Farmer's Association. Patient states he enjoys gardening and fishing.

The patient has two adult children. His son, Raymond, took over management of the tree farm eight years ago. He is in contact with him on a regular basis but rarely gets to see him because Raymond is busy with the farm. Raymond is married and has three children. Patient's daughter, Vanessa, lives in the area and provides most of the support for her father. It is Vanessa who encouraged the patient to move so that they could live closer and take advantage of various support services. Vanessa is married and has two young children.

HISTORY OF PRESENT PROBLEM: Patient is in good general health. He suffers from osteoarthritis in both hips and knees. He has cataracts, kyphosis, and he reported having "ringing in her ears" (tinnitus). The patient takes Metamucil daily, one 81-mg. aspirin per day, and uses Clear Vision eye drops as needed. He is physically strong and was quite active until a fall that occurred February 5th.

On February 13th, his daughter noticed that he was limping as a result of bruising from the recent fall.

On March 15th, the patient experienced a second fall, this time on the walkway outside his home. It appeared nothing was broken, however, there was severe bruising on his left side. On March 21st, the daughter took the patient to her own family physician, Dr. Fidele, because the patient's primary physician had recently retired. According to the daughter, Dr. Fidele assessed the bruising. During the session, he communicated primarily with the daughter who periodically explained what the doctor said to the patient. The doctor recommended physical therapy and wrote an order for home care services. The physical therapist first saw the patient at his home on April 8th.

On April 15th, the patient moved in with his daughter, son-in-law and two grandchildren because he developed a fear of falling again and suffering a more debilitating injury. In addition, it is thought that the daughter can assist with his recovery from his last fall. The son-in-law is not pleased with this situation.

Continued

PE: T 98.1F; B/P 135/90; R 16; P normal. HEENT: unremarkable; CHEST: clear; ABDOMEN: unremarkable; EXTREMITIES: Patient states sharp pain is experienced during dorsiflexion of the left foot. Circulation good.

DX: Achilles tendon contracture

PLAN: Referral for physical therapy; Rx for specialized series of shoes

James Healer, MD

JHW/mg   D: 04/22/08 09:50:16   T: 04/25/08 12:55:01

You Code It!

What are the best, most accurate codes?

_____

_____

_____

ADULT HEALTH ASSOCIATES
720 LONG STREET • ETERNITY, FL 32711 • 407-555-7322

PATIENT: FINN, WILMA
ACCOUNT/EHR #:   FINNWI01
Date: 04/22/08

Attending Physician: James Healer, MD

This patient is an 82-year-old female for care plan oversight services.

She was admitted February 18th via the emergency department after suffering a fall. She sustained a fracture of her right dominant humerus; and bruising along her right shoulder and hip. In the emergency room, she was reluctant to discuss how she fell and she also refused to answer questions about her family or her medical history. There was evidence of significant recent alcohol intake. She was admitted to acute care and underwent internal fixation of the fracture.

After three days in acute care, she was transferred to the nursing facility. It is expected that she will be discharged within the week.

MEDICAL HISTORY: Dr. Patel, her family physician, sent over her records that document a long-standing history of depression. Dr. Patel prescribed Prozac for the depression and Levothyroxine for hypothyroidism diagnosed ten years ago. The record also indicates that the patient is suspected of having an alcohol abuse problem.

Social history documented by Dr. Patel state that the patient's husband divorced her approximately 20 years ago. Family history documented in the record identifies that the patient has a 41-year-old son who lives with her, and who was diagnosed with schizophrenia in his middle twenties. The patient and her son have had periodic involvement with various municipal social service agencies over the past fifteen years.

There is concern that her recent fall could be due to her being under the influence of alcohol. However, there may be evidence that she may have been pushed by her son. There are reports of suspicious bruising in the past, identified by Dr. Patel during annual physicals. Hospital staff raised concerns about the patient's cognitive status because she is such a poor informant and her information is often inconsistent. Staff could not tell whether she could or would not provide information. She is bitter about her son's illness and was angry when questioned about it.

PLAN: After 45 minutes of evaluation and interviews with current and recent care givers, the best course of action at this time is for the patient to be admitted into an assisted living facility upon discharge from the nursing facility. In this environment, she can receive continued PT and be protected from any possible abuse at the hands of her son.

James Healer, MD

JHW/mg   D: 04/22/08 09:50:16   T: 04/25/08 12:55:01

You Code It!

What are the best, most accurate codes?

_____

_____

_____

ADULT HEALTH ASSOCIATES
720 LONG STREET • ETERNITY, FL 32711 • 407-555-7322

PATIENT: ENGLISH, ARTHUR
ACCOUNT/EHR #:   ENGLAR01
Date: 04/22/08

Attending Physician: James Healer, MD

This 87-year-old male patient was brought in to this ED by ambulance after he called 911. Patient stated he awoke and discovered that he was having difficulty walking and speaking.

FAMILY/SOCIAL HISTORY: This patient is a right-handed, 87-year-old, English-speaking widower who lives alone in his own home. His house is a ranch style, single-family home.

    The patient drives his own car. He enjoys reading and sports. He volunteers as a coach for the neighborhood softball league.

    The patient has two adult children. His daughter, Joellyn, lives about 45 minutes away and speaks, by phone, weekly with her father. The patient's son, Mark, lives in another state and is in touch about once or twice per month.

HISTORY OF PRESENT ILLNESS: Patient exhibits some confusion and loss of coordination. His motor and sensory functions appear to be impaired.

PE: Weakness and numbness in leg are evident. CT scan of brain, and EEG are positive for CVA. CBC shows decreased RBC, elevated lactate dehydrogenase (LDH) levels.

DX: Left anterior occlusive cerebral vascular accident (CVA).

PLAN: Admit patient to acute care for additional care.

_____

James Healer, MD

JHW/mg   D: 04/22/08 09:50:16   T: 04/25/08 12:55:01

You Code It!

What are the best, most accurate codes?

_____

_____

_____

ADULT HEALTH ASSOCIATES
720 LONG STREET • ETERNITY, FL 32711 • 407-555-7322

PATIENT: TOWNSEND, MARISSA
ACCOUNT/EHR #:   TOWNMA01
Date: 04/22/08

Attending Physician: James Healer, MD

PATIENT HISTORY: This patient is a 75-year-old female who ran her own doll repair business for 32 years out of a converted garage behind her house. She has been married for over 51 years to Thomas, who is 77 years old. The Townsends have three adult children. The eldest daughter, Jacklyn, aged 49, is a family therapist who lives in Texas. Their other daughter, Laila, aged 45, suffers from developmental disabilities and lives in a group home in a nearby city. Their son, the middle child, Kevin, age 47, is a high school principal who lives in New York with his wife and two children.

MEDICAL HISTORY: The patient has a recent history of angina for which she takes Nitroglycerine tablets sublingually as required. Her vision is deteriorating and she wears bifocals, which were prescribed and fitted within the last four months. She suffers from presbycusis, which was identified three years ago in a full audiometric evaluation as a bilateral, mild-moderate sensorineural hearing loss. She was prescribed a behind-the-ear (BTE) hearing aid for the right ear but does not wear it.

PRESENTING PROBLEM: Currently, the patient is suffering from recent memory problems and confusion, which, according to her husband, have been increasing slowly in severity over the past year or so. She wanders from her home, now more frequently than ever especially during the late afternoon. She gets lost easily. Mr. Townsend has been spending more time watching out for his wife because of this increased wandering. He has not yet sought support from any outside agencies.

Two days ago, while the patient was wandering through the downtown shopping center, she was crossing the street when a car struck her. Her head hit the pavement quite hard. She was not wearing her hearing aid at the time. An ambulance took her to the hospital Emergency department. An x-ray was performed to determine skull fracture, if any, as a result of the head injury. The patient was discharged home in the care of her husband with a diagnosis of multiple bruises and a mild concussion.

Her husband brought her in to our office today because he noted that she was behaving strangely. At first, he figured it was just due to the trauma of the event and concussion-related. Overnight, the patient exhibited confusion. She wandered the house aimlessly, repeatedly searching through the drawers and closets and urinating in a garbage can. When asked by her husband about her behaviors (e.g., 'What are you searching for?'), the patient insisted that she wanted to go home but could not find her way there. She accused her husband of keeping her against her will and kept repeating that she wanted to go home. She became very agitated.

PE: Patient shows unequal papillary response, and decerebrate posturing. CT can shows ischemic tissue and hematoma with no skull fracture.

Continued

DX: Epidural hematoma

PLAN: Admit patient to hospital for further evaluation and treatment.

James Healer, MD

JHW/mg   D: 04/22/08 09:50:16   T: 04/25/08 12:55:01

You Code It!

What are the best, most accurate codes?

_____

_____

_____

ADULT HEALTH ASSOCIATES
720 LONG STREET • ETERNITY, FL 32711 • 407-555-7322

PATIENT: LYNDELL, JACOB
ACCOUNT/EHR #:   LYNDJA01
Date: 04/22/08

Attending Physician: James Healer, MD

This patient is a 75-year-old male, diagnosed with IDDM who was last seen by me almost two years ago. He is a retired fish wholesale worker, married, with 12 children, seven of whom still live in the area. He lives with his wife, Charlotte, in a retirement community.

HISTORY: Patient has peripheral neuropathy with paresthesias of his fingers and feet, diabetic retinopathy, bilateral sensorineural hearing loss (SNHL), and peripheral vascular disease. The patient admits that he still smokes, on average, one pack of cigarettes a day.

PRESENTING PROBLEM: The patient is grossly overweight and denies following the diet given to him by me at our last encounter. He was diagnosed with insulin-dependent diabetes mellitus (IDDM) five years ago and admits that he occasionally forgets to take his insulin.

PE: Decubitus ulcers are evident on the left foot and ankle. Sights of necrotic tissue and the beginnings of gangrene are observed. Decubitus ulcers forming on the right foot require monitoring in hopes of avoiding another amputation. GTT is abnormal.

DX: IDDM, uncontrolled, with peripheral angiopathy and gangrene.

PLAN: Admit to hospital for below the knee (BTK) amputation of left leg.

James Healer, MD

JHW/mg   D: 04/22/08 09:50:16   T: 04/25/08 12:55:01

You Code It!

What are the best, most accurate codes?

_____

_____

_____

ADULT HEALTH ASSOCIATES
720 LONG STREET • ETERNITY, FL 32711 • 407-555-7322

PATIENT: COLLINS, ANDREA
ACCOUNT/EHR #:   COLLAN01
Date: 04/22/08

Attending Physician: James Healer, MD

This patient is an 81-year-old white female that I am meeting for the first time in the hospital where she was admitted following a visit to the ER.

Prior to this hospital admission, she has been living independently in her own suburban house several houses down from her grandson who is very attentive, helping her with yard care and grocery shopping in which she is limited by arthritic pain. The patient is otherwise independent with ADLs (Activities of Daily Living) and other IADLs (Instrumental Activities of Daily Living).

PATIENT HISTORY: The patient lost her husband to cancer two years ago and takes pride in maintaining her independence. She has been relatively healthy throughout her life but did smoke for 35 years. She stopped smoking 10 years ago.

She takes hydrochlorothiazide 25mg daily for hypertension and has an albuterol inhaler that she uses prn for mild emphysema and bronchitis. She only needs the inhaler occasionally, usually in the spring and fall when pollen is in the air, or if she catches a cold. She also takes regular Tylenol about five days out of the week for "arthritis" of her knees. She has never been hospitalized for any reason, other than the birth of her children.

The patient was brought to our office by her grandson, Barney, with a report of maroon stools, that she has been experiencing for the last three days. He states that she has also exhibited a recent onset of dizziness. Patient denies pain or loss of appetite and states she feels well otherwise.

PE: She is a well-developed, well-nourished female who looks younger than her stated age. Her skin looks somewhat pale. Her BP lying down is 130/78 with a pulse of 84. On standing, her BP is 100/63 with a pulse of 124.

Patient is prepped and I perform a flexible sigmoidoscopy to the splenic flexure. A bleeding polyp is identified in the descending colon. The polyp was removed by snare technique. Tissue sent to lab.

DX: Intestinal neoplasm, pending lab report for malignancy.

James Healer, MD

JHW/mg   D: 04/22/08 09:50:16   T: 04/25/08 12:55:01

You Code It!

What are the best, most accurate codes?

ADULT HEALTH ASSOCIATES
720 LONG STREET • ETERNITY, FL 32711 • 407-555-7322

PATIENT: MCLAUGHLIN, RYAN
ACCOUNT/EHR #:   MCLARY01
Date: 04/22/08

Attending Physician: James Healer, MD

It has been eight months since the last time I saw this 67-year-old male. He states that he has been experiencing terrible "knee pain" in both legs.

Patient states that he is taking extra strength Tylenol around the clock (2 tablets every 4 hours) with little or no relief. He has thought about trying Aleve that his neighbor swears by, but he remembers that the doctors at the hospital told him he should not take those types of pills.

PE: He has Heberden's and Bouchard's nodes, and deformity of the knee joints with decreased range of motion. Based on the patient's history and this examination, osteoarthritis is suspected. Patient is taken down the hall to our Imaging department.

AP/Lat X-rays of each knee confirms diagnosis of osteoarthritis. There are no other findings to suggest other diagnoses.

DX: Osteoarthritis, bilateral

Rx: Tripod cane
Patient is advised to begin taking OTC glucosamine plus chondroitin sulfate.
Patient to return prn.

James Healer, MD

JHW/mg   D: 04/22/08 09:50:16   T: 04/25/08 12:55:01

You Code It!

What are the best, most accurate codes?

_____

_____

_____

ADULT HEALTH ASSOCIATES
720 LONG STREET • ETERNITY, FL 32711 • 407-555-7322

PATIENT: EDWARDS, DEACON
ACCOUNT/EHR #:   EDWADE01
Date: 04/22/08

Attending Physician: James Healer, MD

This is a 75-year-old male who recently moved back to the area to be closer to family. He presents to our office for the first time today for his regular annual check-up. He inquires about health prevention and screening. Throughout the years he has remained relatively healthy.

He reports that his current medications consist of 0.15 mg of levothyroxine for treatment of hypothyroidism, and a multivitamin. His only surgeries consist of nonmalignant mole removals.

After retiring from his job as an office manager two years ago, he maintains a very active lifestyle, watching his two preschool age grandchildren, volunteering at the local library and working in his garden. Every morning he and his wife of 42 years go for a three-mile walk in the local park. He has never smoked, limits his alcohol consumption to a glass of wine on special occasions, and drinks 2 cups of coffee a day.

Patient states that his parents are still independent and live locally. His father, age 94, takes medication for HTN; and his mother, age 92, has been on Alendronate for treatment of osteoporosis. Both of his children, a son, aged 41, and a daughter, aged 37, are in perfect health. Unfortunately his sister, age 70, was just diagnosed with breast cancer.

Patient states that neither he nor his wife, Alma, suffers from depression, and that Alma's only medical problem was a gallbladder attack 5 years ago when she was 64.

PE: Patient is a thin, Caucasian male. He is 5′6″ and weighs 121 lb. His BP is 120/70. Heart, lung, chest, and abdominal exam are all within normal limits.

DX: Annual exam – no concerns highlighted

PLAN: Patient to return prn.

_____

James Healer, MD

JHW/mg   D: 04/22/08 09:50:16   T: 04/25/08 12:55:01

You Code It!

What are the best, most accurate codes?

_____

_____

_____

ADULT HEALTH ASSOCIATES
720 LONG STREET • ETERNITY, FL 32711 • 407-555-7322

PATIENT: ARCHER, PENELOPE
ACCOUNT/EHR #:   ARCHPE01
Date: 06/22/08

Attending Physician: James Healer, MD

This 77-year-old female presents with significant memory problems and deficits in functional ability. She is a retired bookkeeper/executive secretary being evaluated for memory loss. As per the referral from her family physician, Dr. Fraiser, her physical examination is normal.

History of Present Illness: The patient's husband mentions that her memory problems have been occurring for about 3 years; the patient thinks it has been only 1 year. According to the husband, the patient's memory loss has been "slow and gradually getting worse." She is having trouble remembering the names of familiar people and misplaces personal belongings such as keys or her glasses. She sets the table for 5 or 6 people when there are only 2 who will be eating. She is mildly depressed and is being treated for her depression by Dr. Fraiser. She does not smoke or drink significant amounts of alcohol. There is a family history of heart disease.

Neurologic Assessment: The patient's physical exam is normal. During the neurologic examination, the patient scores 25 out of 30 on the Functional Activity Questionnaire (FAQ)26, showing difficulty in almost all areas including financial tasks, preparing meals, driving, current events, and ability to follow and understand books, movies or TV programs. Her Mini-Mental State Examination (MMSE)27 score is 21; she is unable to copy a cube.

Neuropsychological Testing: Neuropsychological testing finds moderately severe memory impairment, mild impairment of language comprehension, and borderline impairment in orientation and attention.

Laboratory Evaluation: CT scan shows the brain is slightly atrophied. A complete laboratory workup shows no correctable cause for dementia.

Diagnosis: Senile dementia of the Alzheimer's type.

Treatment: The patient is started on a cholinesterase inhibitor—EXELON (rivastigmine tartrate) 1.5 mg twice daily with full meals. Based on good tolerability, she will be increased to 3 mg of EXELON twice daily with full meals. She is also started on vitamin E 1000 IU twice daily. She is currently being treated for comorbid conditions including depression, hypertension, and hypercholesterolemia, and has been placed on estrogen replacement therapy.

James Healer, MD

JHW/mg   D: 06/22/08 09:50:16   T: 06/25/08 12:55:01

You Code It!

What are the best, most accurate codes?

_____

_____

_____

ADULT HEALTH ASSOCIATES
720 LONG STREET • ETERNITY, FL 32711 • 407-555-7322

PATIENT: ARCHER, PENELOPE
ACCOUNT/EHR #:   ARCHPE01
Date: 09/30/08

Attending Physician: James Healer, MD

This 77-year-old female comes to the office today for a 3-month reassessment.

Both she and her husband feel that she has "significantly improved." She is much more active and feels that "things seem clearer." Her MMSE score has improved to 24. Her FAQ score is 14, and there are dramatic improvements in her ability to shop alone, prepare a meal, and understand her favorite TV shows. She is having much less difficulty with orientation. Up to this point, she has not experienced gastrointestinal side effects or any other difficulties with Exelon treatment.

Diagnosis: Senile dementia of the Alzheimer's type.

Treatment: The Exelon dose is increased to 4.5 mg twice daily with full meals. Return in 4 months for follow-up.

James Healer, MD

JHW/mg   D: 09/30/08 09:50:16   T: 09/30/08 12:55:01

You Code It!

What are the best, most accurate codes?

_____

_____

_____

Neonatal and Pediatrics Cases and Patient Records

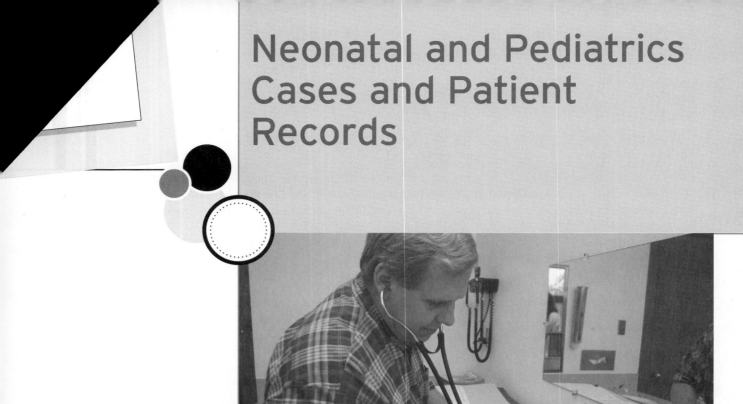

INTRODUCTION

The following case studies are from a neonatology and pediatric practice. In a physician's office of this type, a professional coding specialist is likely to see many different kinds of health situations, especially preventive health care services, relating to the care of children from birth up through the age of 18.

Neonatology is a pediatric subspecialty that deals with the diagnosis and treatment of disorders in newborns. A neonatologist typically consults with neonatal intensive care units (NICU) in hospitals and cares for babies born prematurely; with infections, such as neonatal streptococcal infections; and congenital conditions and concerns, such as heart defects, genetic diseases, and malformations.

Neonatologists are board-certified through the Board of Pediatrics, which is recognized by the American Board of Medical Specialties.

Pediatricians also specialize in caring for children, from birth through 18 years of age. Pediatricians provide preventive health care, as well as treatment of childhood illnesses and diseases. Pediatrics has several subspecialties in addition to neonatology, including:

- Adolescent medicine—health care specifically for teenagers
- Pediatric cardiology—heart problems in children
- Developmental disorders—behavior, communication, and mental disorders
- Pediatric endocrinology—endocrine glands and hormonal difficulties
- Pediatric gastroenterology—digestive system disorders
- Pediatric infectious disease—complex infections, which can include HI and hepatitis
- Pediatric nephrology—malfunction of the urinary system
- Pediatric oncology—treating children diagnosed with malignancy

The Board of Pediatrics certifies pediatricians, and this board certification is recognized by the American Board of Medical Specialties.

You can use these cases to practice coding diagnoses, E/M, procedures, DME, or other HCPCS Level II items, as applicable; code for the physician or the facility; inpatient or outpatient, as applicable:

1. Code for the physician.
2. Code for the anesthesiologist, when applicable.
3. Code for the hospital, when applicable.
4. Code for the pathology and laboratory, when applicable.
5. Code HCPCS Level II codes, when applicable.

PEDIATRIC COMPLETE CARE CENTER
123 BORNE PATH • YOUNGSTOWN, FL 32811 • 407-555-ABCD

PATIENT: VANCE, NICOLE

MRN: VANCNI001

Procedure Performed: Newborn Evaluation

Attending Physician: Pravdah H. Jeppard, MD

The patient is a female, gestational age 39 weeks, 4 days, born vaginally in this facility, 9/1/08, 02:35.

IMPRESSION: Neonate was of a single birth, BWT 2857 grams without significant OR procedures with a normal newborn diagnosis. 19″ long. Head circumference: 32 cm. Amniotic fluid: clear, Cord: 3 vessels. Evidence of a benign tumor of blood vessels due to malformed angioblastic tissues (vascular hamartomas) at right groin. Appears pale, poor skin turgor, mucousy, and transitional stool

APGAR SCORE: 1 min.= 9; 5 min.= 9. Heart rate: >100; Respiratory Effort: Good, Muscle tone: Active, Response to catheter in nostril: Cough, Color: Body pink, extremities blue

MATERNAL HISTORY: 30 year old, G1, blood type O+, spontaneous labor, 16 hr, 24 min., Epidural anesthesia, HIV tested during pregnancy: neg

ADMINISTRATIONS: Hepatitis B, Peds, Vaccine (Recomb) 5 mcg/0.5 ml, given: 9/2/08 NEWBORN HEARING SCREENING: passed.

RECOMMENDATIONS: Follow-up in office 2 days

Pravdah H. Jeppard, MD

PHJ/mg   D: 09/03/08 09:50:16   T: 09/05/08 12:55:01

You Code It!

What are the best, most accurate codes?

_____

_____

_____

PEDIATRIC COMPLETE CARE CENTER
123 BORNE PATH • YOUNGSTOWN, FL 32811 • 407-555-ABCD

PATIENT: GASSLER, CARL

ACCOUNT/EHR #:   GASSCA001

Date: 03/11/08

Attending Physician: Pravdah H. Jeppard, MD

S: Pt is a 2-day-old male who comes in for his first office visit after birth. He was a full-term infant, vaginally delivery. Mother provides prenatal history, family history including the paternal Rh factor and information regarding inherited red cell defects.

O: Wt. 5 lb. 7 ounces, T 98.6. Skin has yellowish skin coloration, including sclerae. Tests, including direct and indirect bilirubin levels, reveal gram-negative bacterial infection and serum bilirubin levels at 7 mg/dl. Blood tests are also performed to test infant and mother both for blood group incompatibilities, hemoglobin level, direct Coombs' test, and hematocrit.

A: Hyperbilirubinemia, due to gram-negative bacterial infection

P: 1. Rx albumin administration (1 g/kg of 25% salt-poor albumin)
      2. Rx antibiotics for infection
      3. Follow-up appointment in three days

Pravdah H. Jeppard, MD

PHJ/mg   D: 03/11/08 09:50:16   T: 03/13/08 12:55:01

You Code It!

What are the best, most accurate codes?

_____

_____

_____

PEDIATRIC COMPLETE CARE CENTER
123 BORNE PATH • YOUNGSTOWN, FL 32811 • 407-555-ABCD

PATIENT: LAGARDIA, LORENA
MRN: LAGALO001
Procedure Performed: Newborn Re-evaluation

Attending Physician: Pravdah H. Jeppard, MD

The patient is a female, gestational age 39 weeks, 5 days, born vaginally in this facility, 7/9/08, 13:15.

IMPRESSION: Neonate was of a single birth, BWT 2927 grams without significant OR procedures with a normal newborn diagnosis. 20″ long. Head circumference: 31 cm. Amniotic fluid: clear, Cord: 3 vessels. PKU test normal at birth

APGAR SCORE: 1 min.= 9; 5 min.= 9. Heart rate: >100; Respiratory Effort: Good, Muscle tone: Active, Response to catheter in nostril: Cough, Color: Body pink, extremities blue

MATERNAL HISTORY: 30 year old, G1, blood type O+, spontaneous labor, 16 hrs, 24 min., Epidural anesthesia, HIV tested during pregnancy: neg; Scottish heritage with family history of phenylketonuria.

ADMINISTRATIONS: Hepatitis B, Peds, Vaccine (Recomb) 5 mcg/0.5 ml, given: 9/2/08 NEWBORN HEARING SCREENING: passed.
   At 36 hours of age, Guthrie screening test on capillary blood sample is positive for PKU.

RECOMMENDATIONS: Restricting dietary intake of amino acid phenylalanine to keep phenylalanine blood levels between 3 and 9 mg/dl. Referral to nutritionist for dietary standards. Follow-up in office 2 days.

Pravdah H. Jeppard, MD

PHJ/mg   D: 07/10/08 09:50:16   T: 07/15/08 12:55:01

You Code It!

What are the best, most accurate codes?

_____

_____

_____

PEDIATRIC COMPLETE CARE CENTER
123 BORNE PATH • YOUNGSTOWN, FL 32811 • 407-555-ABCD

PATIENT: MEEKS, VINCENT

ACCOUNT/EHR #: MEEKVI001

Date: 05/15/08

Attending Physician: Pravdah H. Jeppard, MD

S: Pt is a 9-day-old male who is brought in by his mother because it appears to her that he had some kind of seizure the day before, and again last night. She states that she is frightened.

O: Wt. 6 lb. 11 ounces, T 98.6. Complete blood work, EEG, and ECG ordered.

PE reveals no anomalies.

A: Convulsions in newborn

P: 1. Follow-up appointment once test results are received
   2. Instructions on care given to mother

Pravdah H. Jeppard, MD

PHJ/mg   D: 05/15/08 09:50:16   T: 05/20/08 12:55:01

You Code It!

What are the best, most accurate codes?

_____

_____

_____

PEDIATRIC COMPLETE CARE CENTER
123 BORNE PATH • YOUNGSTOWN, FL 32811 • 407-555-ABCD

PATIENT: BECKMAN, WILLIAM
ACCOUNT/EHR #:   BECKWI001
Date: 10/11/08

Attending Physician: Pravdah H. Jeppard, MD

The patient is a male, gestational age 39 weeks, 4 days, born by cesarean section in this facility, 10/10/08, 17:30.

IMPRESSION: Neonate was of a single birth, BWT 2857 grams without significant OR procedures with a normal newborn diagnosis. 17″ long. Head circumference: 29 cm. Amniotic fluid: clear, Cord: 3 vessels. Head is acrocephalitic and there is evidence of premature cranial suture fusion. The fingers of the right hand are syndactylic, as well.

APGAR SCORE: 1 min.= 7; 5 min.= 8. Heart rate: >100; Respiratory Effort: Good, Muscle tone: Active, Response to catheter in nostril: Cough, Color: Body pink, extremities blue

MATERNAL HISTORY: 41 year old, G1, blood type O+, spontaneous labor, 21 hr, 11 min., Epidural anesthesia, HIV tested during pregnancy: neg

ADMINISTRATIONS: Hepatitis B, Peds, Vaccine (Recomb) 5 mcg/0.5 ml, given: 10/12/08

NEWBORN HEARING SCREENING: passed.

RECOMMENDATIONS: Newborn has acrocephalosyndactyly. Consultation with neonatologist requested.

Pravdah H. Jeppard, MD

PHJ/mg   D: 10/11/08 09:50:16   T: 10/13/08 12:55:01

You Code It!

What are the best, most accurate codes?

_____

_____

_____

PEDIATRIC COMPLETE CARE CENTER
123 BORNE PATH • YOUNGSTOWN, FL 32811 • 407-555-ABCD

PATIENT: WEBSTER, LEOPOLD
ACCOUNT/EHR #:   WEBSLE001
Date: 09/16/08

Attending Physician: Suzanne R. Taylor, MD

Pt is a 7-month-old male brought in by his mother. She states that she picked the child up from their baby sitter's house and he has been listless and unresponsive. There has been no loss of consciousness.

Eyes are glazed and unfocused with petechia showing in sclera. MRI brain confirms shaken infant syndrome with intracranial contusion of brainstem.

Child is admitted to hospital NICU for observation.

Authorities notified of suspected abuse.

Suzanne R. Taylor, MD

SRT/pw   D: 09/16/08 09:50:16   T: 09/18/08 12:55:01

You Code It!

What are the best, most accurate codes?

_____

_____

_____

PEDIATRIC COMPLETE CARE CENTER
123 BORNE PATH • YOUNGSTOWN, FL 32811 • 407-555-ABCD

PATIENT: GARISON, BENJAMIN
ACCOUNT/EHR #:   GARIBE001
Date: 09/16/08

Attending Physician: Suzanne R. Taylor, MD

S: This Pt is a 5-month-old male brought in by his father because of severe rash on Benjamin's buttocks.

O: Ht 35" Wt. 19 lb. T 98.6 Pt appears in minor distress; however, examination shows nothing out of the ordinary.

A: Diaper rash

P: 1. Rx A&D ointment to be applied after each diaper change
     2. Return prn

Suzanne R. Taylor, MD

SRT/pw   D: 09/16/08 09:50:16   T: 09/18/08 12:55:01

You Code It!

What are the best, most accurate codes?

_____

_____

_____

PEDIATRIC COMPLETE CARE CENTER
123 BORNE PATH • YOUNGSTOWN, FL 32811 • 407-555-ABCD

PATIENT: PEA, SWEE T.
ACCOUNT/EHR #:   PEASW002
Date: 07/22/08

Attending Physician: James Healer, MD

S: Pt is a 5-year-old female brought in by her mother for her school vaccinations.

O: Ht 2′5″ Wt. 39 lb. R 15. Child is visibly small for her age. Her teeth show signs of calcification loss and neglect. Her hair is very thin and falls out easily. Eye orbits appear to be slightly sunken. Skin is pale. Complete CBC and urinalysis (dipstick) performed. MMR vaccine, live, sub q and IPV sub q, administered.

A: Nutritional neglect by mother

P: 1. Nutritional guidelines reviewed with mother
     2. School certificate signed
     3. Authorities notified of suspected abuse

James Healer, MD

JHW/mg   D: 07/22/08 09:50:16   T: 07/25/08 12:55:01

You Code It!

What are the best, most accurate codes?

_____

_____

_____

PEDIATRIC COMPLETE CARE CENTER
123 BORNE PATH • YOUNGSTOWN, FL 32811 • 407-555-ABCD

PATIENT: CRUMPET, KARL
ACCOUNT/EHR #:   CRUMKA001
Date: 10/17/08

Attending Physician: James I. Cipher, MD

S: Karl is an 11-month-old male brought in today by his mother. He has been waking up at night and is irritable. Mother states that he has been tugging at his right ear, and has been running a low-grade fever since yesterday. There has been no cough. Pt has a history of problems with his ears and sinuses. Pt is teething.

O: Ht 2′1″ Wt. 25 lb. R 20. T 101.3. HEENT: Purulent nasal discharge, yellow-green in color, is noted. Right TM is erythematous unilaterally, bulging and with purulent effusions. Oropharynx is nonerythematous without lesions. One tooth on the bottom. Tonsils are unremarkable. Neck: Neck is supple with good ROM. Positive cervical adenopathy. Lungs: clear. Heart: Regular rate and rhythm without murmurs.

A: Acute suppurative otitis media, right side.

P: 1. Rx Augmentin 40 mg/kg divided t.i.d. 10 days
     2. Bed rest, lots of fluids.
     3. Follow-up prn or if no improvement in 10 days

James I. Cipher, MD

JIC/mg   D: 10/17/08 09:50:16   T: 10/23/08 12:55:01

You Code It!

What are the best, most accurate codes?

_____

_____

_____

PEDIATRIC COMPLETE CARE CENTER
123 BORNE PATH • YOUNGSTOWN, FL 32811 • 407-555-ABCD

PATIENT: YAMAGUCCI, HANNAH

ACCOUNT/EHR #:   YAMHA001

Date: 10/13/08

S: This is a six year-old female, brought in by her parents with a stated persistent fever. The father reports she has been tired and has a decreased appetite. She was noted to be in her normal state of health until one week ago, at which time she developed conjunctival infection, fever to 103° F, and sore throat. Her parents attributed these symptoms to a recent viral upper respiratory infection that affected several children in Hannah's class. Hannah's mother noted an erythematous rash in her perineal region while bathing her last night and noted peeling of the skin near her fingernails. Hannah has begun to complain of joint pains. Her parents note they initially did not give her any antipyretics, but when they gave acetaminophen yesterday, it did not seem to have any effect. Hannah's parents are worried that a fever of 103°F could be dangerous and cause harm to the child.

O: Hannah does not look "well." She appears tired and disinterested in playing with the toys in the waiting room. She appears to move slowly, saying that it hurts her knees to walk around. At six years old, Hannah is expected to be able to carry on a conversation, but she seems too exhausted to talk for long. Hannah is noted to be an ill-appearing, febrile child. Erythema of the tongue gives it a "strawberry" appearance. Her lips are dry and cracked. Erythema and edema of the feet are noted, and she walks with a slight limp. She has a 1.5 cm palpable cervical lymph node and an erythematous rash of her lower trunk and perineum. Concerned about the possibility of serious illness, the decision is made to admit Hannah to the pediatric floor of the hospital for possible Kawasaki syndrome.

A: Kawasaki syndrome

P: Admit Hannah into the hospital for further tests and treatment. Hannah's parents are upset that they may have waited too long and worry they may have done something to cause the illness. They are concerned that Hannah's playmates will get the disease as well. I reassure them that this is not contagious and is a vasculitis seen in children.

Robert M. Katzman, MD

10/13/08 11:47:39

You Code It!

What are the best, most accurate codes?

_____

_____

_____

PEDIATRIC COMPLETE CARE CENTER
123 BORNE PATH • YOUNGSTOWN, FL 32811 • 407-555-ABCD

PATIENT: MARKOVICH, LISETTE

ACCOUNT/EHR #:   MARLI001

Date: 10/15/08

S: Patient is a 2-month-old Caucasian female, here with her mother for a Well Child Exam. Her mother is a 25-year-old G1P1 woman; whose past medical history is negative. Her mother, Andrea, appears relaxed and states that the baby has been doing well. She is eating and seems to be growing. Mother does state that she is concerned that Lisette may not be getting enough breast milk. She will be returning to work next week and wants to know if she should change to formula feeding. Also she wants to know when she should introduce other foods.

O: Lisette is at the 50th percentile for both weight and length; head circumference is at the 60th percentile. She has been following these growth parameters since birth without dropping off "the curve." Andrea is concerned with how much her baby should be eating and when it is ok to advance her diet. Andrea asks what developmental milestones are expected for a two-month-old infant and what to expect over the next 10 months? We discuss key developmental milestones (gross motor, language, fine motor, social) in a 2-3 month old infant. I reassure the mother that rolling over is achieved between 3-6 months. She should expect to begin to bear weight on her legs and grasp a rattle in the next two months.

PHYSICAL EXAM: Lisette is smiling, playing with her hands, following objects past midline, laughing and cooing. She holds her head up when placed her on her belly. Her exam is normal including primitive reflexes.

IMMUNIZATIONS: The mother would like her to receive vaccines on schedule and would like more information on vaccine safety and necessity. Lisette received Hep B #1 in the nursery. Handouts on each of the vaccines administered today are given to the mother.

ADMINISTERED TODAY: HIB, PCV, and Pediarix (DtAP, IPV and Hep B)

___

Robert M. Katzman, MD

10/15/08 11:47:39

You Code It!

What are the best, most accurate codes?

___

___

___

PEDIATRIC COMPLETE CARE CENTER
123 BORNE PATH • YOUNGSTOWN, FL 32811 • 407-555-ABCD

PATIENT: DELVANEY, TODD
ACCOUNT/EHR #:   DELTO001
Date: 10/13/08

S: Patient is brought in by his mother and father for a Well Child Exam. He is an active 2-year-old male, who was adopted two weeks ago from Thailand. His parents do not have any of his medical records and are not sure if he has had any immunizations. They do know that his birth mother had some limited prenatal care and had a normal delivery at 38 weeks gestation. Todd has been healthy to date, living in a shelter in Thailand. They are concerned because they are not sure if he ever went to a doctor while in Thailand. His parents state that they want to know more about his immunization status, developmental status, and how best to childproof their home. They would also like to be sure his physical exam is normal and that he does not have any underlying medical conditions of which they are not aware. Todd's parents are concerned about him receiving three shots in one day. They are also worried about side effects and wonder if there is any reason he should not receive a vaccine. Mrs. Delvaney notes that she had a sore arm and fever after receiving a flu shot at work—she wonders if this will happen to Todd.

SOCIAL HISTORY: The parents state that their home water supply does not contain fluoride. There is no smoking, alcohol, or drug use in the home. The mother, Lorraine, will care for him during the day for the next year before returning to her job as a nurse. His father, Calvin, is a local high school teacher. While at the shelter, Todd was consuming a diet of soy milk and table foods (predominately rice, meats, and beans). Since coming to the US, his diet has expanded and he drinks whole milk and fruit juice. Parents state that the child has a voracious appetite and particularly enjoys cheese, chicken, apples, and carrots. They do note he only eats when he wants, not necessarily at standard family meal times. They say he seems to have adjusted well over the past 2 weeks.

O: Todd is sitting nervously on his mother's lap. Though he appears thin, he is not believed to be malnourished. When asked, he states his name is "Toddy."

PHYSICAL EXAM: There is a noticeable 3/6 systolic murmur over the child's left lower sternal border (LLSB). There is no way to know if this murmur has been present since birth or changed at all as the boy has been growing. I reassured the parents that this is believed to be a benign murmur, but to be cautious I am going to refer them to a Pediatric Cardiologist to obtain a proper work-up. The remainder of this physical exam is within normal limits. Although he is thin, the child does not appear emaciated or malnourished. He is interactive during the exam and developmentally appears on target, meeting the proper 2-year-old milestones.

PLAN: Refer to Dr. Feld, Pediatric Cardiology Associates. Child to return p.r.n. or for next well child exam.

___

Robert M. Katzman, MD

10/13/08 11:47:39

You Code It!

What are the best, most accurate codes?

___

___

___

PEDIATRIC COMPLETE CARE CENTER
123 BORNE PATH • YOUNGSTOWN, FL 32811 • 407-555-ABCD

PATIENT: MASSADA, CARTER
ACCOUNT/EHR #:   MASCA001
Date: 10/13/08

S: This 3-year-old male is brought in by his mother with a chief complaint of delayed speech. Mother states that he started to babble at about 9 months of age and then learned a few words such as "Dada" and "boo" at 2 years of age. She claims that she and her husband have tried to stimulate the boy's language development by reading to him, interacting with him during television watching, and teaching him to mimic others' speech. They became more concerned as he grew older, noting his speech was less than the other children in his playgroup. They try to engage him in interactive activities, but he does not seem interested. They note that he is very independent and that he is very serious. He likes to play by himself rather than talking with or singing with other children. They worry that he has no playmates or friends because of his speech delay. He has been generally healthy and has had a few ear infections.

PAST MEDICAL HISTORY: Prenatal and past medical histories are otherwise unremarkable and he has not had any serious infections or need for hospitalization.

PHYSICAL EXAM: Vital signs are normal. Height, weight, and head circumference are between the 25th and 50th percentiles. His HEENT, heart, lung, abdominal, skin and neuromuscular portions of the physical exam show no abnormalities. While talking with his parents, it is noted that the child separates from them easily and wanders about the room. He does not seem to notice that everyone is talking about him. He finds some blocks in the corner and sits down to play with them. He did not respond when called to. He starts to sort the blocks by color into groups and lines them up. He seems content playing by himself. I went over to him in the corner and sat down by him. He did not appear to notice that I am there. He continues to line up the blocks (very neatly) and my attempts to interrupt him are unsuccessful. Although he seems content, I notice that he does not laugh or even smile much. Also noted is that he does not look at me or check back to his parents. During the session, he did not say any words.

On developmental screening, his motor development is normal. He is delayed in his language, social, and self-help skills. I administered an audiology evaluation, which shows his hearing to be normal and conducive to speech development. Further evaluation reveals:

1) Social Disturbance: Lack of eye contact, poor attachments, and shows a general lack of social interest.
2) Communicative Disturbance: Failure to develop semantics (word use), failure to develop reciprocity in dialogue, and failure to use language for social interaction.
3) Behavioral Features: Shows a particular attachment to objects. Parents have noted both hand flapping and toe walking.

ASSESSMENT: Autistic Disorder

Robert M. Katzman, MD

10/13/08 11:47:39

You Code It!

What are the best, most accurate codes?

_____

_____

_____

PEDIATRIC COMPLETE CARE CENTER
123 BORNE PATH • YOUNGSTOWN, FL 32811 • 407-555-ABCD

PATIENT: WIRRMAN, BRUCE
ACCOUNT/EHR #: WIRBR001
Date: 10/15/08

This is a 3640 gram newborn male infant born at 39 weeks gestation via normal spontaneous vaginal delivery (NSVD) at Harris Medical Center, to a 17-year-old G3P0 mother who is O+, VDRL NR, Hepatitis B surface antigen (HBsAg) positive, rubella immune, group B streptococcus (GBS) negative, and HIV negative. Artificial rupture of membranes (AROM) occurred 18 hours prior to delivery with clear fluid. Apgar scores were 8 and 9 at 1 and 5 minutes respectively.

Maternal history is remarkable for 1 prenatal visit 1 month ago. An ultrasound performed at that time was consistent with 34 weeks gestation. Toxicology screening at that visit and on admission were negative. Mother is reportedly healthy, with no chronic medical problems and no significant family history. She reports no difficulty during the pregnancy. She denies alcohol, cigarette, medication or drug use. Social history reveals that the mother's support system includes the father of the baby (FOB) and both maternal and paternal grandparents.

EXAM: VS T 37.0 rectal, P 145, R48, BP 49/35. Weight 3640 grams (8 pounds) (75th%), 51 cm (20 inches) (75th%); head circumference 34 cm (13.5 inches) (50th%). This infant is term in appearance, pink and active. Anterior fontanelle is soft and flat. Caput succedaneum is present. Corneas are clear. Ears are normally placed. Nares are patent. Oral mucosa is pink and the palate is intact. Neck is supple without masses. Clavicles are intact. His chest is symmetric and mature breast buds are present. Lungs are clear with equal aeration. Heart is regular with no murmurs heard. Abdomen is flat and soft with no masses. Three vessels are visible within the umbilical cord. Femoral and brachial pulses are symmetric and 2+. Hips demonstrate full range of motion, no tightness, no clicks. Ortolani and Barlow signs are negative. Perineal creases are symmetric. Anus is patent. Male genitalia are normal, with both testes descended. His skin is pink with a few facial petechiae. He moves all extremities well. His Moro reflex is intact. His grasp response is symmetrical. His suck reflex is strong.

By 7 hours of age, he has passed meconium once, has had no urine output, and has nippled 15 cc of infant formula from a bottle. His mother does not want to breastfeed because she says she has no milk and will be returning to school soon. Besides, she read that formula makes your baby grow just as well as breast milk.

Robert M. Katzman, MD

10/15/08 11:47:39

You Code It!

What are the best, most accurate codes?

_____

_____

_____

PEDIATRIC COMPLETE CARE CENTER
123 BORNE PATH • YOUNGSTOWN, FL 32811 • 407-555-ABCD

PATIENT: SIZEMORE, KYLE
ACCOUNT/EHR #: SIZKY001
Date: 10/15/08

This two-day-old male infant was referred from a community hospital for bilious vomiting and a heart murmur. The baby was born at 37 weeks gestation to a G4P3 39-year-old woman who had no prenatal care.

EXAM: VS T37.1 (ax), P150, R45, BP 75/50, oxygen saturation 99% in room air. Height, weight and head circumference are at the 50th percentile. He appears jaundiced, and has a flat facial profile; short, upslanting palpebral fissures; a flat nasal bridge with epicanthal folds; a small mouth with protruding tongue; and single palmar creases. His lungs are clear to auscultation. His heart is tachycardic with a loud holosystolic murmur. His abdomen is non-distended. Generalized hypotonia is present.

Abdominal radiograph shows a "double-bubble sign." Duodenal atresia is suspected. A nasogastric tube is placed and IV fluids are administered. A duodenoduodenostomy is performed. An echocardiogram demonstrates a ventricular septal defect, which is medically managed. A chromosomal abnormality is suspected and a karyotype is done. Trisomy 21 is diagnosed.

Ds: Trisomy 21 (Down syndrome)

PLAN: Discuss details of condition with both parents. Informational brochures are provided, along with contact information for a local support group.

Robert M. Katzman, MD

10/15/08 11:47:39

You Code It!

What are the best, most accurate codes?

_____

_____

_____

PEDIATRIC COMPLETE CARE CENTER
123 BORNE PATH • YOUNGSTOWN, FL 32811 • 407-555-ABCD

PATIENT: NEWBERRY, DANIEL

ACCOUNT/EHR #:   NEWDA001

Date: 10/15/08

This is a 14-month-old male infant who is brought in by his parents with a chief complaint of high fever and no response to antipyretic therapy. This illness started suddenly with the abrupt onset of fever early yesterday morning. He then developed a severe cough and increased work of breathing. No other symptoms are noted. The patient was born in a refugee camp and lived in Texas before moving here 3 months ago. The mother reports that he is frequently ill. No reports from earlier health care visits are available, but his mother reports he was also seen as an outpatient frequently and he was hospitalized at least once in Texas. He was hospitalized 2 months ago for pneumococcal pneumonia (right upper lobe consolidation and pneumococcal bacteremia).

EXAM: VS T 40.3, P 145, R 55, BP 100/60, oxygen saturation 98%, weight 7 kg (<5th percentile). He is listless, tired, and small for age. He is lying on the examination table, moving little and whimpering slightly to stimulation with tachypnea and chest retractions. His head is normocephalic, without signs of trauma. Both ear canals contain purulent drainage. Mouth exam is unremarkable. His heart is tachycardic with no murmurs heard. His chest shows mild retractions, tachypnea, dullness to percussion over the posterior upper chest, decreased breath sounds in the area of dullness with occasional fine crackles. His abdomen is scaphoid and soft, with active bowel sounds, no masses, and no hepatosplenomegaly. His extremities are slender and wasted with decreased muscle mass and strength. Neurological exam is normal.

A blood culture is positive for pneumococcus. Because of his recurrent infections and the failure to meet normal growth expectations, an immunologic work-up is done. He is found to have markedly elevated IgM, undetectable IgG and IgA with diminished total B lymphocytes (CD19). His clinical picture is consistent with hypogammaglobulinemia with high IgM or Hyper-IgM syndrome.

DIAGNOSIS: Pneumocystis carinii pneumonia (PCP)

PLAN: Admit into hospital for intravenous antibiotics and IVIG replacement therapy with trimethoprim-sulfamethoxazole prophylaxis for Pneumocystis carinii pneumonia (PCP).

Robert M. Katzman, MD

10/15/08 11:47:39

You Code It!

What are the best, most accurate codes?

_____

_____

_____

PEDIATRIC COMPLETE CARE CENTER
123 BORNE PATH • YOUNGSTOWN, FL 32811 • 407-555-ABCD

PATIENT: WASHINGTON, JERMAINE
ACCOUNT/EHR #:   WASJE001
Date: 10/13/08

This is a 4-week-old male who has been brought in by his father and mother with a one-week history of "noisy breathing." His parents note that his noisy breathing is worse when they lay him down or with crying. It is most noticeable when he takes a breath in. There has been no history of fever, coughing, runny nose, change in his cry, apnea, or feeding difficulties. He has been gaining weight appropriately. Prenatal course was uneventful and he was delivered at 38 weeks gestation by spontaneous vaginal delivery without complications. Family History is unremarkable.

EXAM: VS T 37.0, P 120, R 48, oxygen saturation 98% in room air. Weight and height are at the 50%ile. He is alert, active, in no acute distress. There is audible inspiratory stridor noted in the supine position, which is improved with extension of his neck. His anterior fontanel is soft and flat. His eyes and ears are normal. No nasal flaring is visible and his nares appear patent. His throat shows no erythema or lesions. His lips are moist and pink. There are no retractions or pectus abnormalities. His lungs are clear to auscultation throughout once the stridor clears with airway repositioning (no wheezes or rales). Aeration is good. He has noisy referred upper airway sounds when he is supine with his neck flexed. His heart is regular without murmurs. His color, perfusion, capillary refill and pulses are good.

    A flexible fiberoptic laryngoscopy confirms the diagnosis of mild laryngomalacia.

DIAGNOSIS: Mild laryngomalacia

PLAN: Come back in two weeks for recheck

_____

Robert M. Katzman, MD

10/13/08 11:47:39

You Code It!

What are the best, most accurate codes?

_____

_____

_____

PEDIATRIC COMPLETE CARE CENTER
123 BORNE PATH • YOUNGSTOWN, FL 32811 • 407-555-ABCD

PATIENT: EVERSON, ADIN
ACCOUNT/EHR #:   EVEAD001
Date: 10/15/08

This is a newborn male infant born at 0415 on this date to a 23-year-old G2P1 mother at 39 weeks gestation via NSVD (normal spontaneous vaginal delivery).

Appropriate antenatal care and monitoring occurred throughout the pregnancy. As there were no significant antenatal problems, no prenatal ultrasonography was done. Immediately following delivery, the baby looks "normal." He cries immediately, however, at 1 minute of age, he remains very cyanotic. The neonatal resuscitation team is called to the delivery room. At 5 minutes of age, the baby remains very cyanotic, tachypneic and dyspneic, despite 100% oxygen via mask. The resuscitation team starts bag-mask positive pressure ventilation with 100% oxygen, but the baby becomes bradycardic; therefore he is intubated and ventilated. Auscultation of the lungs reveal good breath sounds in the right chest, but no breath sounds in the left. The heart sounds seemed loudest in the right chest, and the abdomen appears scaphoid. Ventilation is continued through the endotracheal tube, while an NG tube is inserted and suction is applied. A STAT chest x-ray is done, which reveals bowel (and the NG tube tip) in the left chest cavity.

DX: Congenital diaphragmatic hernia presenting in the delivery room
The baby is transferred to the NICU.

Robert M. Katzman, MD

10/15/08 11:47:39

You Code It!

What are the best, most accurate codes?

_____

_____

_____

PEDIATRIC COMPLETE CARE CENTER
123 BORNE PATH • YOUNGSTOWN, FL 32811 • 407-555-ABCD

PATIENT: ABBOTT, JALEEL
ACCOUNT/EHR #:   ABBJA001
Date: 10/15/08

This is a 3-month-old male brought to this clinic by his parents with a chief complaint of decreased activity, poor feeding and constipation.

PAST MEDICAL HISTORY: The infant was born at 39 weeks gestation, with no complications during the pregnancy or birth. The infant is exclusively breast fed, up-to-date on immunizations and has suffered from no previous illness. On further questioning, his mother reports her son has not been himself for the past week. He has had no fever and there are no sick contacts. He has been less active, with a weak cry during this time. His mother also notes the infant has not been as interested in feeding and has suffered from constipation. His urine output is decreased with only four wet diapers in the last 24 hours. Typically, he has 3-4 soft stools per day, usually after feeds, but has had no bowel movement in the past 5 days.

EXAM: VS 37.0, P 114, R 22, BP 98/62, Wt. 5.3 kg (75%), Ht. 57cm (50%). He is awake, non-toxic appearing, with expressionless facies and a weak cry. His anterior fontanel is flat and soft. He has poor head control. He has diminished pupillary reflexes, absent corneal reflexes, bilateral ptosis, and decreased tearing. He has a weak suck and gag reflexes with increased oral secretions. His neck is supple without adenopathy. Heart and lungs are normal. Aeration is good. His abdomen is soft, full, non-tender, with decreased bowel sounds throughout. No hepatosplenomegaly. Rectal exam shows no stool in the rectal vault and decreased anal sphincter tone. His extremities are slightly cool, with delayed capillary refill. His skin shows no rash or petechiae. He has decreased muscle tone throughout and diminished deep tendon reflexes.

    A sepsis work up is done and he is started on IV fluids and empiric antibiotics for sepsis. Stool samples are sent for Clostridium botulinum toxin assays. His cultures are subsequently negative. His clinical condition worsens such that he cannot feed and he eventually develops hypoventilation and respiratory insufficiency requiring mechanical ventilation. An electromyography study is done which shows brief, small, abundant, motor unit potentials, known by the acronym BSAP, a characteristic pattern associated with infant botulism. His stool assay returns positive for botulism toxin.

    He is hospitalized for infant botulism.

Robert M. Katzman, MD

10/15/08 11:47:39

You Code It!

What are the best, most accurate codes?

_____

_____

_____

PEDIATRIC COMPLETE CARE CENTER
123 BORNE PATH • YOUNGSTOWN, FL 32811 • 407-555-ABCD

PATIENT: CARDONE, DAPHNE
ACCOUNT/EHR #: CARDA001
Date: 03/15/08

This is a 16-year-old female brought in by her father, with the chief complaint that he thinks his daughter is using drugs and wants her to get treatment. The father reports that she has often been acting "high," with sleeplessness for several days in a row, unusual euphoria, pressured speech, increased activity (e.g., cleaning the bathroom), suspiciousness, and some aggressive behaviors.

HPI: After requesting that the father wait outside, she admits that she uses "ice," or "batu," roughly 2-3 times per week, smoking it by pipe. She obtains the drug from her friends. She admits to occasional marijuana use and weekend drinking of alcohol, without any history of blackouts, hallucinations, or incapacitating withdrawal symptoms. Although previously an above-average student, she has, for the past year, been truant from school and is failing most of her classes. She has also run away from home on several occasions. She gives vague answers when asked about sexual history.

    Her past medical history is otherwise negative. Family history is significant for a history of alcoholism and a possible psychotic illness. Her parents are divorced. There is no history of abuse or domestic violence.

EXAM: VS T 37.5, P 110, R 18, BP 130/80. She is somewhat restless and guarded, with poor eye contact and brief answers. HEENT significant for slightly dilated pupils. Heart shows regular rhythm and elevated rate. Pelvic examination is performed, although she has agreed reluctantly. The remainder of physical examination is normal.

LABS: Urine toxicology positive for methamphetamine, negative for others, including alcohol. Electrocardiogram is significant for sinus tachycardia, otherwise normal.

DIAGNOSES: Methamphetamine dependence and Chlamydia cervicitis.

PLAN: Pt is referred for admission to an adolescent substance abuse treatment program.

Robert M. Katzman, MD

03/15/08 11:47:39

You Code It!

What are the best, most accurate codes?

_____

_____

_____

Neurology Cases and Patient Records

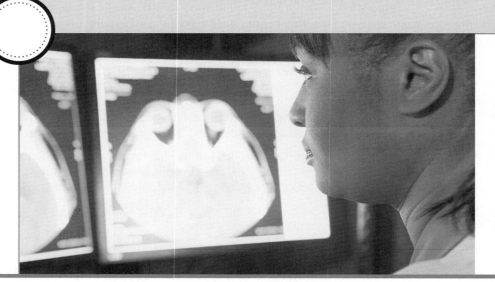

INTRODUCTION

The following case studies are from a neurologist's practice. In a neurologist's office, a professional coding specialist is likely to see many different types of health situations.

Physicians who specialize in the diagnosis and treatment of conditions of the nervous system including the brain and the spinal cord are called neurologists. These health care professionals identify, diagnose, and treat such diseases as Parkinson's disease, Alzheimer's disease, meningitis, and stroke. Neurosurgery is a sub-specialty for physicians who diagnose and treat conditions affecting the neurological system, such as brain tumors or hydrocephalus. These professionals may also work with patients for pain management.

The Board of Psychiatry and Neurology bestows board certification to neurologists who qualify. The certification is recognized by the American Board of Medical Specialties.

You can use these cases to practice coding diagnoses, E/M, procedures, DME, or other HCPCS Level II items, as applicable; code for the physician or the facility; code inpatient and outpatient services, as applicable:

1. Code for the physician.
2. Code for the anesthesiologist, when applicable.
3. Code for the hospital, when applicable.
4. Code for the pathology and laboratory, when applicable.
5. Code HCPCS Level II codes, when applicable.

FRAISER, HARROLD, & YAWZI, Neurology
81 BAYER BOULEVARD • SENSATION, FL 32811 • 407-555-5852

PATIENT: KELLO, JOAN
ACCOUNT/EHR #:   KELJO001
Date: 09/16/08

Attending Physician: Suzanne R. Taylor, MD

The patient is a 25-year-old female with a history of recurrent sinus infections who was well until five days ago. She presents with fever, severe frontal headache, facial pain, and runny nose. Patient states she has been having difficulty concentrating.

T 101.5° HEENT: Tenderness over frontal and left maxillary sinuses. Nasal congestions visible.
    CT scan reveals opacification of both frontal and left maxillary, sphenoid sinuses and a possible large non-enhanced lesion in the brain.
    Parasagittal MRI and axial MRI show a large (7cm) well-circumscribed epidural collection compressing the left frontal lobe.

DX: Epidural abscess with frontal lobe lesions caused by significant compression on frontal lobe
    Recommendation for surgery to evacuate the abscess
    Rx antibiotics and pseudoephedrine

_____

Suzanne R. Taylor, MD

SRT/pw   D: 9/16/08 09:50:16   T: 9/18/08 12:55:01

You Code It!

What are the best, most accurate codes?

_____

_____

_____

FRAISER, HARROLD, & YAWZI, Neurology
81 BAYER BOULEVARD • SENSATION, FL 32811 • 407-555-5852

Patient Name: Robbins, Mark
Admission Date: 11/09/08

Attending Physician: Carrie L. Sutton, MD

HPI: This is a male patient who was recently in the hospital. He was diagnosed at the time with a malignancy in the cerebral area. Patient has been undergoing outpatient radiation. The son called me and told me that the patient was having some difficulty breathing and mental status seemed to have deteriorated in a rather rapid nature. I discussed this with the nurse at the extended care facility where he resides and we did give him a Lasix injection 40 mg. He did not respond very much and they brought him to the emergency room. Initial tests basically were negative, but after discussion with this internist, it was decided to go ahead and admit patient for further neurological evaluation.

PMH: Significant for the malignancy in the cerebral area, hypertension, gastritis, diabetes, secondary to steroids. He also has osteoarthritis.

Medications: Patient has been maintained on Prevacid 30 mg po bid, Bumex 0.5 mg po q day prn, Captopril 100 mg q 12, Norvasc 10 mg po q day, insulin siding scale. He has been on Decadron per the radiation/oncologist. Depakote 250 mg qid and Diflucan recently 150 mg po q day. He received Phenergan on prn basis for nausea, Tylenol grains 10 q 4-6 prn pain, Darvocet one q 4-6 prn pain. Chloraseptic spray to the mouth. His diet is thick and liquid as tolerated, diabetic diet.

Social History: Noncontributory at this time.

Family History: Noncontributory at this time.

Vital signs: Stable

General Appearance: Somewhat lethargic-appearing white male, he has always been somewhat quiet with a flat affect.

HEENT: Normal

Cervical and Cardiopulmonary Exam: Unchanged

Lungs: Clear

Heart: Heart rate regular

Abdomen: No obvious pain, normal bowel sounds

Extremities: Trace edema bilaterally

Continued

Chapter 12   Neurology Cases and Patient Records

Impression: The patient is admitted with a known brain tumor, he has been undergoing radiation, he has an oncologist and he is admitted at this time by the neurologist for further evaluation regarding his mental changes.

Carrie L. Sutton, MD

CLS/pw   D: 11/09/08 09:50:16   T: 11/15/08 12:55:01

You Code It!

What are the best, most accurate codes?

_____

_____

_____

FRAISER, HARROLD, & YAWZI, Neurology
81 BAYER BOULEVARD • SENSATION, FL 32811 • 407-555-5852

Patient Name: Robbins, Mark
Admission Date: 11/10/08

Attending Physician: Carrie L. Sutton, MD

Findings & recommendations of consultant: PT is an 84-year-old male who is known to have brain tumor which I believe is a glioblastoma multiforme. Apparently he has been receiving radiation therapy, but has begun to go downhill and was admitted with pneumonia several days ago. Despite treatment, because of his obtunda-tion, the patient's pneumonia has progressed. He is having respiratory distress, apparently more yesterday than today. A chest x-ray today has shown a small, approximately 10% right pneumothorax. Today the patient has not evidenced any respiratory distress and in fact has been either sleeping or obtunded and apparently only slightly responding. He is no code and is receiving palliative therapy only with no intubation or CPR to be given in the case of an arrest. The family's intentions are that he be made comfortable and not to try to prolong his life. He has apparently not been complaining of any pain when he was able to state his complaints. His temperature is 100.0 at maximum, respirations are currently very unlabored at approximately 18 per minute, blood pressure 174/104, heart rate 116 with regular rhythm. His O2 saturations on a non-rebreather mask are in the mid 90s. The patient's most recent chest x-ray today shows the pneumonia to be worsening and the development of a small pneumothorax, as previously mentioned.

PMH: Discloses that he has hypertension and has glucose intolerance, apparently provoked at least partly by corticosteroids. An echogram was within normal limits. He apparently has been in reasonably good health. He has had hand surgery before and has history of enlarged prostate.

Family History: Noncontributory

Social History: Noncontributory

ROS: Unobtainable

PE: Reveals an elderly gentleman who appears to be sleeping, and I did not try to arouse him. His vital signs show that he is afebrile. His blood pressure is 162/95, respirations are unlabored at 16-18, heart rate is 116 and temperature is currently 99.2. Head and neck examination: I do not find any acute abnormality, no JVD is seen, no palpable abnormal lymphadenopathy. His chest reveals a few coarse breaths sounds and a few rhonchi, no wheezes, no rubs. Breath sounds are fairly good on both sides. Heart reveals a tachycardia with a regular rhythm, no rub, murmur, gallop. Abdomen is soft, nontender. Normal bowel sounds. No hepatosplenomegaly. GU/Rectal: Not done. Extremities show no acute changes. The patient's chest x-ray, as described previously.

Continued

Overall Impression: Pt appears to be quite comfortable at this time. The patient is not having any distress that I can observe, and I think that his prognosis is probably terminal. At this point in time, I would not recommend putting in a chest tube as he does not seem to be having any respiratory compromise or discomfort from having the pneumothorax and given its small size, I suspect that it would be unlikely to afford him any improvement in symptoms. However, it is something that we could monitor, and should it progress or his symptoms become worse, this could always be re-evaluated. I discussed this in detail with the patient's son who I believe understands all of the options and is in agreement with taking this course at this time. I also discussed this with Dr. Moore so he is informed.

Carrie L. Sutton, MD

CLS/pw   D: 11/10/08 09:50:16   T: 11/17/08 12:55:01

You Code It!

What are the best, most accurate codes?

_____

_____

_____

Patient Name: HARPER, VAN

Admission Date: 11/10/08

Attending Physician: Carrie L. Sutton, MD

This is the first visit for this 89-year-old, right-handed male who comes for evaluation of possible normal pressure hydrocephalus.

The patient's family has been noting that the patient has symptoms consistent with normal pressure hydrocephalus and apparently were made aware of this in recent publications. The patient has had mental deterioration. He has a history of urinary urgency and has been seen by Dr. Reine for this. Problems with his gait, which he describes as "vertigo in his legs" and he "minces his steps." His primary care physician is Dr. Torman.

The patient has allergies to pollen and hayfever. His medications include Plavix, Aspirin, Lipitor, Avodart, Uroxatral, Hyzaar, Calcium 600 = Vitamin D and multivitamins.

PERTINENT MEDICAL HISTORY: The patient does not smoke cigarettes or drink alcohol.

SOCIAL HISTORY: He is married and is a retired optometrist.

FAMILY HISTORY: His mother died at the age of 96 of "dementia" and possible stroke. His father died at the age of 96 of an unknown cause.

REVIEW OF SYSTEMS: The patient has had several transient ischemic attacks in January, April, and July 2004. He is status post cataract surgery. He is status post a syncopal episode in January of 2004. He has a history of hypertension, asthma, bronchitis, and a history of bilateral inguinal hernia repairs forty-five years ago. In January of 2004, he had a urinary tract infection and also had a cardiac evaluation, which was negative. Otherwise, his review of systems is negative for cardiac, pulmonary, gastrointestinal, genitourinary, or musculoskeletal disease.

PHYSICAL EXAMINATION: This is a well-developed, well-nourished elderly white male in no acute distress who appears to be awake, alert, and oriented. His blood pressure is 170/70. His pulse is 70. His respiration is 16. His head is atraumatic, normocephalic. He is status post cataracts. He has dentures. His neck is subtle without jugular venous distention or bruits. His lungs are clear to auscultation. His heart is regular rhythm. His abdomen is soft. His extremities are without clubbing, cyanosis, or edema. Examination of his spine does not demonstrate any direct cervical spine tenderness. The patient has kyphoscoliosis of the thoracolumbar spine. Neurologic examination of cranial nerves II – XII demonstrate a decrease in upward gaze and a decrease in hearing. He wears hearing aids. Otherwise, they appear to be grossly unremarkable. Motor function is 5/5 = in all major motor groups. Sensory examination appears to be grossly intact in all extremities. Deep tendon reflexes are 0 = for the biceps, triceps, and brachioradialis. In the lower extremities, the patellas, suprapatellars, and hamstrings are 0 =. The right Achilles is 2 +, the left is absent. The toes are downgoing bilaterally. The patient's cerebellar testing is intact for finger to nose function. On regular gait testing, the patient has a magnetic/shuffling gait. Station testing does not demonstrate any drift or Romberg's sign.

REVIEW: There are no x-rays available for review.

IMPRESSION: The patient has possible normal pressure hydrocephalus versus ischemic cerebrovascular disease.

Continued

RECOMMENDATIONS: The patient should have an MRI scan, MR Angiogram of the brain, and MR Angiogram of the carotid and vertebral arteries and then return to see me in the office.

Carrie L. Sutton, MD

CLS/pw   D: 11/10/08 09:50:16   T: 11/17/08 12:55:01

You Code It!

What are the best, most accurate codes?

_____

_____

_____

FRAISER, HARROLD, & YAWZI, Neurology
81 BAYER BOULEVARD • SENSATION, FL 32811 • 407-555-5852

Patient Name: HARPER, VAN
Admission Date: 12/15/08

Attending Physician: Carrie L. Sutton, MD

The patient was last seen on November 10. The MRI scan of the brain demonstrates that the patient has hydrocephalus with transependymal edema.

IMPRESSION: The patient has either normal pressure hydrocephalus or a low pressure communicating hydrocephalus.

RECOMMENDATIONS: In either case, he requires a ventricular shunt placement. I have explained to the patient and his family the shunt procedure, its indications, risks, benefits, and alternatives in detail including the risk of bleeding, infection, injury to the brain tissue with hemorrhages, stroke, paralysis, blindness, coma, or even death. All of their questions have been answered. No guarantees have been given. I have advised that the patient will need to have medical clearance from his primary care physician, Dr. Torman. Once we have the medical clearance, we can schedule him for surgery.

Carrie L. Sutton, MD

CLS/pw   D: 12/15/08 09:50:16   T: 12/21/08 12:55:01

You Code It!

What are the best, most accurate codes?

_____

_____

_____

FRAISER, HARROLD, & YAWZI, Neurology
81 BAYER BOULEVARD • SENSATION, FL 32811 • 407-555-5852

Patient Name: HARPER, VAN

Attending Physician: Carrie L. Sutton, MD
Admission Date: 11 January 2008
Discharge Date: 15 January 2008

Operative Report:
Preoperative Diagnosis: Normal pressure hydrocephalus
Postoperative Diagnosis: Normal pressure hydrocephalus
Operation: Right parieto-occipital ventriculoperitoneal shunt placement with cerebro-spinal fluid manometry and Hakim valve programming.

Surgeon: Carrie L. Sutton, MD

Anesthesia: General endotracheal
Anesthesiologist: Carter H. Beauman, MD
Estimated Blood Loss: Less than 10 cc.
Complications: None

Procedure: This 89-year-old gentleman had progressive urinary, gait, and memory problems with MRI study demonstrating significant ventriculomegaly consistent with normal pressure hydrocephalus. Because of the patient's deterioration, he was offered the option of ventriculoperitoneal shunt placement to try to stop the downward deterioration of his mental faculties.

    Following the obtaining of informed consent, the patient was taken to the operating table for the procedure. The patient was placed supine on the operating table, inducted under general anesthesia and intubated. His right parieto-occipital scalp was shaved, and then the scalp, neck, chest, and abdomen on the right side were washed with alcohol and prepped with DuraPrep solution and then draped with sterile drapes with additional Ioban dressing. The skin incision was marked out with a skin marker for the right parieto-occipital scalp, centered on a point approximately 3 cm lateral to and 8-to-9 cm rostral to the inion, and in the right upper quadrant of the abdomen at the mid-costal line. These incisions were then infiltrated with 1/2% lidocaine with 1:200,000 epinephrine solution. The skin incision was then made in the scalp with a #10 blade and hemostasis was obtained with Bovie cauterization. A pneumatic perforator was used to drill a hole in the cranium and then the margins of the bur hole were waxed with bone wax for hemostasis. Blunt dissection of the occipital scalp was used to create a subcutaneous cul-de-sac for placement of the value system and following this, a subcutaneous passer was used to create a track for passing the distal Bactocill peritoneal catheter between the two incisions. The abdominal incision was also opened with a #10 blade to facilitate passage.

    Once the distal catheter was in place, the dura was cauterized using the Bovie cautery bayonet technique, and then a ventricular catheter was passed into the ventricles without difficulty. The cerebrospinal fluid pressure was measured to be approximately 9 cm of water and cerebrospinal fluid was also sent for routine culture and Gram stain. Once the cerebrospinal fluid pressure had been measured, the Hakim valve was programmed to a pressure resistance of 60 mm of water. The valve was then connected to the ventriculostomy catheter, which was 10 cm in length. It was a Bactocill catheter that was used for this also. The connection was made with a 2-0 silk ligature. The valve was also connected to the distal peritoneal catheter with a 2-0 silk ligature. The valve was then pulled underneath the scalp and anchored to the pericranium with 3-0 Prolene anchoring sutures to prevent migration of the valve. There was good spontaneous flow of cerebrospinal fluid from the distal portion of the peritoneal catheter. Excess length of the peritoneal cavity was removed and then several slits were made in the sides of the peritoneal catheter to provide additional egress points for cerebrospinal fluid as needed.

Continued

Once this was done, the abdominal incision was opened further with a Bovie cautery and cutting current. The anterior abdominal fascia was divided with a Bovie cautery, and then blunt dissection with a hemostat was used to split the fibers of the rectus abdominus muscles. The posterior abdominal fascia was then identified and lifted up with hemostats and then divided with Metzenbaum scissors. The peritoneum was then identified, lifted up with hemostats, and again divided with Metzenbaum scissors. Following this, the peritoneal cavity was easily visualized. A hemostat and then a peritoneal trocar were able to be passed into the peritoneal cavity without difficulty. Following this, the distal portion of the ventriculoperitoneal shunt was passed into the peritoneal cavity without difficulty, after once again ascertaining that there was spontaneous flow of spinal fluid. Once the catheter was in the peritoneal cavity, #0 Vicryl sutures were used to reapproximate the posterior abdominal fascia, and then the anterior abdominal fascia. The Scarpa's fascia was then closed with #0 Vicryl interrupted sutures with inverted knots. Gelfoam soaked in Thrombin was placed overlying the point of insertion of the ventriculostomy catheter, and then the galea was closed with #0 Vicryl interrupted sutures with inverted knots. The areas were irrigated with Bacitracin irrigation solution during the closure process, and then the skin incisions were closed with 3-0 nylon simple running sutures with good skin approximation. The skin incisions were then washed again with Bacitracin irrigation solution, and then dressed with triple antibiotic ointment and coverlet dressings. The patient was awakened from general anesthesia, extubated, and taken to the recovery room for further observation. Estimated blood loss from the entire procedure was less than 10 cc. The patient appeared to have tolerated the procedure well.

Carrie L. Sutton, MD

CLS/pw   D: 01/11/08 09:50:16   T: 01/27/08 12:55:01

You Code It!

What are the best, most accurate codes?

_____

_____

_____

FRAISER, HARROLD, & YAWZI, Neurology
81 BAYER BOULEVARD • SENSATION, FL 32811 • 407-555-5852

PATIENT NAME: HARPER, VAN
MRN: HARVA001

Attending Physician: Carrie L. Sutton, MD
Admission Date: 11 January 2008
Discharge Date: 15 January 2008

FINAL DIAGNOSIS: Normal pressure hydrocephalus. History of hypertension. History of benign prostatic hypertrophy. History of asthma. History of hypercholesterolemia.

HISTORY OF PRESENT ILLNESS: This 89-year-old male developed symptoms of normal pressure hydrocephalus, including gait problems and urinary problems as well as decreased mentation. He had outside studies, which demonstrated that the patient had large ventricles consistent with normal pressure hydrocephalus and the patient was offered the option of ventricular shunt procedure. The patient agreed and was admitted for surgery.

The patient has a history of allergies to pollen. His medications: the patient had home medications delineated in the order sheets. His social history: he did not smoke cigarettes or drink alcohol. He was a retired optometrist. Family history was positive for dementia and stroke. Review of systems was positive for transient ischemic attacks, hypertension, history of asthma and bronchitis, history of cataract surgery, and history of hernia repairs.

On physical examination, this was a well-developed, well-nourished, elderly white male who was awake, alert, and in no acute distress. His head was atraumatic and normocephalic. His heart was regular rhythm. Lungs were clear to auscultation. Abdomen was soft and nontender. On neurologic examination, he had a magnetic gait. Extremities without clubbing, cyanosis, or edema.

HOSPITAL COURSE: The patient was admitted for surgery on January 11, 2008, and underwent a right parietooccipital ventricular peritoneal shunt placement with a Hakim valve, which was programmed to 60 mm after CSF manometry demonstrated higher pressures. The procedure was uneventful. Postoperatively, the patient was seen in consultation by Internal Medicine. He was awake, alert, and conversant. His postoperative CT scan demonstrated excellent position of the ventriculostomy catheter and the ventricles without the evidence of hemorrhage. The patient was noted to have a marked improvement in his gait according to his family within 48 hours of surgery. He had no headaches, and by January 15, 2008, he was felt to be sufficiently stable. He was able to be discharged home for outpatient follow-up. His condition at discharge was stable/improved.

Carrie L. Sutton, MD

CLS/pw   D: 01/11/08 09:50:16   T: 01/27/08 12:55:01

You Code It!

What are the best, most accurate codes?

_____

_____

_____

PATIENT NAME: CARMICHAEL, ABNER

MRN: CARAB001

Attending Physician: Carrie L. Sutton, MD

Admission Date: 11 January 2008

Discharge Date: 15 January 2008

This is a left-handed male admitted for sudden onset of memory loss.

HISTORY OF PRESENT ILLNESS: AT 5:15 p.m.+pt took a nap. When he woke up, he could not remember anything, according to his wife. No loss of consciousness. No slurred speech. No motor or sensory loss in limbs. Presented to the ER.

PAST MEDICAL HISTORY: 2 CVAs 1988 and 1995. Right hand weakness persisted. TIA 12/95. Syncope 6/95. Cardiac pacemaker. Seizure disorder. On Dilantin and Neurontin for a while, then discontinued by neurologist last several months (Dr. Promat). Penile implant. Inguinal herniorrhaphy. Hay fever.

SOCIAL HISTORY: Married. Nonsmoker for years.

FAMILY HISTORY: Noncontributory

MEDICATIONS: Tylenol 250 mg bid

ALLERGIES: Sulfa

ROS: As per HPI

EXAM: Afebrile, BP 163/86, HR: 71 (paced)

HEENT: Atraumatic. No lesions.

NECK: Without carotid bruits, supple

CHEST: Clean

HEART: No arrhythmia, Pacer

ABDOMEN: Soft, non-tender

EXTREMITIES: No swelling, 4+ pedal pulses

NEURO: Awake, alert, but not oriented. He answers questions glibly and tangentially. Can't tell date, but knows his name and address. Does not know MD's name who are following him. Does not seem to retain new information. Speech fluent.

     CN: II – VII intact
     MOTOR: Diminished dexterity, right hand and fingers
     SENSORY: No deficiency
     COORDINATION: No limb dysmetria

Continued

CAT SCAN (No C): Old left hemisphere infarct frontal, parietal and posterior temporal lobes. No mass effect. Atrophy diffuse.

EKG: Paced rhythm

Lab: Chol 242

Carrie L. Sutton, MD

CLS/pw   D: 01/11/08 09:50:16   T: 01/27/08 12:55:01

You Code It!

What are the best, most accurate codes?

_____

_____

_____

FRAISER, HARROLD, & YAWZI, Neurology
81 BAYER BOULEVARD • SENSATION, FL 32811 • 407-555-5852

PATIENT NAME: FLETCHER, LACY
MRN: FLELA001

Attending Physician: Carrie L. Sutton, MD
Admission Date: 11 January 2008

This is a 2-year-old female who appears to be recovering from an upper respiratory infection when she develops vomiting. Her grandmother may have given her aspirin but she was supposed to have taken acetaminophen. She initially presents to the emergency department with irritability and restlessness. She subsequently develops convulsions which are treated with anticonvulsants and she is admitted to the PICU.

EXAM: VS T 37.8, P 100, R 50, BP 110/70, oxygen saturation 99% in room air. Height, weight, head circumference are at the 50th percentile. She is agitated and not cooperative. Head shows no signs of external trauma. Pupils are equal and reactive to light. Conjunctiva are clear, sclera non-icteric. EOMs cannot be fully tested, but they are conjugate. TMs are normal. Mouth is not easily examined. Neck reveals no adenopathy. She is agitated so it is not possible to be certain that her neck is supple. Heart regular without murmurs. Lungs are clear. Abdomen is flat with normal bowel sounds. It is difficult to tell if she has any hepatosplenomegaly. No definite tenderness. No inguinal hernias are present. She moves all extremities. Reflexes are not testable because of her agitation.

LABS: Serum bilirubin: Normal. Serum AST and ALT: increased. Serum ammonia: increased. Prothrombin time: prolonged. A CT scan of the brain is obtained which shows cerebral edema.

    Her neurologic symptoms rapidly worsen and she becomes unresponsive. She is intubated and put on mechanical ventilation.

    Reye's syndrome is suspected. A confirmatory liver biopsy reveals diffuse, small lipid deposits in the hepatocytes (microvesicular steatosis) without significant necrosis or inflammation. These findings are consistent with the diagnosis of Reye's syndrome.

Carrie L. Sutton, MD

CLS/pw   D: 01/11/08 09:50:16   T: 01/27/08 12:55:01

You Code It!

What are the best, most accurate codes?

_____

_____

_____

FRAISER, HARROLD, & YAWZI, Neurology
81 BAYER BOULEVARD • SENSATION, FL 32811 • 407-555-5852

PATIENT NAME: BRUMM, CARLO
MRN: BRUCA001

Attending Physician: Carrie L. Sutton, MD
Admission Date: 11 January 2008

HISTORY OF PRESENT ILLNESS: This is a five year-old male, referred by his pediatrician, Dr. Raul Boles, with an abnormal gait. He was adopted from another country about a year ago, and his adopting parents have noticed that he is clumsy when he runs and he falls often. He runs on his tiptoes, which has occurred since they started taking care of him. Otherwise, he has no other problems. He is doing well in kindergarten despite his language difficulty. His teacher notes that he has trouble getting up from a sitting position at school. His parents deny any chronic fevers, leg pain, weight loss, seizures, skin rash, urinary or bowel incontinence, or frequent colds.

PAST MEDICAL HISTORY, DEVELOPMENTAL HISTORY, FAMILY HISTORY, BIRTH HISTORY are unknown. His immunizations are up-to-date and his PPD this year has been negative.

EXAM: His vital signs are normal. His height, weight and head circumference are at the 50th percentile. He is alert, active, shy, well-nourished, slim, and in no distress. His skin shows no neurocutaneous stigmata. His head is normocephalic and atraumatic. His pupils are equal, round, reactive to light. No nystagmus is evident. His fundi are normal with sharp disk margins. His TMs are clear. His throat is normal with a uvula midline. His lungs, heart, and abdomen are normal. His back shows no sacral dimples.

NEUROLOGIC EXAM: A standard cranial nerve exam reveals no deficits. His strength is +4/5 in his deltoids, knee flexors and extensors; +5/5 in his biceps and triceps. His calves are visibly enlarged with a firm, rubbery feeling. He gets up to a standing position using a Gowers' maneuver. No dysdiadochokinesia. Negative Romberg sign. Sensation to light touch is intact. His reflexes are +2/4 in his biceps, triceps, brachioradialis, patella and ankle. His plantar reflex is downgoing (negative Babinski sign). No clonus is elicited. Normal anal wink and abdominal reflexes are present. His gait is best described as a wide-based waddling. When running, he tends to run on his toes. He is unable to jump.

LABS: CBC w/differential

PROCEDURES: Muscle biopsy to be performed.

DIAGNOSIS: Duchenne muscular dystrophy (DMD)

Carrie L. Sutton, MD

CLS/pw   D: 01/11/08 09:50:16   T: 01/27/08 12:55:01

You Code It!

What are the best, most accurate codes?

_____

_____

_____

FRAISER, HARROLD, & YAWZI, Neurology
81 BAYER BOULEVARD • SENSATION, FL 32811 • 407-555-5852

PATIENT NAME: GREENE, JEFFREY
MRN: GREJE001

Attending Physician: Carrie L. Sutton, MD
Admission Date: 11 January 2008

HISTORY OF PRESENT ILLNESS: Two days ago, this 6-month-old male infant was sitting in an infant carrier, which was placed on top of a stroller. The carrier accidentally fell approximately 3 feet onto the ground. He hit his head on the plastic portion of the car seat. There was an immediate cry and no loss of consciousness. His behavior, activity, and feeding pattern are reported as normal. Two days later (today) his mother notes a boggy swelling in the right temporal area of the head and because of this, she brought him to the emergency room for evaluation. He continues to have normal activity and no vomiting.

PAST MEDICAL HISTORY: He has been previously healthy. There is no history of substance use, or child protective services (CPS) involvement in the family.

EXAM: VS T 36.9, P 120, R 18, BP 92/50, oxygen saturation 100% in room air. Height, weight and head circumference at the 25th to 50th percentiles. He is alert, active, easily arousable on exam and clean in appearance. He has a 9 by 7 cm swelling over the right temporal/parietal region that is soft, possibly tender, with no palpable bony deformity. No lacerations or wounds are noted. His anterior fontanel is soft and flat. Pupils are 3 mm bilaterally and reactive to light. EOMs are conjugate. There is no hemotympanum, no nasal discharge, and his mucus membranes are moist. His heart, lung, and abdomen exams are normal. Neurologic and extremity exams are normal.
    A head CT scan shows a subgaleal hematoma (hematoma under the aponeurosis of Galen), a non-depressed linear skull fracture, and a normal brain.
He is discharged home to the care of his parents. He followed up with his pediatrician the next day without sequelae.

_____

Carrie L. Sutton, MD

CLS/pw   D: 01/11/08 09:50:16   T: 01/27/08 12:55:01

You Code It!

What are the best, most accurate codes?

_____

_____

_____

FRAISER, HARROLD, & YAWZI, Neurology
81 BAYER BOULEVARD • SENSATION, FL 32811 • 407-555-5852

PATIENT NAME: ROMERO, ANGELA
MRN: ROMAN001

Attending Physician: Carrie L. Sutton, MD
Admission Date: 11 January 2008

HISTORY OF PRESENT ILLNESS: This is a 10-month-old girl whose parents bring her into the emergency room for tonic-clonic seizures lasting a few minutes. This baby girl is a product of a normal pregnancy and was delivered full-term by normal spontaneous vaginal delivery. There were no postnatal complications and this infant was discharged from the hospital at 48 hours of life. Her history is significant for jerking movements (onset at 5 months of age) described as sudden flexion of the neck, arms, and legs onto the trunk preceded by a cry. Her parents were not too worried about this behavior since the child would return back to normal and they attributed it to colic or "gas." There is no history of fever, coughing, vomiting or diarrhea. She has been gaining weight appropriately and eating normally. She is on solid foods and formula, which the parents prepare correctly. Her immunizations are up to date. She is on no medications and her development has been normal. She is able to sit up, crawl, cruise with both hands, and combines syllables.

FAMILY HISTORY: Unremarkable in that there is no history of seizures, mental retardation, or consanguinity.

EXAM: VS T 37.0, P 100, R 26, BP 90/60, O2 sat 100% on RA, weight 9.0 kg (50%ile), length 73 cm (50%tile), HC 44.5 cm (50%tile). She is alert, active, and in no distress. She is not toxic. She tracks well. She has good bonding with her mother. She has multiple small 1-2 cm oval, irregular hypopigmented macules on her trunk and extremities. HEENT is normal. Her neck is supple without lymphadenopathy. Heart, lungs and abdomen are normal.
NEURO: She has no facial asymmetry. She moves all her extremities well. There are no focal deficits. She does not exhibit cortical thumbing or scissoring of her lower extremities. She tracks well. She has good head control and is able to support herself on her legs.

     A head CT scan revealing cortical tubers in the cerebral cortex and multiple subependymal nodules in the lateral ventricles. She is admitted to the floor where an EEG shows "hypsarrhythmia." A complete echocardiogram and a complete renal ultrasound are also done showing tumors in both the heart and kidneys. A diagnosis of tuberous sclerosis is made. She is started on ACTH, unfortunately her condition fails to improve and she continues to have intractable seizures in addition to being mentally retarded.

Carrie L. Sutton, MD

CLS/pw   D: 01/11/08 09:50:16   T: 01/27/08 12:55:01

You Code It!

What are the best, most accurate codes?

_____

_____

_____

FRAISER, HARROLD, & YAWZI, Neurology
81 BAYER BOULEVARD • SENSATION, FL 32811 • 407-555-5852

PATIENT NAME: BINYON, ROSE
MRN: BINRO001

Attending Physician: Carrie L. Sutton, MD
Admission Date: 11 January 2008

HISTORY OF PRESENT ILLNESS: This patient is a 6-month-old female brought into the office as a new patient for a well baby visit. Her family moved here recently from Asia, where she was born. There were no prenatal or postnatal complications, and she has had no significant medical problems since birth.

FAMILY HISTORY: Positive for her father who has a condition in which his body is covered with fleshy small growths, similar to skin tags, and on the father's side, there are several family members with the same warty growths, seizures, and high blood pressure.

EXAM: VS are normal. Her growth parameters are in the 25–50th percentiles. Her examination is otherwise unremarkable except for multiple coffee colored spots on her trunk and abdomen.

DIAGNOSIS: Neurofibromatosis.
Schedule parents for a follow-up visit tomorrow to discuss this further.

_____

Carrie L. Sutton, MD

CLS/pw   D: 01/11/08 09:50:16   T: 01/27/08 12:55:01

You Code It!

What are the best, most accurate codes?

_____

_____

_____

FRAISER, HARROLD, & YAWZI, Neurology
81 BAYER BOULEVARD • SENSATION, FL 32811 • 407-555-5852

PATIENT NAME: TINDER, JENNIFER
MRN: TINJE001

Attending Physician: Carrie L. Sutton, MD
Admission Date: 11 January 2008

HISTORY OF PRESENT ILLNESS: The patient is a 16-year-old female, G1P0 mother at 37 weeks, scheduled for a C-section. Prenatal care was not sought until 32 weeks gestation. Mother did not take any vitamins or folate supplements prior to that time. Initial prenatal lab studies were significant for an elevated alpha fetoprotein. A prenatal ultrasound done at 34 weeks demonstrated a meningomyelocele. No hydrocephalus was noted at that time. A neurosurgeon was consulted. A C-section is scheduled to deliver the infant as non-traumatically as possible with the availability of the neurosurgeon close by.

At delivery, the infant is delivered with Apgar scores of 7 and 8. Birthweight is 3.2 kg. A translucent membrane sac overlying the mid-lumbar region is noted. It is leaking xanthochromic fluid. Upper extremity movement is noted to be good, but lower extremity movement is not as vigorous. The infant is transferred to the NICU where vascular access is obtained and initial stabilization measures are performed. Five hours later, the infant is taken to the operating room where a neurosurgeon closes the meningomyelocele defect over the lower back. Post-operative recovery in the NICU is unremarkable. Lower extremity movement is moderate. A head ultrasound study shows mild hydrocephalus.

_____

Carrie L. Sutton, MD

CLS/pw   D: 01/11/08 09:50:16   T: 01/27/08 12:55:01

You Code It!

What are the best, most accurate codes?

_____

_____

_____

FRAISER, HARROLD, & YAWZI, Neurology
81 BAYER BOULEVARD • SENSATION, FL 32811 • 407-555-5852

PATIENT NAME: LEWIS, COLLETTE
MRN: LEWCO001

Attending Physician: Carrie L. Sutton, MD
Admission Date: 11 January 2008

HISTORY OF PRESENT ILLNESS: This is a 10-year-old female who is brought into the office by her parents with a chief complaint of clumsiness and blurred vision. She had been well until approximately 2 weeks ago when she noticed a loss of sensation and strength in her left leg, a rapid deterioration in vision, and a decrease in coordination. There is no history of fever, vomiting, or seizures. One year prior to this event, she presented to the hospital with poor coordination, dizziness and headaches. A left hemiplegia was noted as well as an asymmetric gait. A full recovery was made 5 days later, and she was discharged from the hospital without further treatment or a definite diagnosis.

EXAM: VS are normal. Her weight, height, and head circumference are all at the 50th percentile. She is alert but subdued. Her HEENT exam is notable for severe visual loss and pale optic discs on funduscopy. Her heart, lungs, and abdomen are normal. She is noted to have a hyporeflexive paraparesis noted on the left.

    I admitted her into the hospital. A CT scan shows slightly enlarged ventricles, and an MRI scan shows multiple lesions in the periventricular white matter and cerebellum. Pattern visual evoked responses showed markedly delayed latencies. She is treated with corticosteroids and a full recovery within a few weeks is expected.

DIAGNOSIS: Multiple sclerosis (MS)

_____

Carrie L. Sutton, MD

CLS/pw   D: 01/11/08 09:50:16   T: 01/27/08 12:55:01

You Code It!

What are the best, most accurate codes?

_____

_____

_____

FRAISER, HARROLD, & YAWZI, Neurology
81 BAYER BOULEVARD • SENSATION, FL 32811 • 407-555-5852

PATIENT NAME: MILLER, NATASHA
MRN: MILNA001

Attending Physician: Carrie L. Sutton, MD
Admission Date: 11 January 2008

HISTORY OF PRESENT ILLNESS: This is a 12-year-old Caucasian female brought to the emergency room by her mother with a chief complaint of leg weakness. One week prior, she had a fever of 101.4 with vomiting and diarrhea. After 3 days, the vomiting and diarrhea resolved. She was doing well until this morning when she fell while trying to get out of bed and could not stand or walk without support. She denies headache, blurred vision, tinnitus, vertigo, dysphagia, or incontinence. There is no history of toxic ingestion. Her immunizations are up to date. While in the ER she complains that her arms feel weak.

EXAM: VS T 37.0, P 84, R 24, BP 102/64. Height and weight are at the 25th percentile. She is alert, slightly fearful but cooperative. HEENT: She has no nystagmus and no papilledema. Her extraocular movements are intact. Pupils are equal and reactive to light. No facial weakness or asymmetry is present. Heart, lung and abdomen exams are normal. NEURO: Strength 4/5 in the upper extremities, 3/5 in the lower extremities. DTRs 1-2+ in the upper extremities and absent in the lower extremities. Sensation is intact in all extremities. Cerebellar function is normal except for the weakness. No cranial nerve abnormalities are noted. She refuses to walk.

    CBC, electrolytes, BUN, creatinine, glucose, calcium and liver function tests are normal. Urine toxicology screen is negative. A lumbar puncture is performed. Opening pressure is normal. CSF analysis shows protein 146 mg/dL (high), glucose 70 mg/dL, 5 WBC per cu-mm, 1 RBC per cu-mm, and gram stain shows no WBCs and no organisms.

    An MRI of the brain and spinal cord is normal. She is started on IVIG and over the next few days, she slowly regains strength in her arms and legs. However, she still requires assistance with walking at the time of discharge.

DIAGNOSIS: Guillain-Barre syndrome (GBS)
    She is referred to a rehabilitation hospital to continue outpatient physical therapy.

Carrie L. Sutton, MD

CLS/pw   D: 01/11/08 09:50:16 T: 01/27/08 12:55:01

You Code It!

What are the best, most accurate codes?

_____

_____

_____

Obstetrics and Gynecology Cases and Patient Records

INTRODUCTION

The following case studies are from an obstetrics and gynecology practice. In a physician's office of this type, a professional coding specialist is likely to see many different kinds of health situations, including preventive health care services.

Gynecologists are physicians who specialize in women's health. These health care professionals provide routine care for women, including Pap smears or breast examinations, as well as help patients with such age-appropriate concerns as the onset of menses, birth control, family planning, and menopause. Subspecialties of gynecology include gynecologic oncology (the care and treatment of women with cancers of the reproductive organs), reproductive endocrinology (the care and treatment of women and men who have infertility problems), and surgery (diagnostic and therapeutic procedures such as hysterectomy or oophorectomy).

Gynecologists may also practice obstetrics, which is a subspecialty focusing on the care of women during pregnancy—from conception through labor and delivery and through the postpartum period. An obstetrician may further specialize in perinatology (maternal-fetal medicine), caring for women with high-risk pregnancies.

Gynecologists and obstetricians can be board-certified through the Board of Obstetrics and Gynecology, which is recognized by the American Board of Medical Specialties.

You can use these cases to practice coding diagnoses, E/M, procedures, DME, or other HCPCS Level II items, as applicable; code for the physician or the facility; code inpatient and outpatient services, as applicable:

1. Code for the physician.
2. Code for the anesthesiologist, when applicable.
3. Code for the hospital, when applicable.
4. Code for the pathology and laboratory, when applicable.
5. Code HCPCS Level II codes, when applicable.

THE WOMEN'S HEALTH CENTER
671 SENORA LANE • LOVELAND, FL 32772 • 407-555-8541

PATIENT NAME: REMARNI, SOPHIA
MRN: REMSO01
Admission Date: 13 September 2008
Discharge Date: 13 September 2008

Operative Report
Date: 13 September 2008

Preoperative DX: Status post delivery, undesired fertility, multiparity
Postoperative DX: Same
Operation: Laparoscopic bilateral tubal cauterization using Kleppingers

Surgeon: Rodney L. Cohen, MD
Assistant: None
Anesthesia: General endotracheal per Dr. Morrison
Complications: None
Findings: See body of dictation
Specimens: None
Disposition: See body of dictation

PROCEDURE: The patient was taken to the OR, and was placed in the dorsal lithotomy position and was prepped and draped in a sterile manner. A speculum was inserted into the vagina and a single-tooth tenaculum used to grasp the anterior lip of the cervix. A Hulka tenaculum was used to grasp the cervical lip and manipulate the uterus. Once this was done, an infraumbilical incision was made with the knife, and a Veress needle inserted through the incision site. CO2 gas was instilled after saline via syringe was checked for position. CO2 gas, approximately 2 L, was instilled into the abdominal cavity. Once this was done, the Veress was removed, and a 5mm trocar was inserted through the incision site. The laparoscopic camera was then placed through the sleeve.

Under direct visualization and transillumination, after Trendelenburg position, a second incision site was made with the knife suprapubically in the midline, and a 5mm trocar inserted through the incision site. First, a blunt probe was used to identify the fallopian tubes. They were easily visible, so the Kleppingers were then used to cauterize full thickness burns on each fallopian tube approximately five-to-six adjacent times until good cautery and using the monitor to perform this was done. Once this was finished and thought to be satisfactory, the instruments were removed. The CO2 gas was allowed to passively escape. The incision sites were closed with 4-0 Vicryl in an interrupted manner. Approximately 10 cc total of 1.25% Marcaine was injected subcutaneously for pain relief. The Hulka tenaculum was removed and a silver nitrate stick was used to cauterize one of the puncture sites on the cervix. This was the end of the procedure. The patient tolerated it well and went to the recovery room in good condition.

9/13/08 10:37:10

You Code It!

What are the best, most accurate codes?

_____

_____

_____

THE WOMEN'S HEALTH CENTER
671 SENORA LANE • LOVELAND, FL 32772 • 407-555-8541

PATIENT: SANDERS, MARLENE
MRN: SANMA01
Admission Date: 19 September 2008
Discharge Date: 19 September 2008
Date: 19 September 2008

Preoperative DX: High-grade squamous intraepithelial lesion of the cervix
Postoperative DX: Same
Operation: Loop electrosurgical excision procedure (LEEP) and ECC (endocervical curettage)

Surgeon: Rodney L. Cohen, MD
Assistant: None
Anesthesia: General by LMA
Findings: Large ectropion, large non-staining active cervix essentially encompassing the entire active cervix
Specimens: To pathology
Disposition: Stable to recovery room

PROCEDURE: The patient was taken to the OR where she was placed in the supine position and administered general anesthesia. She was then placed in cane stirrups and prepped and draped in the usual fashion. Her vaginal vault was not prepped. The coated speculum was then placed and the cervix exposed. It was then painted with Lugol and the whole entire active cervix was non-staining with the clearly defined margins where the stain began to be picked up. The cervix was injected with approximately 7 cc of lidocaine with 1% epinephrine. Using a large loop, the anterior cervix was excised and then the posterior loop was excised in separate specimens. Because of the size of the lesion one piece in total was not accomplished. Prior to the excision, the endocervical curettage was performed and specimen collected. All specimens sent to pathology. The remaining cervical bed was cauterized and then painted with Monsel for hemostasis. The case was concluded with this. Instruments were removed. The patient was taken down from candy cane stirrups, awakened from the anesthesia and taken to the recovery room in stable condition.

9/19/08 19:38:17

You Code It!

What are the best, most accurate codes?

_____

_____

_____

THE WOMEN'S HEALTH CENTER
671 SENORA LANE • LOVELAND, FL 32772 • 407-555-8541

PATIENT:	CALLMAN, LOUISE
MRN:	CALLO01
Admission Date:	7 September 2008
Discharge Date:	8 September 2008
Date:	7 September 2008
Preoperative DX:	Stenotic cervical os with hematometrium
Postoperative DX:	Same
Operation:	Cervical dilatation with release of old blood. This was done under ultrasound guidance followed by endometrial curettage.
Surgeon:	Rodney L. Cohen, MD
Assistant:	None
Anesthesia:	General by LMA
Complications:	None
Findings:	See body of dictation
Specimens:	Endometrial curettings to pathology
Disposition:	Stable to recovery room

PROCEDURE: The patient was taken to the OR where she was placed in the supine position and administered general anesthesia per LMA. She was then placed in candy-cane stirrups and prepped and draped in the usual sterile fashion. A weighted speculum was placed in the vagina and with the aid of a Deaver retractor, the anterior portion of the cervix was grasped with single-toothed tenaculum. There were no evident holes or dimples or scenes suggestive of where the external cervical os might be, as the cervix had completely agglutinated across the entire surface. Using lacrimal ducts and gentle tension, the area of suspicion was gently poked until a perforation gave way. This tract was followed with serial dilators until ultimately brown old blood was released ensuring that I was in the right place. This was done with the aid of abdominal ultrasound guidance for the risk of false tracking and missing the endocervical canal uterus was real. The uterus was emptied. The cervix was dilated up to approximate 8 mm. This allowed for free flow of the contained old blood. This was followed by sharp curette of all the uterine lining surfaces. This specimen was captured and sent to pathology. Lastly a small 7 size suction catheter was inserted to ensure the remainder of any old captured blood that may be sitting in the deep recesses of this severely retroverted uterus was obtained and this concluded the case. The instruments were removed. The patient was taken down from cane stirrups. The patient was awakened from anesthesia and taken to the recovery room in stable condition.

9/7/08 11:47:39

You Code It!

What are the best, most accurate codes?

_____

_____

_____

THE WOMEN'S HEALTH CENTER
671 SENORA LANE • LOVELAND, FL 32772 • 407-555-8541

PATIENT NAME: CAVELLI, JUDY
MRN: CAVJU01
Admission Date: 4 September 2008
Discharge Date: 5 September 2008
Operative Report
Date: 4 September 2008

Preoperative DX: 1. Chronic pelvic pain; 2. History of endometriosis;
                             3. Right adnexal mass, probable endometrioma
Postoperative DX: Same
Operation: Total abdominal hysterectomy with bilateral salpingo-oophorectomy and
                             lysis of pelvic adhesions with procedure of unusual difficulty secondary to
                             endometriosis

Surgeon: Rodney L. Cohen, MD
Assistant: None
Anesthesia: General endotracheal intubation by Dr. Kastorman
Complications: None
Findings: See body of dictation
Specimens: None
Disposition: See body of dictation

PROCEDURE: The patient was taken to the operating room and she was placed supine on the table. Underwent general anesthesia with endotracheal intubation without complication. The patient had Foley catheter inserted. Was prepped and draped in a sterile fashion for abdominal procedure. Scalpel was used to make a vertical midline incision in elliptical fashion removing the previously noted dense abdominal scar, taken down through subcutaneous tissue to the level of the anterior rectus sheath, nicked in its midline and extended the length of the incision. Blunt dissection through the midline rectus muscles exposing the peritoneum, sharply entered the midline, extended the length of the incision down to the bladder. Balfour self-retaining retractor was put into place, elevated with blue towels with care taken to avoid posterior nervous injury. Initial attempts to pack the bowel off the field were difficult as there were significant adhesions between the colon and the previous area of the left adnexectomy and the endometrioma that was on the right side. Through an extensive and lengthy dissection, the bowel was carefully dissected from the pelvis with both blunt and sharp dissection with care to avoid bowel injury. The right adnexa was then carefully dissected by both blunt and sharp dissection off the side wall to avoid ureteral injury. After freeing up all tissue, the packing was removed from the abdomen, and the bowel was again repacked away from the operative site and then the hysterectomy was proceeded with in the usual fashion. Bilaterally, the uteroovarian ligaments were cross clamped with Kelly clamp for traction. The uterus was elevated. Bilaterally, the round ligaments were identified, cross clamped with Heaney clamps, severed with pelvic scissors and ligated with 0-Vicryl suture in a Heaney ligature type fashion. The bladder was sharply dissected of the lower uterine segment. Bilaterally, the uterine arteries were skeletonized, cross clamped with Heaney clamps, severed with pelvic scissors and then ligated with 0-Vicryl suture. The remaining portion of the cardinal ligaments were then cross clamped with Heaney clamp, severed with pelvic scissors, and ligated with 0-Vicryl suture in Heaney ligature type fashion. At the upper most portion of the vagina, the angles were cross clamped with Heaney clamp, severed with pelvic scissors, and the uterus, cervix, and remaining right adnexa were then removed from the vaginal cuff.

Bilaterally, the angles were ligated with 0-Vicryl suture in Heaney ligature type fashion and the central portion of the vaginal cuff was closed with a 0-Vicryl suture in a running interlocking fashion. The pelvis was copiously irrigated and inspected, noted to be clean and dry with the exception of some small bleeding sites overlying the region of the right ureter in the region of the extensive dissection. These were cauterized and clipped with care taken to avoid a ureteral injury. There was a small tissue ooze due to the extensive dissection and Gelfoam

Continued

was placed in the site. Prior to this, the pelvis was copiously irrigated and inspected and noted to be clean and dry. All instrumentation was removed. Prior to this, a look at all operative sites revealed good hemostasis. All pedicles revealed good hemostasis. All instrumentation was removed. The fascia and peritoneum were closed in a bulk fashion using 0-PDS suture in a running mixed simple interlocking fashion starting from the superior margin of the incision and running to the midline, starting from the inferior margin of the incision and running to the midline.

Subcutaneous tissue was irrigated and inspected and noted to be clean and dry. It was drawn together in the midline with 3-0 plain suture in a running simple fashion and then the skin was reapproximated with a 4-0 Vicryl suture in subcuticular fashion. Steri-Strips and overlying pressure dressing was applied. The patient was awakened on her own, breathing on her own in good condition and transferred to the recovery room.

9/4/08 12:43:45

You Code It!

What are the best, most accurate codes?

_____

_____

_____

THE WOMEN'S HEALTH CENTER
671 SENORA LANE • LOVELAND, FL 32772 • 407-555-8541

PATIENT NAME: OPPENHEIM, OLIVIA
MRN: OPPOL01
Admission Date: 9 September 2008
Discharge Date: 10 September 2008

Operative Report
Date: 10 September 2008

Preoperative DX: 1. Menometrorrhagia refractory to medical treatment;
    2. Endometrial mass; 3. Adnexal masses with normal CA-125
Postoperative DX: Same
Operation: Supracervical hysterectomy, bilateral salpingo-oophorectomy

Surgeon: Rodney L. Cohen, MD
Assistant: None
Anesthesia: General endotracheal
Complications: None
Findings: See body of dictation
Specimens: None
Disposition: See body of dictation

PROCEDURE: The patient was taken to the OR, was placed supine position and was prepped and draped in the usual sterile manner. A Foley catheter was inserted into the bladder to drain the urine. A Pfannenstiel skin incision was made with a knife and carried down to the fascia. The fascia was nicked in the midline and extended bilaterally. Kochers were used to grasp the superior portion of the fascia that was separated sharply and bluntly in the midline. Kochers were then used to grasp the inferior portion of the fascia that was separated sharply and bluntly. The rectus muscles were separated. Hemostats were used to grasp the peritoneum and extend superiorly under direct visualization and inferiorly under translumination. The bladder flap was developed and pushed well of the low uterine segment. The Balfour self-retaining retractor was placed and the bowel packed with warm moist laps. Two curved Kelly clamps were placed across the corneal area of the uterus on each side. The right round ligament was placed on stretch. A 0-Vicryl was used to suture ligate this ligament. The anterior and posterior leaves of the broad ligament were then opened. The same procedure was done to the left. The infundibulopelvic ligament on the right was then identified. The ureter was found to be well out of the way, and a curved Heaney clamp x 2 was placed across the infundibulopelvic ligament and this ligament excised. A 0-Vicryl free tie, as well as a 0-Vicryl suture ligation was performed with good hemostasis. Next, the same procedure was done on the left obtaining the left round ligament and infundibulopelvic ligament in the same manner. Next, the bladder flap was dissected off the low uterine segment and cervix. Once this was done appropriately, the uterine artery on the left side was skeletonized and curved Heaney clamps were used to obtain these. Suture ligation was performed with 0-Vicryl. The uterine artery was then obtained on the right. Straight Heaney used in succession to obtain the cardinal ligaments. The patient was noted to have endometriosis on her ovaries, as well as a lot oozing with aberrant blood vessels at this time and it was decided to go ahead with a supracervical hysterectomy due to the nature of the patient's tissue and difficulty, and going any deeper into the pelvis. A Bovie was used to cauterize and remove the fundal portion of the uterus and lower uterine segment, and a portion of the cervix as well. The remaining cervical stump was cauterized en mill and 0-Chromic was first used to reapproximate the inside edges of the cervix, then 0-Vicryl was used on the outside through the cervix in a running locking manner for hemostasis. Once this was done, all areas were inspected for any further bleeding. Bovie cautery or figure-of-eight sutures were placed as necessary. The bladder flap was placed over the cervical stump in the mid portion.

Continued

A 2-0 Chromic was used to anchor this. The right ureter was identified and found to be peristalsing normally. The left ureter could not be seen but was palpated low in the pelvis. Irrigation was performed. No further bleeding was noted, so all the instruments were removed, counts are correct, the rectus muscles were reapproximated with 0-Chromic in an interrupted manner. The fascia was closed with 0-Vicryl in the running manner. The subcutaneous tissue was thoroughly irrigated and the skin was closed with staples. This ended the procedure. The patient tolerated it well and went to recovery room in good condition.

9/09/08 09:24:26

You Code It!

What are the best, most accurate codes?

_____

_____

_____

PATIENT NAME: Lefferty, Loretta
MRN: LEFLO01
Admission Date: 15 September 2008
Discharge Date: 16 September 2008

Operative Report
Date: 15 September 2008

Preoperative DX: Pelvic mass
Postoperative DX: Peritoneal inclusion cyst with involvement of the left fallopian tube and a portion of the left ovary
Operation: Laparoscopy, exploratory laparotomy, removal of mass

Surgeon: Rodney L. Cohen, MD
Assistant: None
Anesthesia: General
Complications: None
Findings: See body of dictation

INDICATIONS: The patient is a 47-year-old Latin-American female status post total abdominal hysterectomy with pelvic mass on ultrasound, mildly symptomatic.

PROCEDURE: The patient was taken to the operating room after the induction of adequate general anesthesia, prepped and draped in the dorsolithotomy position. A catheter was introduced into her bladder. Bimanual exam revealed a fullness near the vaginal cuff.

Small subumbilical incision was made to the skin and the Veress needle was inserted. Peritoneal cavity was insufflated with 2 L of carbon dioxide. 10mm trocar sleeves were placed in through this and it was noted that the omentum which was adherent to the anterior abdominal wall had been perforated with the trocar and sleeve. There was no evidence of bleeding during the course of the initial scope; however, later as the scope was removed there was noted to be a small amount of bleeding where the omentum and the abdominal wall fused.

Examination with laparoscopy revealed a 5-6 cm multiloculated pelvic mass which was encapsulated with bowel and which was plastered against the vaginal cuff. There was no evidence of any pedicles and it was not felt that this would be amenable to laparoscopic therapy.

The trocar sleeves were removed. The incision was closed with a single fascial 0-Chromic suture and 4-0 skin sutures.

Attention was then turned, a Pfannenstiel incision was made and extended to be subcutaneous tissue and fascia. The muscle and fascia were bluntly separated and the peritoneal cavity was entered atraumatically. The mass was seen to be arising from the left adnexal area. The right ovary was identified and was plastered against the sidewall, was normal in size and without evidence of visible abnormalities other than being plastered against the sidewall. The mass had bladder adherent over the anterior portion and bowel adherent over the posterior portion. Tedious and careful dissection was accomplished to separate the mass from all of these. The mass appeared to have clear fluid within it and seemed to be in at least three different loculations. The infundibulopelvic ligament was identified running into the mass. Thus it was felt to be ovarian and tubular in complex nature. The left ureter was dissected away from the mass and just as the mass was beginning to be almost completely isolated, it ruptured and poured forth clear fluid, but this allowed access to the inside portion of the mass. The mass was then removed along with what appeared to be the entire portion of the tube. There was a portion of the left ovary which was still plastered against the superior portion of the vagina and this was left intact in light of there being no pathology at that point. The pelvic sidewall had been opened and there were multiple small bleeding points that were coagulated. The infundibulopelvic ligament that had been isolated, clamped and cut, was provided with complete hemostasis. There was a small rent in the ligamentous tissue which was adherent to the mass and multiple small figure-of-eight sutures using 2-0 Chromic or coagulation were used to provide hemostasis.

Continued

Tedious examination of all cut surfaces revealed no evidence of bleeding at this point. Irrigation was accomplished and reexamination revealed the area to be dry. Examination of the omentum where the initial laparoscopy had been performed revealed a small amount of bleeding and coagulation was used to provide hemostasis and a single figure-of-eight suture was used to secure the fascia from the underneath portion to prevent any future hernia formation. The self-retaining retractor which had previously been placed was then removed. The laps were removed. The bowel was allowed to return to the peritoneal cavity but prior to this a single sheet was placed over all of the cut surfaces on the left adnexal and superior bladder area to attempt to provide further reduction of adhesion formation.

Having removed all the instruments, the muscles were reapproximated across the midline with a 0-Chromic suture and sub-fascia hemostasis were achieved. The fascia was closed with 0-Vicryl. Subcutaneous irrigation and hemostasis were achieved and the skin was closed with skin staples.

The urine was clear throughout the procedure. The sponge, needle, and instrument counts were correct. The mass was sent to pathology and felt to be involving apportion of the infundibulopelvic ligament, fallopian tube, some peritoneal reflection, and possibly a small portion of the ovary.

The patient is being awakened and prepared for transfer to the recovery room.

9/15/08 07:58:10

You Code It!

What are the best, most accurate codes?

_____

_____

_____

THE WOMEN'S HEALTH CENTER
671 SENORA LANE • LOVELAND, FL 32772 • 407-555-8541

PATIENT NAME:	TAYLOR, THOMASINA
MRN:	TAYTH01
Admission Date:	5 September 2008
Discharge Date:	6 September 2008

Operative Report
Date:	5 September 2008
Preoperative DX:	1. First trimester missed abortion; 2. Undesired fertility
Postoperative DX:	Same
Operation:	1. Dilation and curettage with suction;
	2. Laparoscopic bilateral tubal ligation using Kleppinger bipolar cautery
Surgeon:	Rodney L. Cohen, MD
Assistant:	None
Anesthesia:	General endotracheal anesthesia
Complications:	None
Findings:	The patient had products of conception at the time of dilatation and curettage. She also had normal-appearing uterus, ovaries, fallopian tubes, and liver edge.
Specimens:	Products of conception to pathology
Disposition:	To PACU in stable condition

PROCEDURE: The patient was taken to the operating room and she was placed in the dorsal supine position. General endotracheal anesthesia was administered without difficulty. The patient was placed in dorsal lithotomy position. She was prepped and draped in the normal sterile fashion. A red rubber tip catheter was placed gently to drain the patient's bladder. A weighted speculum was placed in the posterior vagina and Deaver retractor anteriorly. A single-tooth tenaculum was placed in the anterior cervix for retraction. The uterus sounded to 9 cm. The cervix was dilated with Hanks dilators to 25 French. This sufficiently passed a #7 suction curet. The suction curet was inserted without incident and the products of conception were gently suctioned out. Good uterine cry was noted with a serrated curet. No further products were noted on suctioning. At this point, a Hulka tenaculum was placed in the cervix for retraction. The other instruments were removed.

Attention was then turned to the patient's abdomen. A small vertical infraumbilical incision was made with the knife. A Veress needle was placed through that incision. Confirmation of placement into the abdominal cavity was made with instillation of normal saline without return and a positive handing drop test. The abdomen was then insufflated with sufficient carbon dioxide gas to cause abdominal tympany. The Veress needle was removed and a 5mm trocar was placed in the same incision. Confirmation of placement into the abdominal cavity was made with placement of the laparoscopic camera. Another trocar site was placed two fingerbreadths above the pubic symphysis in the midline under direct visualization. The above noted intrapelvic and intraabdominal findings were seen. The patient was placed in steep Trendelenburg. The fallopian tubes were identified and followed out to the fimbriated ends. They were then cauterized four times on either side. At this point, all instruments were removed from the patient's abdomen. This was done under direct visualization during the insufflation. The skin incisions were reapproximated with 4-0 Vicryl suture. The Hulka tenaculum was removed without incident.

Continued

The patient was placed back in the dorsal supine position. Anesthesia was withdrawn without difficulty. The patient was taken to the PACU in stable condition. All sponge, instrument, and needle counts were correct in the operating room.

9/5/08 10:40:36

You Code It!

What are the best, most accurate codes?

_____

_____

_____

THE WOMEN'S HEALTH CENTER
671 SENORA LANE • LOVELAND, FL 32772 • 407-555-8541

PATIENT NAME: GAULT, IONA
MRN: GAUIO01
Admission Date: 5 September 2008
Discharge Date: 6 September 2008

Operative Report
Date: 5 September 2008
Preoperative DX: Multiparity, desiring permanent sterilization
Postoperative DX: Same
Operation: Postpartum bilateral tubal ligation

Surgeon: Gary Rothman, MD
Assistant: None
Anesthesia: General endotracheal anesthesia
Complications: None
Findings: Normal postpartum anatomy

PROCEDURE: After appropriate consents were signed, the patient was explained the risks and alternatives of the surgery and the patient agreed to the operation. The patient was taken to the operating room, was given general endotracheal anesthesia, was prepped and draped in the usual fashion. Through a transverse infraumbilical incision, peritoneal cavity was entered. Army-Navy retractors were placed. The right fallopian tube was picked up with Babcock, followed all the way to the fimbria for identification. Then, in the mid-ampullary portion two times of 0 chromic were placed and tube was cut and sent to pathology for identification. A similar thing was done on the left side. Then, fascia was closed with 0 Vicryl in a running locking fashion. The skin was closed with 4-0 Vicryl in a subcuticular fashion and was infiltrated with Marcaine 0.5%. The patient was extubated in the operating room and taken to the recovery room in stable condition.

D: 09/05/08 12:51:41   T: 09/07/08 01:16:18

You Code It!

What are the best, most accurate codes?

_____

_____

_____

THE WOMEN'S HEALTH CENTER
671 SENORA LANE • LOVELAND, FL 32772 • 407-555-8541

PATIENT NAME: PHELPS, MAXINE
ACCOUNT #:   PHEMA01
Date: 13 December 2008

Attending Physician: Yamira E. Newadha, MD
Location: Office

HISTORY OF PRESENT ILLNESS: This is a 40-year-old female who a month ago noted a lump in her right breast (8 o'clock position of the right breast just outside the areola). This prompted bilateral screening mammography. The mammo demonstrated a linear area of increased density and architectural distortion at the 12 o'clock position in the right periareolar region.

    This was suspicious mammographically and a biopsy of this was recommended. The patient had follow-up ultrasound as well. The ultrasound demonstrated a lobulated cyst of 6mm at the 8 o'clock position corresponding to the patient's area of palpable abnormality. NO other lesions were noted.

    Due to the mammogram, the patient has an incidental finding of an area of increased density at the 12 o'clock position and requires biopsy. This is not appreciable on examination and requires needle localization and excisional biopsy for which she is here today.

    The patient has no family history of breast cancer. Age of menarche: 13. She was pregnant three times with one child, first child born at age 20.

Past Medical History: No coronary disease, hypertension, or diabetes

Past Surgical History: None

Medications: None

Allergies: None

Social History: The patient does not smoke, does not drink. No history of drug use.

Physical Examination:

Breasts: The patient examined in erect and supine. Both breast are symmetric. There is no skin dimpling. There is no nipple inversion. There is no mass appreciated in either breast with careful attention paid to the right breast overlying the 8 o'clock region as well as the 12 o'clock region. Again, no mass was appreciated. She has no axillary, cervical, supraclavicular, or infraclavicular adenopathy notes.

Lungs: Clear

Heart: Regular rhythm

Impression: Right breast mass

Continued

This is a 40-year-old who has an incidental finding of an area of increased density at the 12 o'clock position of the right breast. This cannot be appreciated on physical examination. She will require needle loc/excisional biopsy. The indication, alternatives, and complications of the procedure have been discussed with this patient. She understands and wishes to proceed.

Yamira E. Newadha, MD

YEM/mg   D: 12/13/08 12:51:41   T: 12/15/08 01:16:18

You Code It!

What are the best, most accurate codes?

_____

_____

_____

THE WOMEN'S HEALTH CENTER
671 SENORA LANE • LOVELAND, FL 32772 • 407-555-8541

PATIENT NAME: TOMLINSON, THERESA
ACCOUNT #: TOMTH01
Date: 15 December 2008

Preoperative Diagnosis: Right breast mass
Postoperative Diagnosis: Same (pending pathology)
Operation: Excision of right breast mass, intermediate wound closure – 4 cm

Surgeon: Roweena L. Macomba, MD
Assistant: None
Anesthesiologist: Terence Abnernathy, MD
Anesthesia: MAC/1% lidocaine diluted 50% with Bicarbonate (10cc)

HISTORY: This is a 51-year-old female admitted to the minor surgery suite for excision of a 1 cm palpable nodule in the superficial aspect of the right breast in the 12 o'clock axis near the periphery. The indications, alternatives and possible complications were reviewed and consent was obtained.

PROCEDURE: With the patient in the supine position, the area in question was prepped and draped in the usual sterile fashion using Betadine. After adequate IV sedation, 1% lidocaine without epinephrine was used to infiltrate the soft tissues at that level to create a field block.

An elliptical incision was made about the lesion itself, considering its intimate association with the overlying skin. The 4 cm incision was deepened into the subcutaneous space. The mass was excised in its entirety with a rim of normal appearing breast, fat, and surrounding skin. Adequate hemostasis was secured within the depths of the wound. The wound was closed in layers. The deeper breast tissue was approximated using interrupted 3-0 chromic sutures. The subcuticular layer was approximated using interrupted 4-0 Biosyn sutures. The skin edges were closed using 4-0 Vicryl in the subcuticular space in a continuous fashion. Mastisol and Steri-Strips were applied. A dressing was applied. The procedure was terminated. Needle, sponge and instrument counts were correct. Estimated blood loss was minimal.

DISPOSITION: The patient tolerated the procedure and was discharged from the minor operating department in satisfactory condition.

Roweena L. Macomba, MD

RLM/mg   D: 12/15/08 12:55:01   T: 12/18/08 09:50:16

You Code It!

What are the best, most accurate codes?

_____

_____

_____

THE WOMEN'S HEALTH CENTER
671 SENORA LANE • LOVELAND, FL 32772 • 407-555-8541

PATIENT NAME: OSGOOD, BENITA
ACCOUNT #:   OSGBR01
Date: 15 September 2008

Attending Physician: Roland F. LaScala, MD

INTERVAL HISTORY: The patient is a 29-year-old female G1 P0 who presents at term with regular uterine contractions. The patient's antepartum course has been uncomplicated to date. Sonogram and amniocentesis were normal. GBS culture was negative.

PHYSICAL EXAMINATION:
HEENT:	Unremarkable
Neck:	Supple
Chest:	Clear
Abd:	Guarded, soft
Contractions:	Q3 – 4 minutes, 40 – 50 seconds duration
Membrane:	Ruptured @ 21:45 with clear fluids
Vaginal discharge:	"Show"
Vaginal Exam:	3 cm dilated Eff: 80%, Sta: -2
Vital Signs:	T98.7, P82, R20, FHR 130s, Location LLQ
Fetal Status:	Reassuring
Assessment:	Term pregnancy, in spontaneous labor
Plan:	Admit, Expectant management for delivery

Roland F. LaScala, MD

RFL/mg   D: 9/15/08   T: 9/20/08

You Code It!

What are the best, most accurate codes?

_____

_____

_____

THE WOMEN'S HEALTH CENTER
671 SENORA LANE • LOVELAND, FL 32772 • 407-555-8541

PATIENT NAME:	OSGOOD, BENITA
ACCOUNT #:	OSGBR01
Date:	16 September 2008
Attending Physician:	Roland F. LaScala, MD
Anesthesia:	Epidural
Type of Delivery:	NSVD
Condition of Perineum:	MLE
Episiotomy:	Midline performed
Vagina/Cervix:	Intact
Delivered:	Live, single born, female, weight 6 lb. 4 oz.@01:05
Type of Stimulation:	Mouth suction
Condition:	Good
Birth Injury:	None
Apgar Rating:	1 min. = 9
	5 min. = 9

Roland F. LaScala, MD

RFL/mg   D: 9/16/08   T: 9/20/08

You Code It!

What are the best, most accurate codes?

THE WOMEN'S HEALTH CENTER
671 SENORA LANE • LOVELAND, FL 32772 • 407-555-8541

PATIENT NAME: HARRIS, ROSEANNE
ACCOUNT #:   HARRO01
Date: 1 October 2008

In the 41st week of her first pregnancy, a 37-year-old woman arrived at Labor and Delivery at 6:30 a.m. for a planned induction of labor due to mild, pregnancy-induced, hypertension.

After intra-vaginal placement of misoprostol, the nurse observed her briefly and, at 11:00 a.m., discharged her from the unit. She went for a walk with her husband in a park next to the hospital.

Patient's membranes spontaneously ruptured and she returned to the labor and delivery unit. A recently hired, new graduate, nurse admitted the patient, took her vital signs, and checked the fetal heart rate. The mother's blood pressure was 176/95 but the nurse thought this was related to nausea, vomiting, and discomfort from the contractions.

The resident examined the mother, determined that her cervix was 5-6 cm, 90 percent effaced and the vertex was at 0 station. An internal fetal heart monitor was placed because the mother's vomiting and discomfort caused her to move around too much in the bed, making it hard to record the fetal heart rate with an external monitor. The internal monitor revealed a steady fetal heart rate of 120 and no decelerations.

The mother continued to complain of painful contractions and requested an epidural. Shortly after placement of the epidural, the monitor recorded a prolonged fetal heart rate deceleration. The heart rate returned slowly to the baseline rate of 120 as the nurse repositioned the mother, increased her intravenous fluids and administered oxygen by mask.

An epidural analgesia infusion pump was started. The fetal heart rate strip indicated another deceleration that recovered to baseline. The nurse informed the resident who checked the tracing and told her to "keep an eye on things."

The primary nurse noted in the labor record that the baseline fetal heart rate was "unstable, between 100-120" but she did not report this to the resident.

The nurse recorded that the fetal heart rate was "flat, no variability." As the nurse was documenting this as a non-reassuring fetal heart rate pattern, the patient expressed a strong urge to push and the nurse called for an exam.

A resident came to the bedside, examined the mother and noted that she was fully dilated with the caput at +1. A brief update was written in the chart, but the clinician who had performed the exam was not noted.

The mother was repositioned and began pushing.

The fetal heart rate suddenly dropped and remained profoundly bradycardic for 11 minutes. The resident was called and attempted a vacuum delivery since the fetal head was at +2 station. The attending then entered and attempted forceps delivery.

An emergency cesarean delivery was performed; the baby was stillborn. The physician identified a uterine rupture that required significant blood replacement.

Roland F. LaScala, MD

RFL/mg   D: 10/01/08   T: 10/03/08

You Code It!

What are the best, most accurate codes?

THE WOMEN'S HEALTH CENTER
671 SENORA LANE • LOVELAND, FL 32772 • 407-555-8541

PATIENT NAME: JOCQUIN, YASMINE
ACCOUNT #:   JOCYA01
DATE: 1 October 2008

This is a 26-year-old, G1P0, O+, VDRL NR, rubella immune, HBsAg negative female at 27 weeks gestation presents to labor and delivery with a 2 day history of headache and facial swelling. Maternal history is remarkable for a single prenatal visit in the first trimester.

EXAM: VS T 37, P 75, RR 14, BP 170/100. Her exam is remarkable for facial and pretibial edema and hyperreflexia.

LABS: Urine dipstick positive for 3+ protein. Ultrasound demonstrates decreased amniotic fluid. The fetus is in the breech position and no fetal abnormalities are noted. Estimated fetal weight is 650 grams.
     A decision is made to deliver the infant by cesarean section following maternal treatment with betamethasone.
     Labor and delivery occurs without incident.
     Infant taken to NICU. Neonatologist paged.
     Mother taken to recovery in good condition.

Roland F. LaScala, MD

RFL/mg   D: 10/01/08   T: 10/03/08

You Code It!

What are the best, most accurate codes?

_____

_____

_____

Oncology Cases and Patient Records

CHAPTER
14

INTRODUCTION

The following case studies are from an oncology practice. In a physician's office of this type, a professional coding specialist is likely to see patients with different kinds of malignant tumors.

Oncologists are physicians who specialize in the diagnosis and treatment of malignancies, the second greatest cause of mortality (death) in the United States. They may be involved in determining the type and extent of cancer and providing such treatments as surgery, radiation, or chemotherapy.

These health care professionals may be board-certified in medical oncology through the Board of Internal Medicine, which is recognized by the American Board of Medical Specialties.

You can use these cases to practice coding diagnoses, E/M, procedures, DME, or other HCPCS Level II items, as applicable; code for the physician or the facility; code inpatient and outpatient services, as applicable:

1. Code for the physician.
2. Code for the anesthesiologist, when applicable.
3. Code for the hospital, when applicable.
4. Code for the pathology and laboratory, when applicable.
5. Code HCPCS Level II codes, when applicable.

SWANSON ONCOLOGY
969 TURNABOUT LANE • REMISSION, FL 32811 • 407-555-9573

PATIENT: BACHELDER, JEFFREY
MRN: BACJE001
Admission Date: 13 October 2008
Discharge Date: 13 October 2008
Date: 13 October 2008

Preoperative DX: Malignant neoplasm, scrotum, CA in situ
Postoperative DX: Same
Procedure: Resection of scrotum, needle biopsy of testis, laparoscopy with a ligation of spermatic veins

Surgeon: Daniel Macintosh, MD
Assistant: None
Anesthesia: General

INDICATIONS: The patient is a 59-year-old male with a recent diagnosis of malignancy of the scrotum.

PROCEDURE: The patient was placed on the table in supine position. General anesthesia was administered by Dr. Cattan. He was placed in proper position. A needle biopsy was taken of the testis, and then a surgical resection of the scrotum was performed. Before closing, a surgical laparoscopy with a ligation of the spermatic veins was performed, as well.

10/13/08 11:47:39

You Code It!

What are the best, most accurate codes?

_____

_____

_____

SWANSON ONCOLOGY
969 TURNABOUT LANE • REMISSION, FL 32811 • 407-555-9573

PATIENT: MARSHALL, BARRY
ACCOUNT/EHR #:   MARBA001
Date: 11/09/08

Attending Physician: Willard B. Reader, MD

S: Pt is a 51-year-old male who comes in concerned about a sore he noticed on his left temple, directly at the hairline. He states that his mother died six years ago from melanoma, and his brother was diagnosed with pre-cancerous cells of the epidermis. Pt states he is the captain of a beach volleyball team, and volunteers at the local YMCA as a water aerobics instructor. He says that he tries to be diligent about sunscreen, but sometimes he forgets.

O: Ht 5'11" Wt. 189 lb. R 20. T 98.6. BP 120/95 Cultures of lesion were taken and sent to our in-house lab. The pathology report confirms the lesion is malignant. I discussed options with the patient and recommended surgical removal of the lesion as soon as possible.

A: Malignant melanoma of skin of scalp

P: Pt to call to make appointment for surgical procedure

_____

Willard B. Reader, MD

WBR/pw   D: 11/09/08 09:50:16   T: 11/13/08 12:55:01

You Code It!

What are the best, most accurate codes?

_____

_____

_____

SWANSON ONCOLOGY
969 TURNABOUT LANE • REMISSION, FL 32811 • 407-555-9573

PATIENT: UNDERWOOD, PRICILLA
MRN: UNDPR001
Date: 25 September 2008

Diagnosis: Medulloblastoma
Procedure: Central Venous Access Device (CVAD) insertion

Physician: Frank Vincent, MD
Anesthesia: Conscious sedation

PROCEDURE: Patient is a 4-year-old female, with a recent diagnosis of malignancy. Due to an upcoming course of chemotherapy, the CVAD is being inserted to ease administration of the drugs. The patient was placed on the table in supine position. The patient is given Versed to achieve conscious sedation. The incision was made to insert a central venous catheter, centrally. During the placement of the catheter, a short tract (non-tunneled) is made as the catheter is advanced from the skin entry site to the point of venous cannulation. The catheter tip is set to reside in the subclavian vein. The patient was gently aroused from the sedation and was awake when transported to the recovery room.

Frank Vincent, MD

FV/mg   D: 9/25/08 09:50:16   T: 9/25/08 12:55:01

You Code It!

What are the best, most accurate codes?

_____

_____

_____

SWANSON ONCOLOGY
969 TURNABOUT LANE • REMISSION, FL 32811 • 407-555-9573

PATIENT: TRANSIL, BRENDA
ACCOUNT/EHR #:   TRABR001
Date: 9/29/08

Attending Physician: Benjamin L. Johnston, MD

Referring Physician: James I. Cipher, MD

HPI: The patient is well known to me from her earlier hospitalization. This is a 71-year-old female with a past history of metastatic follicular carcinoma of the thyroid who had been recently retreated at this medical center for superior vena cava syndrome and obstruction with anticoagulation. At that time, she developed a febrile illness, at which time infectious disease was consulted.

It turned out that an infectious disease workup was negative and it was felt that she had an underlying autoimmune type basis for her fever and was put on prednisone. On the prednisone, her fever resolved and all the other symptoms resolved, and she had been doing quite well.

In the interim, it was determined that she did have metastatic thyroid carcinoma disease and so, she was admitted today for radioactive iodine therapy. However, during the physical examination at the clinic yesterday, Dr. Radner discovered an abdominal mass. She denied any history of trauma; denied fevers, chills, sweats, or other systemic symptoms. She had been doing quite well actually since going home on low-dose maintenance prednisone therapy.

A CT was done that showed a retroperitoneal mass and a CT-guided biopsy was done this morning that revealed frank pus. She subsequently underwent drainage of 500 cc of grossly purulent material, described as pea-green soup. We are now asked to consult to help with the antibiotic management. The fluid did not apparently appear to be foul smelling but did look green and thick.

The patient, again, continues to deny any fevers, chills, sweats, or systemic symptoms. At the time the subsequent drainage was done today, two drainage catheters were placed into the abscess. She experienced hypotension, nausea, and diaphoresis, which resolved with some fluid boluses. She is now in the IMC for further management because of the episode of hypotension and a concern of sepsis.

Again, on talking to the patient, she denies any history of trauma to the area. She denies any history of abdominal pain, fevers, chills, sweats, nausea, vomiting, diarrhea, or systemic symptoms. She has no past history of diverticulitis or diverticular diseases. She has not had any diarrhea or abdominal pain.

The preliminary Gram stain results shows a few white blood cells; no organisms. Cultures are pending.

Her white count at this time was 12,800, with a left shift but she is on oral prednisone. The sedimentation rate was 42. The PT was 12.4 and the PTT is 25. The chemistries are remarkable for a glucose of 115, albumin of 3.6, cholesterol of 235, and the liver function tests were normal.

PAST MEDICAL HISTORY: As stated, the past medical history is significant for follicular cell carcinoma of the thyroid, status post subtotal thyroidectomy, 03/07/96; status post right internal jugular repair from tumor invasion into the jugular; and biopsy of mediastinal metastatic disease. The patient is also status post carcinoma. She is status post mastectomy for breast carcinoma in 07/05. She has post-thoracotomy syndrome in 03/07, with fever and effusion, which resolved. She has a history of a small clot at the site of the venogram entry of the left leg. She had been on Coumadin and may possibly have had a retroperitoneal bleed. She also has a history of hypocalcemia secondary to her thyroidectomy and is on calcium maintenance.

MEDICATIONS: Her medications at this time include Nolvadex 10 mg po bid; Os-Cal 1000 mg po tid; Rocaltrol 0.25 mcg po bid; and prednisone 10 mg po qam

ALLERGIES: She is ALLERGIC TO PENICILLIN and SULFA.

REVIEW OF SYSTEMS: As stated, the review of systems is essentially unremarkable. She denies fevers, chills, sweats, abdominal pain, nausea, vomiting, and diarrhea. The fevers had resolved on the prednisone.

PHYSICAL EXAM: BP 100/60; P 90; T 98.4

Continued

APPEARANCE: Alert, oriented, in no acute distress.

HEAD: Normocephalic, atraumatic.

EYES: Pupils are equal, round, and reactive to light and accommodation. Extraocular movements full.

MOUTH/TONGUE/PHARYNX: Throat clear. No thrush or exudates.

NECK: Supple. No stiffness.

LUNGS: Few crackles at both bases. Scattered rhonchi bilaterally. Good air exchange.

CARDIVASC: Regular rhythm. Normal S1 and S2. No murmurs.

ABDOMEN: Soft. Some tenderness in the right middle quadrant, with drainage catheters in place and no definite mass appreciated at this time.

EXTREMITIES: No joint effusions or deformities. Trace edema of the ankles.

SKIN: Some scattered ecchymoses. No significant rashes or lesions noted.

NEURO: Grossly normal. No focal deficits.

IMPRESSION:
1. Retroperitoneal mass appears to be an abscess; may possibly have been secondary to a possible bleed that secondarily got infected. She has had no preceding systemic signs of infection or trauma to the area. Other etiologies would be some type of relationship to possible abdominal disease but she has no history of diverticular disease and this would be less likely. The most likely organisms to consider, again, would be Staphylococcus, Streptococcus, anaerobes, and gut flora.
2. Metastatic thyroid follicular carcinoma; to receive radiation therapy.

PLAN/RECOMMENDATIONS:
1. Will start her empirically on intravenous antibiotic therapy with clindamycin and Cipro, which should cover Staphylococcus, Streptococcus, anaerobes, and gram-negatives, until more culture results are known.
2. Monitor vital signs carefully and supportive care if she becomes hypotensive again.
3. Will check blood cultures as well as urine culture.
4. Would not give radioactive iodine at this time until we have cleared up her infection.

Thanks for the consultation. Will follow.

Benjamin L. Johnston, MD

BLJ/mg   D: 9/29/08 09:50:16   T: 10/1/08 12:55:01

You Code It!

What are the best, most accurate codes?

SWANSON ONCOLOGY
969 TURNABOUT LANE • REMISSION, FL 32811 • 407-555-9573

PATIENT: ABERNATHY, CARTER
ACCOUNT/EHR #:   ABECA001
Date: 10/15/08

Attending Physician: Valerie R. Victors, MD

S: Pt is a 45-year-old male diagnosed with carcinoma of the inner cheek three months ago. He has chewed tobacco for the last twenty years. Pt states he quit chewing 6 weeks ago. He presents today for his therapeutic injection.

O: Pt is brought into the examining room, and given an injection of Interferon Alfa-2a, 3 million units, IM.

A: Malignant carcinoma, cheek, internal

P: Series of injections to continue on daily basis

___

Valerie R. Victors, MD

VRV/mg   D: 10/15/08 09:50:16   T: 10/17/08 12:55:01

You Code It!

What are the best, most accurate codes?

___

___

___

SWANSON ONCOLOGY
969 TURNABOUT LANE • REMISSION, FL 32811 • 407-555-9573

PATIENT: LANGER, DENNY
ACCOUNT/EHR #:   LANDE001
Date: 10/15/08

Attending Physician: Valerie R. Victors, MD

Diagnosis on Admission: History of Ewing's sarcoma with recurrent chemotherapy for progressive disease

Final Diagnosis: Known Ewing's sarcoma with pulmonary metastases, with apparent resolution of thoracic and vertebral involvement

Consultations and Procedures during course of hospital stay:

                                      Routine imaging studies, including 1. Chest x-ray; 2. CT scan of the thorax; 3. Nucleotide bone scan

History of present illness and brief hospital course by system: Briefly, the patient is a 32-year-old male with a known history of Ewing's sarcoma of the left lower extremity, first diagnosed in 1998. The patient was subsequently found to have pulmonary metastases. He has been seen previously in the hematology/oncology clinic for routine chemotherapy consisting of vincristine, cyclophosphamide, Doxorubicin, and routine bone marrow rescue with GCSF therapy. Current therapy includes a regime of Cytoxan, Cyclophosphamide and Topotecan which corresponds to pediatric oncology group protocol #9354.

     Current admission at presentation, patient was well appearing with no significant medical problems, except for his known Ewing's. He was hydrated as per protocol and tolerated the chemotherapy routine well. Serum chemistries remained stable during the course of the hospital stay. Significant findings during the course of the hospital stay included the results of the imaging studies alluded to previously. 1. Routine chest x-ray obtained 7/28/08 showed the presence of a port-a-cath well positioned in the superior vena cava. In addition, there appeared to be an improving pattern of pulmonary metastases from the known Ewing's sarcoma when compared to films from 6/11/00. 2. Computerized spiral tomography of the thorax obtained 7/28/08, when compared to similar films from 5/9/00, showed significant interval improvement of metastatic disease, involving both the pulmonary parenchyma and the mediastinum of known Ewing's sarcoma. There were persistent small numerous pulmonary nodules which appeared to be in resolution when compared to earlier films. 3. Nucleotide-99 HTP bone scan obtained 7/28/08, compared to a previous study of 6/12/00, showed a) a persistent left posterior skull and possible left side of the L2 vertebra to have activity; however, these were less intense than on the previous study. B) There was an expansile lesion present in the distal left femur which was a similar distribution of activity, but again it seemed to be less intense. C) There had been resolution of activity which had previously been noted on the right side of the T8 vertebra and the sixth costal rib posteriorly had resolved.

     Patient is admitted to begin a chemotherapeutic regime.

Valerie R. Victors, MD

VRV/mg   D: 10/15/08 09:50:16   T: 10/17/08 12:55:01

You Code It!

What are the best, most accurate codes?

_____

_____

_____

PATIENT: ALLMAN, SERITA
ACCOUNT/EHR #:   ALLSE001
Date: 10/15/08

Attending Physician: Matthew Saunders, MD

CC: Patient with Ewing's sarcoma, routine chemotherapy

HPI: This is a 10-year-old female with Ewing's sarcoma of the left lower extremity diagnosed in 2005. The patient was scheduled for radiation in 2006 when significant pulmonary metastases were found. Last admission was July 6, 2006, for chemotherapy consisting of vincristine, cyclophosphamide, doxorubicin, mesna and G-CSF. Previous admission was June 11, 2006, for ifosfamide, cyclophosphamide, and etoposide chemotherapy. Previous sick hospital admission was May 8, 2006 for a pleural effusion. The patient has had no intercurrent illnesses, no nausea, vomiting, diarrhea, or constipation since the last admission. No fevers. The patient has noted some mucositis following the past chemotherapy which resolved with Miles Magic mouthwash eight days ago.

Past Medical History: Is as above for Ewing's sarcoma of left lower extremity, the patient has received chemotherapy. Last chemotherapy consisting of pediatric oncology group #9354, regime A with ICE, the patient is currently starting. Birth history: The patient was born at 34 weeks gestation, birth weight of six pounds, no complications following delivery. Developmental history: The patient had normal milestones. Immunizations are up to date to three years of age. Past surgical history: The patient had multiple catheter replacements and a bone marrow biopsy.

Allergies: Phenergan

Medications: None

Social history: The patient lives with her mother, father, two brothers, and one sister. They have no pets. There are no smokers in the home.

Family history: Paternal grandmother with breast cancer.

ROS:

PE:

Vital Signs: Temperature 98.1, pulse 115, respirations 20, blood pressure 110/61, height 143.5 cm, weight 28.1 kilos.

General: The patient is a female with alopecia in no acute distress.

HEENT: Complete alopecia, normocephalic, atraumatic. Pupils are equal and reactive to light, fundi are visualized without lesions. TMs are gray bilaterally with good landmarks. Pharynx is clear, mucous membranes are without lesions.

Neck: No lymphadenopathy is noted.

Lungs: Clear to auscultation bilaterally.

Chest: There is a PermCath in the right chest which is intact without tenderness.

Heart: Cardiac exam is with regular rate and rhythm without murmurs or rubs.

Abdomen: Positive bowel sounds, nontender, nondistended with no hepatosplenomegaly noted, the patient's abdomen is soft.

Pelvic/Rectal: GU deferred.

Continued

Extremities: No clubbing, cyanosis or edema. Pulses are 2+ femorals, distal posterior tibial pulses, dorsalis pedis and radial pulses. Capillary refill is less than two seconds.

Neuro: The patient was alert and oriented and responds to questions appropriately. Cranial nerves II-XII are grossly intact. Sensation is intact bilaterally. The patient's muscle strength is 5/5 bilaterally. Deep tendon reflexes are 2+ in all groups.

Assessment: This is a 10-year-old patient with metastatic Ewing's sarcoma here for routine chemotherapy. Pediatric Oncology Group #9464 consisting of cyclophosphamide, topotecan chemotherapy.

1. Oncology. The patient will have lab drawn, CBC with diff, retic count, complete metabolic profile, LDH, and UA prior to starting chemotherapy. Other labs: The patient will have chest x-ray, AP and lateral, CT scan, bone scan during hospital stay. The patient will be prehydrated with 550 cc of D5 1/4 normal saline over 30 minutes q.d. times five days. The patient will receive Zofran 4mg IV q8h times five days. The patient will receive cyclophosphamide 275 mg. in 55 cc of normal saline IV over 30 minutes q.d. times five days. The patient will received topotecan 0.8 mg in 50 cc D5W IV over 30 minutes q.d. times five days. The patient will continue hydration post chemotherapy D5 1/4 normal saline at 75 cc/hour until next day of chemo, q.d. times five days. On day six, the patient will be on G-CSF 140 mcg subcu q.d. times 10-14 days post nadir of absolute neutrophil count greater than or equal to 5,000.
2. Hematologic. The patient will have type and cross on parents' blood for direct donated white blood cells if needed; the patient will be sent to the Blood Bank for type and donation.
3. ID. The patient will be observed for fever.
4. Social. Patient plan discussed with parents with me present. The parents agree to chemotherapy.
5. The patient will have a regular diet, routine vital signs, and activity as tolerated.

Matthew Saunders, MD

MS/mg   D: 10/15/08 09:50:16   T: 10/17/08 12:55:01

You Code It!

What are the best, most accurate codes?

_____

_____

_____

SWANSON ONCOLOGY
969 TURNABOUT LANE • REMISSION, FL 32811 • 407-555-9573

PATIENT: GARRISON, THEODORE
ACCOUNT/EHR #:   GARTH001
Date: 10/15/08

Attending Physician: Matthew Saunders, MD

1. Metastatic colon carcinoma, on palliative systemic chemotherapy with second line chemotherapy combination at this time.
2. Obstructive uropathy, status post replacement of internal ureteral stent.

Complications: None

Special Procedures: Replacement of ureteral stent by Dr. Surikian on 6/30/08; port placement by Dr. Madison on 6/26/08.

Discharge Medications: OxyContin 40 mg p.o. q12 hours, Neurontin 300 m g p.o. t.i.d., Vicodin one or two every 4 hours as needed for breakthrough pain, Zantac 150 mg p.o. b.i.d., Magic mouth wash one or two teaspoons for symptomatic sore mouth and sore throat.

Disposition: The patient will be followed by the MD Anderson Cancer Center in two weeks' time, at which time restaging studies will be scheduled.

Hospital Course: Patient is a pleasant 38-year-old unfortunate black male with progressive metastatic colon carcinoma, having failed first line chemotherapy with Camptosar, 5FU, and Leucovorin and is currently on 5FU infusion therapy at monthly intervals with Mitomycin added to every odd numbered cycle of same. He was admitted on 6/26/08 for cycle #3 of 5 FU with Mitomycin this time. He tolerated the chemotherapy quite well. To facilitate ongoing therapy, a port was placed at my request on the day of admission by Dr. Madison, and also at the patient's request, a urology consultation with Dr. Surikian was requested for replacement of the internal ureteral stent which was accomplished on 6/30/08.

    The patient remained stable with good performance status at 70% or better on a Karnofsky scale throughout the hospital course.

    Vital signs have remained stable and he is being discharged in stable condition with the above follow up instructions.

Matthew Saunders, MD

MS/mg   D: 10/15/08 09:50:16   T: 10/17/08 12:55:01

You Code It!

What are the best, most accurate codes?

_____

_____

_____

SWANSON ONCOLOGY
969 TURNABOUT LANE • REMISSION, FL 32811 • 407-555-9573

PATIENT: HAWAN, MARILYN
ACCOUNT/EHR #:   HAWMA001
Date: 10/15/08

Preop DX: Right ureteral obstruction secondary to colon cancer
Postop DX: Same
Operation: 1. Cystoscopy
                                   2. Right retrograde pyelogram
                                   3. Removal and replacement of double-J stent

Surgeon   Michael Surikian, MD
Anesthesia: General

HISTORY/INDICATIONS: This is a 28-year-old black female with a history of colon cancer and secondary right ureteral obstruction who had a stent inserted a number of months ago. At this time, she is in the hospital and it is time for a stent change. Consequently, the patient presents for the procedure.

PROCEDURE: The patient was taken to the operating room and there she was given general anesthetic, positioned in the dorsal lithotomy position, the genitalia scrubbed and prepped with Betadine. Sterile towels and sheets were utilized to drape the patient in the usual fashion. A cystoscope was introduced into the bladder. The ureteral catheter was identified. It was grabbed and removed without any difficulty. Subsequently, the cystoscope was reinserted into the bladder and the right ureteral orifice was identified over a Pollack catheter. A glide wire was inserted into the right collecting system. Some contrast was injected and a hydronephrotic right side was noted. Then, the wire was placed through the Pollack catheter. With the wire in position, over the wire a 7 French 26 cm double-J stent was inserted. Excellent coiling was noted fluoroscopically in the kidney and distally with a cystoscope. The bladder was then drained and again it was inspected prior to removal. There was no evidence of any tumors or lesions in the bladder. The stent was in good position. The cystoscope was removed and the patient was taken to the recovery room awake and in stable condition.

Michael Surikian, MD

MS/mg   D: 10/15/08 09:50:16   T: 10/17/08 12:55:01

You Code It!

What are the best, most accurate codes?

_____

_____

_____

SWANSON ONCOLOGY
969 TURNABOUT LANE • REMISSION, FL 32811 • 407-555-9573

PATIENT:	LIGHTFOOT, WANITA
ACCOUNT/EHR #:	LIGWA001
Date:	10/15/08

Preop DX:	Cervical cancer
Post op DX:	Same
Operation:	Examination under anesthesia and placement of tandem for afterloading radiation

Surgeon:	Jacob Sapperstein, MD/David Buckman, MD
Assistant:	Caroline Blythe, MD
Anesthesia:	General anesthesia

PROCEDURE: After adequate induction of general anesthesia, the patient was placed in the dorsal lithotomy position and she was prepped and draped in the usual sterile manner for vaginal surgery. An exam under anesthesia was performed. The patient has had a significant response to her external beam radiation and chemotherapy. Initially, she had a large 3B lesion with tumor extending from side wall to side wall. Today she has fibrosis in both parametria. The right parametria is free from the side wall and there is some movement allowed there. The left side is not as free, but again it mostly feels like smooth fibrosis as opposed to nodular tumor. The upper vagina is very small due to the radiation changes and there is no viable-appearing tumor on the cervix. We could not identify cervix today. There was an os uterus. After exam under anesthesia, she was prepped and draped and a weighted speculum was placed in the vagina. A Deaver retractor was utilized to identify the upper vagina. A sound was used, the os was identified, and the uterus sounded to 7 cm. We dilated the cervix then and allowed placement of a tandem. The vaginal walls were too small and too close together to allow placement of even the smallest ovoid we had available, and so Dr. Buckman decided to just place the tandem in, so the tandem was packed. Foley catheter was placed. Five cc of radiopaque dye were placed in the Foley bulb. After packing the tandem in place, we then sutured the labia to the tandem so that it would not move during treatment. The patient tolerated the procedure well. Blood loss was minimal and she was taken to recovery in stable condition.

10/15/08 11:47:39

You Code It!

What are the best, most accurate codes?

_____

_____

_____

SWANSON ONCOLOGY
969 TURNABOUT LANE • REMISSION, FL 32811 • 407-555-9573

PATIENT: FLICKER, PHOEBE
ACCOUNT/EHR #:   FLIPH001
Date: 10/15/08

H&P

CC: The patient is a 70-year-old woman admitted from the outpatient department with a chief complaint of bloating and gas for one week.

HPI: The patient had been on a cruise and had about a one-week history of bloating, gas per rectum as well as burping, early satiety, and indigestion. These symptoms were similar to what she had prior to her cholecystectomy, as well as when she first diagnosed with gastroparesis. The symptoms are worse after eating meat. The patient also has been noticing increased swelling of her ankles, which is usually very mild, and some shortness of breath. She denies cough, paroxysmal nocturnal dyspnea, palpitations, chest pain or diaphoresis.

    In the Outpatient department, she had an electrocardiogram done, which showed a new right bundle branch block, and she was transferred here to rule out a myocardial infarction.

Past medical history: Hypercholesterolemia; hypertension; diabetes, insulin requiring; gastroparesis; stress test two years ago, which was normal; endoscopy three years ago

Past surgical history: Cholecystectomy

Medications: At home, Dyazide 1 tablet a day; Vasotec 5.0 mg a day; Mevacor 20 mg a day; Prilosec 20 mg a day; Reglan 20 mg twice a day; insulin 70/30, 35 Iu in the morning, and 20 Iu in the evening

Allergies: No known drug allergies

Social history: The patient does not smoke and drinks about one to two shots of whiskey every night to help her sleep. She is recently retired and lives with her husband and is active.

Review of systems: The review of systems is also positive for weight gain, occasional loose stool without blood or diarrhea, and chronic sleeplessness. Her diabetes is well controlled.

PE

BP: 127/70; Pulse 88; Resp 16; T: afebrile

Appearance: The patient looked well, is obese, and has good skin.

Head: Clear

Eyes: Clear

Ears: Clear

Nose: Clear

Mouth/Tongue/Pharynx: Clear

Neck: She has a mild goiter.

Lungs: Good bilateral air entry, resonant, with a few bibasilar crackles

Cardiovasc: Regular rate and rhythm, with a normal jugular venous pressure. Heart sounds 1 and 2, with no rubs, murmurs, or gallops, and no carotid bruits.

Abdomen: Obese but soft, nontender, with a large cholecystectomy scar. Bowel sounds were very active.

Continued

Extremities: The lower extremity examination was remarkable for 2+ pitting edema and 3+ pulses, with no evidence of deep venous thrombosis.

Neurological: Grossly normal

Electrocardiogram: The electrocardiogram showed sinus rhythm with right bundle branch block but no acute or old myocardial infarction and no ischemic changes.

Diagnoses:
1. This is a 70-year-old female with abdominal symptoms and a new right bundle branch block. Possible myocardial infarction but is very unlikely, although this needs to be ruled out.
2. Probable diabetic gastroparesis worsening but also exacerbated by excesses on the cruise.
3. Fluid retention due to increased sodium/water intake.
4. Pulmonary embolus is very unlikely.

Plan/Recommendations:
1. Admit to telemetry.
2. Check SMA-20, CBC, urinalysis, TSH, and serial cardiac enzymes and electrocardiograms.
3. Also, check chest x-ray and KUB.
4. She has been started on aspirin and topical nitroglycerin.
5. She will be started on Propulsid 10 mg t.i.d. and gastroesophageal reflux disease precautions.
6. She will also be seen by the dietician for weight reduction.
7. We will continue to control her diabetes.

Robyn Bennito, MD

10/15/08 11:47:39

You Code It!

What are the best, most accurate codes?

_____

_____

_____

SWANSON ONCOLOGY
969 TURNABOUT LANE • REMISSION, FL 32811 • 407-555-9573

PATIENT: MC SWAIN, WILMA
ACCOUNT/EHR #:   MCSWI001
Date: 10/15/08

HPI: The patient is a 45-year-old woman who was readmitted from the outpatient department. She came in complaining of bloating and swelling of her ankles. The patient was in on 3/20/08, with the above symptoms and was diagnosed with worsening gastroparesis and gastroesophageal reflux disease. She was symptomatically improved on Propulsid, but the symptoms did not totally abate. She was seen in the outpatient department on follow up and had an ultrasound of the abdomen. This showed ascites, small liver and large spleen. The patient was admitted for further workup.

    The patient's alcohol consumption is one to two drinks every night to help her sleep. Occasionally, she has none for a week, but usually no more.

PMH: The patient's past medical history includes hypercholesterolemia, hypertension, diabetes type II insulin requiring, gastroparesis, cholecystectomy and obesity.

Medications:
Lasix 20 mg a day
Potassium chloride
Vasotec 5 mg a day
Mevacor 20 mg a day
Prilosec 50 mg a day
Propulsid 10 mg t.i.d.
Insulin 70/30, 20 in the morning and 10 in the evening

PE

Vital Signs: Stable

Head: Clear

Eyes: Clear

Ears: Clear

Nose: Clear

Mouth/Tongue/Pharynx: Clear

Chest: Clear

Cardiovasc: Regular rate and rhythm. Heart sounds S1, S2. Jugular venous pressure was normal. No S3.

Abdomen: The abdomen is obese and very distended. It was difficult to ascertain splenomegaly and there was ascites on percussion.

Extremities: The lower extremities showed 2+ edema and good pulses.

Electrocardiogram: The electrocardiogram showed a sinus rhythm with no changes to previous one.

Laboratory: The Chem-7 was normal with a creatinine of 1, glucose was 174. The liver function tests were totally normal as they were on the previous admission.
    The CBC was normal with a hemoglobin of 12.5 and a normal differential.

Continued

                      Chapter 14   Oncology Cases and Patient Records

Diagnosis:

1. Ascites and edema, probably secondary to cirrhosis and portal hypertension. The differential for this is ovarian cancer, gastrointestinal malignancy or other intra-abdominal malignancy.
2. Cirrhosis due to alcohol – autoimmune hepatitis – medications – heart failure.

Plan/Recommendations:

1. The plan is to admit.
2. The patient will undergo paracentesis.
3. We will check for cytology, culture, cell count and albumin.
4. Check a 2-D echocardiogram for left ventricular failure.
5. CT scan for the abdomen and pelvis for malignancy.

We will start on spironolactone for her ascites and edema.

Robyn Bennito, MD

10/15/08 11:47:39

You Code It!

What are the best, most accurate codes?

_____

_____

_____

SWANSON ONCOLOGY
969 TURNABOUT LANE • REMISSION, FL 32811 • 407-555-9573

PATIENT: REESE, REBECCA
ACCOUNT/EHR #:   REERE001
Date: 10/15/08

Rebecca is an 18-month-old female brought by her parents to the office on referral from Dr. Herrin, her pediatrician. He noted something during the ophthalmoscopy exam during her last well-baby exam.

PAST MEDICAL HISTORY: There is no history of weight loss, anorexia, crossed eyes, fever, or irritability.

EXAM: VS T 37.0, P 110, R 26, BP 92/42. Height, weight, head circumference are all at the 40th percentile. She is alert and active. On a routine ophthalmoscopy exam, Dr. Herrin noted that the child does not have a red reflex in the right eye. Leukocoria is present in the right eye. A normal red reflex observed in the left eye. The ophthalmoscopy exam performed today reveals a tumor in the posterior pole of the right eye. An orbital CT demonstrates that the tumor is confined to the globe (i.e., no spread outside the eye). Pupils are equal and reactive. The eyes are conjugate. Facial function is good. The remainder of the physical examination is negative.

DIAGNOSIS: Tumor, posterior pole, right eye

CLINICAL COURSE: Since the tumor is small it is treated with laser photoablation. Careful follow-ups are scheduled to monitor for recurrences or development of secondary tumors.

Robyn Bennito, MD

10/15/08 11:47:39

You Code It!

What are the best, most accurate codes?

_____

_____

_____

SWANSON ONCOLOGY
969 TURNABOUT LANE • REMISSION, FL 32811 • 407-555-9573

PATIENT: LUCAS, MORGAN
ACCOUNT/EHR #: LUCMO001
Date: 10/15/08

Morgan is a 10-year-old boy, brought into the ED by his parents, with epistaxis for two hours and hematemesis. He complains of nausea, constipation, severe hip pain and headache. He has a history of recurrent Stage IV neuroblastoma, initially diagnosed two years ago, treated with chemotherapy and a bone marrow transplant. He received chemotherapy again when his cancer recurred six months ago. Initially his tumor responded, but eventually it progressed and includes bone marrow involvement. He has started experimental chemotherapy at the request of his parents, with his assent. He has multiple metastatic bone lesions, most pronounced on his head and right hip. He has required increasing doses of pain medications. He has been attending school a few hours a day, but this week he has been increasingly tired with increased pallor. This morning, he woke up with epistaxis that would not stop with pressure. About 1 hour later he started vomiting bright red blood. He is currently taking 8 mg of hydromorphone (Dilaudid) orally every 6 hours around the clock for pain. He rates his current pain level as a 6 on a scale of 10.

EXAM: VS T 37, P 120, RR 18, BP 100/50. His skin is pale and dry with multiple bruises. He has multiple lumps on his scalp. Dried blood, blood clots and some oozing blood is noted in both nares. Subconjunctival hemorrhages and pallor are noted. His neck is supple with no lymphadenopathy. Heart regular rate without murmurs. Lungs are clear. A central venous catheter is present in his left anterior chest. His abdomen is soft with no hepatosplenomegaly. There is mild tenderness. Exam of his extremities is significant for bruising and pallor. He has moderate tenderness over his back, hips and pelvis.

LAB: WBC 2.4, 70% neutrophils, Hgb 6.2, Hct 19.6, platelet count 3,000.

HOSPITAL COURSE: He receives packed RBC transfusions to correct his anemia (which may also improve his stamina) and platelet transfusions which stop his epistaxis. He is started on MS Contin (slow release morphine) 60 mg PO q12 hr with morphine 15 mg PO for breakthrough pain as needed which controls his pain well. His physician discusses the future use of IV morphine on a patient controlled analgesia (PCA) pump. He is started on Senokot (senna) to prevent constipation. Since he seems to improve, or at least remain stable, with the experimental chemotherapy, this is continued.

Linda F. Rasmussen, MD

10/15/08 11:47:39

You Code It!

What are the best, most accurate codes?

_____

_____

_____

Ophthalmology Cases and Patient Records

INTRODUCTION

The following case studies are from an ophthalmology practice. In an ophthalmology office, a professional coding specialist is likely to see many different types of health conditions, including preventive health care services.

When it comes to caring for the eyes of a patient, there may be three different types of eye care specialists involved.

Ophthalmologists are trained to diagnose and treat eye diseases, such as macular degeneration, conjunctivitis, and ophthalmia neonatorum. In addition, they care for patients with injuries to the eye, such as a foreign body in the eye or a detached retina; and perform surgery, such as cataract removal, glaucoma correction, or LASIK surgery.

An optometrist is a health care professional who is trained and licensed to perform eye examinations and to prescribe eyeglasses and contact lenses. While an ophthalmologist may also prescribe eyeglasses or contact lenses in addition to other services, an optometrist is limited to this work.

The eye care specialist who will typically provide those glasses or lenses is called an optician. Opticians are not permitted to examine the eyes or prescribe glasses or lenses. They are professionals trained in grinding and forming lenses.

Ophthalmologists may decide to maintain a subspecialty, such as a retina specialist or a pediatric ophthalmologist.

Ophthalmologists are board-certified by the Board of Ophthalmology, which is recognized by the American Board of Medical Specialties.

You can use these cases to practice coding diagnoses, E/M, procedures, DME, or other HCPCS Level II items, as applicable; code for the physician or the facility; code inpatient and outpatient services, as applicable:

1. Code for the physician.
2. Code for the anesthesiologist, when applicable.
3. Code for the hospital, when applicable.
4. Code for the pathology and laboratory, when applicable.
5. Code HCPCS Level II codes, when applicable.

OPHTHALMOLOGY CARE CENTER
6481 SIGHT BOULEVARD • ANYTOWN, FL 32719 • 407-555-5137

PATIENT: PORTLAND, BROOKE
ACCOUNT/EHR #:   PORTBR002
Date of Operation: 06/17/08

Preoperative Diagnosis: Nuclear sclerosis 2+ with a 2+ posterior subcapsular cataract, right eye
Postoperative Diagnosis: Same
Operation: Phacoemulsification of cataract with posterior chamber intraocular lens
                                 implantation, right eye

Surgeon: Julian Gallagher, MD
Assistant: Cindy Morse, MD
Anesthesia: Local

DESCRIPTION OF OPERATIVE PROCEDURE: Local anesthesia was obtained with retrobulbar and modified Van Lint injection using a 50-50 mixture of 4 percent Lidocaine and 0.75 percent Marcaine with Wydase. A Honan balloon was placed for approximately 15 minutes. The patient was positioned, prepped and draped in the usual sterile fashion. A wire lid speculum was inserted, and the operating microscope was brought into position. A temporal limbal corneal incision was made with a 2.75 mm keratome, and Viscoat was injected into the anterior chamber. Using a cystotome and Utrata forceps, a continuous tear capsulorrhexis was performed. A limbal paracentesis stab incision was made at 6 o'clock with a diamond blade. Hydrodissection and hydrodelineation of the lens was accomplished with balanced salt solution via cannular injection. Phacoemulsification of the lens proceeded as the lens was sectioned into quadrants with each quadrant removed. Residual lens cortex was removed with irrigation and aspiration. The posterior capsule was polished with an irrigating Graether collar button. Viscoat was injected into the capsular bag, and the cataract incision was opened with the keratome. Using lens-folding forceps, an Alcon, Model MA60VM, 6.0 mm optic, 21.5 diopter posterior chamber intraocular lens was inserted into the capsular bag. A Sinskey hook was used to facilitate rotation and centration of the lens. Residual anterior chamber Viscoat was removed with irrigation and aspiration. Balanced salt solution was injected into the anterior chamber, and the wound was observed to be watertight. Subconjunctival Celestone and Cefazolin were injected. Topical Iopidine solution and Maxitrol ophthalmic ointment were instilled. Dressing included eye pad and Fox shield. The patient tolerated the procedure well without complications.

Julian Gallagher, M.D.

JG/mg   D: 06/17/08 09:50:16   T: 06/19/08 12:55:01

You Code It!

What are the best, most accurate codes?

_____

_____

_____

OPHTHALMOLOGY CARE CENTER
6481 SIGHT BOULEVARD • ANYTOWN, FL 32719 • 407-555-5137

PATIENT: WESTERBY, ELMO
ACCOUNT/EHR #:   WESTEL001
Date: 09/16/08

Attending Physician: Suzanne R. Taylor, MD

Preoperative DX: Orbital mass, OD
Postoperative DX: Herniated orbital fat pad, OD
Procedure: Excision of mass and repair, right superior orbit

Surgeon: Raul Sanchez, MD
Anesthesia: Local

PROCEDURE: After proparacaine was instilled in the eye, it was prepped and draped in the usual sterile manner and 2 percent Lidocaine with 1:200,000 epinephrine was injected into the superior aspect of the right orbit. A corneal protective shield was placed in the eye. The eye was placed in down-gaze.

The upper lid was everted and the fornix examined. The herniating mass was viewed and measured at 0.75 cm in diameter. Westcott scissors were used to incise the fornicele conjunctiva. The herniating mass was then clamped, excised, and cauterized. It appeared to contain mostly fat tissue, which was sent to pathology.

The superior fornix was repaired using running suture of 6-0 plain gut. Bacitracin ointment was applied to the eye followed by an eye pad. The patient tolerated the procedure well and left the operating room in good condition.

_____

Suzanne R. Taylor, MD

SRT/pw   D: 9/16/08 09:50:16   T: 9/18/08 12:55:01

You Code It!

What are the best, most accurate codes?

_____

_____

_____

OPHTHALMOLOGY CARE CENTER
6481 SIGHT BOULEVARD • ANYTOWN, FL 32719 • 407-555-5137

PATIENT: GROENENDAL, PETER
ACCOUNT/EHR #:   GROEPE001
Date: 09/16/08

The patient is a 61-year-old male who came into the office due to progressive right eye swelling and loss of vision. He was diagnosed with Type 2 diabetes approximately 5 years ago. Patient complained about severe headaches, on the right side of his head, which began about 1 week ago. He also had a fever and blurred vision during that time period. There is a personal history of frequent nasal congestion and sinus tenderness for which he took over-the-counter decongestants and blew his nose forcibly. During this same week he had been admitted to the hospital for erythema and swelling over the right eye and received IV antibiotics for 5 days. WBC 18,600 with 72% PMN and 11% band forms, glucose 364, lumbar puncture 8 WBC, protein 90 mg% and glucose 130 mg%. CT scan suggested right retrobulbar density and maxillary sinusitis.

    On PE, severe proptosis of the right eye with conjunctival and scleral edema and minimal eye movement. No vision or light perception. Bilateral frontal and ethmoid sinus tenderness (RT>LT): otherwise PE within normal limits. Patient placed on nafcillin, ceftazidime and Flagyl for orbital cellulites versus cavernous sinus thrombosis. Mucormycosis entertained but amphotericin B not administered. Multiple cultures (blood, superficial, operative) negative. Surgery included orbitotomy, ethmoidotomy and sphenoidotomy.

    CT with contrast revealed marked proptosis of the right orbit, thrombosis and enlargement of the right superior ophthalmic vein as well as increased density and prominence of the right cavernous sinus. There was opacification of the sphenoid and ethmoid sinuses and the left maxillary sinus. Changes suggesting chronic sinusitis also observed in the right maxillary sinus and both frontal sinuses.

Suzanne R. Taylor, MD

SRT/pw   D: 9/16/08 09:50:16   T: 9/18/08 12:55:01

You Code It!

What are the best, most accurate codes?

_____

_____

_____

OPHTHALMOLOGY CARE CENTER
6481 SIGHT BOULEVARD • ANYTOWN, FL 32719 • 407-555-5137

PATIENT: ROBINET, RENAY
ACCOUNT/EHR #:   ROBIRE001
Date: 10/7/08

Attending Physician: Walter P. Henricks, MD
Referring Physician: Valerie Victors, MD

This new Pt is a 36-year-old female who lost her right eye in a skiing accident. She presents today for the prescription, fitting, and placement of her ocular prosthesis (artificial eye).

P: Follow-up in one month.

_____

Walter P. Henricks, MD

WPH/mg   D: 10/7/08 09:50:16   T: 10/9/08 12:55:01

You Code It!

What are the best, most accurate codes?

_____

_____

_____

OPHTHALMOLOGY CARE CENTER
6481 SIGHT BOULEVARD • ANYTOWN, FL 32719 • 407-555-5137

PATIENT: DENTMER, BARNEY
ACCOUNT/EHR #:   DENTBAR001
Date: 10/7/08

Attending Physician: Walter P. Henricks, MD

This is a 4-week-old male infant born to a 26-year-old G2P2 O+, rubella immune, group B strep negative, HBsAg negative, VDRL negative, GC and Chlamydia negative married female at 40 weeks gestation via spontaneous vaginal delivery with Apgar scores of 8 and 9 at 1 and 5 minutes. Pregnancy, delivery and postpartum hospital course were uncomplicated. He presents with his mother to our office with a two-day history of bilateral eye drainage. He had been in good health until two days ago when he developed yellow drainage and mild periorbital swelling.

    Review of systems is negative except for the recent development of a cough that he "probably caught from his older brother."

EXAM: VS T 37.5, P 120, RR 60, BP 60/40, oxygen saturation 94% in room air, weight 4.0 kg (50%ile). He is a well developed, well nourished, non-toxic male infant with mild tachypnea and staccato cough, but in no acute distress. His upper and lower eyelids are edematous. There is mild conjunctival infection with moderate amounts of mucopurulent drainage bilaterally. Pseudomembranes are seen with eversion of the upper eyelids. Coarse breath sounds are appreciated bilaterally with occasional rales and fine expiratory wheezes. The remainder of his exam is unremarkable.

    The conjunctiva is swabbed for gram stain, culture and chlamydia direct fluorescence antibody staining. Complete blood count is remarkable for eosinophilia. Chest radiograph reveals bilateral patchy infiltrates with hyperinflation. After receiving positive chlamydia DFA results, I informed the mother of the diagnosis. Initially shocked, she admits that six months ago, she and her husband had separated briefly, but are now back together.

DX: Ophthalmia neonatorum, due to Chlamydia trachomatis

Plan: Order written for testing for other STDs in the infant. In addition, both parents are urged to be tested for STDs by their own physicians. Parents are counseled regarding a reported association between oral erythromycin and infantile hypertrophic pyloric stenosis. Retesting for C. trachomatis is not indicated once treatment has been completed unless symptoms persist. The mother is informed that, if left untreated, chlamydia conjunctivitis will subside within 2-3 weeks, but chronic infection is common.

Rx: Oral erythromycin (50mg/kg/day in 4 divided doses) for 14 days

---

Walter P. Henricks, MD

WPH/mg   D: 10/7/08 09:50:16   T: 10/9/08 12:55:01

You Code It!

What are the best, most accurate codes?

OPHTHALMOLOGY CARE CENTER
6481 SIGHT BOULEVARD • ANYTOWN, FL 32719 • 407-555-5137

PATIENT: ULTON, SOPHIA
ACCOUNT/EHR #:   ULTOSO001
Date: 10/7/08

Attending Physician: Walter P. Henricks, MD

This is a 6-month-old female who is brought to my office, by her parents, for a well child examination. She has had no problems in the past with her eyes and, according to her parents, she tracks well and reaches for objects. Her parents deny any crossing of the eyes when she looks at objects from a distance; however, her mother mentions that she had a lazy eye when she was a child and needed to be operated on.

EXAM: Vital signs are normal for age. Her red reflex and corneal light reflex tests are normal. Cover test is negative for strabismus. Her extraocular movements appear intact and she is able to follow objects 180 degrees.

DX: Normal eye examination

PLAN: Next appointment at 9 months old or earlier prn

_____

Walter P. Henricks, MD

WPH/mg   D: 10/7/08 09:50:16   T: 10/9/08 12:55:01

You Code It!

What are the best, most accurate codes?

_____

_____

_____

OPHTHALMOLOGY CARE CENTER
6481 SIGHT BOULEVARD • ANYTOWN, FL 32719 • 407-555-5137

PATIENT: AMBRO, MEGAN
ACCOUNT/EHR #:   AMBRME001
Date: 10/7/08

Attending Physician: Walter P. Henricks, MD

A 6-month-old female infant is brought to our office, referred by her pediatrician, Dr. Houseman, due to a concern regarding her crossed eyes. Her parents say her eyes have been crossed since birth, and the left eye seems to cross more than the right. They deny any problem with her vision. They report that she plays with toys and recognizes people across the room. She was a full term infant without perinatal complications, and has no known medical problems.

EXAM: She is alert and playful.

External: Her left eye is clearly esotropic (crossed inward). There is no facial hemiparesis.

Vision: She tracks toys well using both eyes. With the left eye covered, she fixes and follows easily. However, she fusses when the right eye is covered and has more trouble following with this left eye (i.e., she is fussing when the right eye is covered because she can't see as well with her left eye). Motility: Full extraocular movements. There does not seem to be any retraction of the globe on adduction. No nystagmus.

Pupils: Equally round and reactive to light; no afferent pupil defect. No leukocoria. Corneal reflection test (Hirschberg test): A penlight is directed toward the cornea, and the reflected image is located temporal to the center of the left pupil. Cover-uncover test: On covering the right eye, there is an outward shift of the left eye. When the eye is uncovered, the left eye shifts back inward. Alternate-cover test: On switching the cover to the left eye, there is an outward shift of the right eye. When the cover is alternated from one eye to the other, there is always an outward shift of the opposite eye.
  No structural ocular abnormalities are found, and there is no significant refractive error.

DX: Infantile esotropia; amblyopia, left eye

PLAN: Parents are told to have her wear a patch 6 hours a day over the right eye for a month, to effect improvement of vision in her left eye.
  Once this has been accomplished, we will schedule surgery to correct her strabismus.

___

Walter P. Henricks, MD

WPH/mg D: 10/7/08 09:50:16 T: 10/9/08 12:55:01

You Code It!

What are the best, most accurate codes?

___

___

___

PATIENT: BROOKSTONE, FREDERICK
ACCOUNT/EHR #:   BROOFR001
Date: 10/7/08

Attending Physician: Walter P. Henricks, MD

A 28-month-old male is referred to our office by his pediatrician, Dr. Katzman, with a swollen right upper eyelid for one day. His mother states that the eyelid had a small red lump two days prior, but the eyelid became progressively swollen. The patient has a low-grade fever, but he is otherwise still playful.

    The pediatrician had diagnosed the patient with right upper eyelid cellulitis and prescribed oral antibiotics and warm compresses. After two days of antibiotics, the eyelid is still swollen and red. At this point, the patient is referred here.

EXAM: T 102F. Edema, erythema, warmth and pain of the eyelid are observed at the right upper eyelid. Visual acuity, eye motility, and pupillary reaction are all normal. There appears to be very little pain on eye movement.

DX: Preseptal eyelid cellulitis (periorbital cellulitis), caused by Haemophilus influenzae type B

PLAN: Admit into the hospital pediatrics ward for intravenous antibiotics

---

Walter P. Henricks, MD

WPH/mg   D: 10/7/08 09:50:16   T: 10/9/08 12:55:01

You Code It!

What are the best, most accurate codes?

_____

_____

_____

OPHTHALMOLOGY CARE CENTER
6481 SIGHT BOULEVARD • ANYTOWN, FL 32719 • 407-555-5137

PATIENT: SWANKLEE, CLAUDIA
ACCOUNT/EHR #:   SWANCL001
Date: 10/7/08

Attending Physician: Walter P. Henricks, MD

An 8-year-old female is brought in to the emergency department by her parents with moderately severe right eye pain six hours after riding her bicycle through some low hanging leaves from a tree. She didn't notice the tree branches until a few leaves hit her in the face. She has no bleeding wounds. I was called in for the ophthalmological consultation by the attending physician, Dr. Morgan.

EXAM: VS are normal. She does not want to open her right eye because of discomfort. Some anesthetic eye drops are instilled into her right eye. She complains that this burns a lot and she begins to cry. After 10 minutes (topical anesthetic usually works within minutes), she is able to open her eye. Her visual acuity was 20/20 in the left eye and 20/30 in the right eye. Her pupils are equal and reactive. Her conjunctiva is slightly infected. No hyphema is visible. A drop of saline is placed on a fluorescein paper strip. This drop is then touched to her lower eyelid so fluorescein dye flows over the surface of her eye. With an ultraviolet light, a 0.5 cm linear abrasion is seen in the lateral aspect of her right cornea.

DX: Corneal abrasion

PLAN: Her eye is rinsed with saline to remove excess fluorescein. A single drop of homatropine (a cycloplegic agent) is instilled into her right eye. Antibiotic ointment is instilled into her eye and a pressure eye patch is applied. She is instructed to take over-the-counter analgesics for pain.

Walter P. Henricks, MD

WPH/mg   D: 10/7/08 09:50:16   T: 10/9/08 12:55:01

You Code It!

What are the best, most accurate codes?

_____

_____

_____

OPHTHALMOLOGY CARE CENTER
6481 SIGHT BOULEVARD • ANYTOWN, FL 32719 • 407-555-5137

PATIENT: BRUCE, LLOYD
ACCOUNT/EHR #:   BRUCLL001
Date: 10/7/08

Attending Physician: Walter P. Henricks, MD

This is an 80-year-old male who was referred by Dr. Tellmon due to recurrent episodes of blurry vision and hyphema in his left eye. Each episode was associated with high intraocular pressures.

PAST MEDICAL HISTORY: Significant for bilateral cataract extraction and lens implantation 19 years ago.

EXAM: His BCVA was 20/20 OU and pressures were 20 OU. In the left eye, he had 2+ cells (mostly rbc's), a patent PI, a sulcus PCIOL in the vertical position, an intact posterior capsule, and an area of blood staining between optic and capsule. In the right eye, there was no cell or flare, two patent PI's, an ACIOL in the vertical position, and an open posterior capsule. There was no rubeosis, transillumination defects OU, pseudophakodonesis or pseudoexfoliation OU. Gonioscopy revealed open structures 360 degrees OU with no PAS. A UBM revealed the inferior haptic of the left eye sulcus IOL pressing on the ciliary body / iris junction. The superior haptic was OK.

DX: Uveitis-glaucoma-hyphema (UGH) syndrome OS

PLAN: Treatment of UGH Syndrome is discussed with patient. He requests time to discuss this with his daughter who lives in another state. He will return in one week.

Walter P. Henricks, MD

WPH/mg D: 10/7/08 09:50:16 T: 10/9/08 12:55:01

You Code It!

What are the best, most accurate codes?

_____

_____

_____

PATIENT: ROTHSTEIN, PHIL
ACCOUNT/EHR #: ROTHPH001
Date: 10/7/08

Attending Physician: Walter P. Henricks, MD

This is a 32–year-old male being evaluated for repair of LUL ptosis.

HPI: Patient noted progressive ptosis of the LUL for 3 years, which now blocks his vision. He has no other complaints or problems.

POH/PMH: Healthy, no history of eye problems.

EXAM: Vision 20/20 OU without correction. Extraocular motility with -2 elevation defect OU. VF full OD, VF with ~20% superior VF cut OS.
    Pupils: 5 mm in the dark, 3 mm in the light, no RAPD, equally reactive
    IOP 18 mmHg OU
    Anterior segment normal. DFE normal.
    Pt is able to maintain chin-up position. RUL retraction and marked ptosis OS is evident. Palpebral fissures are 10 mm OD and 5 mm OS with palpebral function of 15 mm OD and 10 mm OS. There is a twitching of the LUL when the patient looks up after looking down.

DX: Myasthenia gravis

TREATMENT
    1. Refer patient for neurology consultation.
    2. Rx pyridostigmine bromide 60 mg PO 4X/day with dosage adjustment according to response.
    3. Monitoring with consideration for surgery to remove the thymoma.

Walter P. Henricks, MD

WPH/mg   D: 10/7/08 09:50:16   T: 10/9/08 12:55:01

You Code It!

What are the best, most accurate codes?

_____

_____

_____

OPHTHALMOLOGY CARE CENTER
6481 SIGHT BOULEVARD • ANYTOWN, FL 32719 • 407-555-5137

PATIENT: GRAYSON, WALLACE
ACCOUNT/EHR #: GRAYWA001
Date: 10/7/08
Attending Physician: Walter P. Henricks, MD

This is a 49-year-old male who has been on Amiodarone therapy. At this time, the patient denies visual problems. He present to our office today for a routine ophthalmological examination.

HPI: Patient has a history of atrial fibrillation and hypertension. He has been on Amiodarone therapy for several years. Patient reports that, six weeks ago, his primary care doctor, Dr. LaBelle, made a change in his cardiac medications that included the removal of amiodarone from his medication regimen.

PMH: Atrial fibrillation and hypertension. No other ocular or health problems.

OCULAR EXAM:
• VA 20/20 OD and OS
• Intraocular Pressures and Confrontation Visual Fields normal
• DFE normal OU
• EOM Full OU
• SLE notable for corneal deposits in the cornea at the level of the basal epithelium, inferiorly OU. Deposits form a faint golden-brown whorl pattern evident in both corneas.

DX: Corneal Verticillata

TREATMENT
Depositing drugs are stopped with the expectation that the condition will eventually self-correct.

Walter P. Henricks, MD

WPH/mg   D: 10/7/08 09:50:16   T: 10/9/08 12:55:01

You Code It!

What are the best, most accurate codes?

_____

_____

_____

OPHTHALMOLOGY CARE CENTER
6481 SIGHT BOULEVARD • ANYTOWN, FL 32719 • 407-555-5137

PATIENT: WARREN, BONITA
ACCOUNT/EHR #:   WARRBO001
Date: 10/7/08

Attending Physician: Walter P. Henricks, MD

This new patient is a 44-year-old female with a lesion on her left lower lid.

HPI: The patient noted that the lesion has been present for the last 18 months. She states that it occasionally becomes inflamed, and then heals but it always comes back. She has not noted any change in the size of the lesion over the course of this time frame.

PAST EYE HISTORY: No previous ocular history. No eye surgery nor eye trauma.

PAST MEDICAL HISTORY: Hypothyroidism

CURRENT MEDICATIONS: Levothyroxine

FAMILY AND SOCIAL HISTORY: Noncontributory. Patient is a non-smoker and occasionally consumes alcohol.

OCULAR EXAM:
• Visual Acuity, with correction: OD, OS—20/20
• Pupils, Motility, and Intra-ocular pressure: normal, OU
• External and anterior segment examination:
• OD: normal; OS: normal but for the eyelid lesion on the left lower lid, as noted (see Figure 1). The lesion is 3x5 mm in size, with central ulceration and rolled, pearly borders with telangiectatic vessels. There are lashes missing (madarosis) in the area of the lesion.

DX: Nodular Basal Cell Carcinoma (BCC)

TREATMENT: An excisional biopsy is performed and demonstrates skin with central ulceration of the epidermis and multiple islands of basophilic neoplastic cells in the superficial dermis. The neoplastic cells appear to arise from surface epidermis. The diagnosis was consistent with basal cell carcinoma.
    Mohs surgery with oculoplastic reconstruction is planned.

Walter P. Henricks, MD

WPH/mg   D: 10/7/08 09:50:16   T: 10/9/08 12:55:01

You Code It!

What are the best, most accurate codes?

_____

_____

_____

OPHTHALMOLOGY CARE CENTER
6481 SIGHT BOULEVARD • ANYTOWN, FL 32719 • 407-555-5137

PATIENT: RODRIQUEZ, IMANI
ACCOUNT/EHR #:   RODRIM001
Date: 10/7/08

Attending Physician: Walter P. Henricks, MD

This patient is a 4-year-old female who presents with a dog bite to left side of face.

HPI: Approximately three hours ago, patient was playing with a pit bull, the pet of a neighbor. Family witnessed the dog make a single lunge at the girl's face. Due to the adults' attempts to intervene, only the top jaw made contact. The dog did not attack further, and the incomplete bite to the left face was the only injury sustained.

POH/PMH/SH: No past ocular history. No past medical history. No current medications or allergies. Well-adjusted preschool child lives at home with both parents. Childhood immunizations are up-to-date, according to the mother.

OCULAR EXAM:
• VA 20/25 OD and OS without correction
• Extraocular motility and IOP were normal, OU
• CVF: Full OD, OS
• Lids: Right side - Normal
• Lids: Left side - 2 lacerations on the left upper lid, the larger and deeper of the laceration passes just medial to the upper punctum. Initial exploration of laceration raises concerns for probable canalicular involvement, but further detailed examination in this anxious pediatric patient was unable to be accomplished.
• Continuation of the examination in the operating suite revealed that the remainder of the anterior segment examination and DFE were normal.

TREATMENT: Primary surgical repair of the lacerated or avulsed canaliculus using pigtail probes is performed immediately. The patient was taken to the operating suite for examination under anesthesia (EUA) and laceration repair, likely to include canalicular repair.

DX: Superior canalicular laceration

Walter P. Henricks, MD

WPH/mg   D: 10/7/08 09:50:16   T: 10/9/08 12:55:01

You Code It!

What are the best, most accurate codes?

_____

_____

_____

OPHTHALMOLOGY CARE CENTER
6481 SIGHT BOULEVARD • ANYTOWN, FL 32719 • 407-555-5137

PATIENT: HARDY, DERRICK
ACCOUNT/EHR #:   HARDDE001
Date: 10/7/08

Attending Physician: Walter P. Henricks, MD

This 25-year-old male comes into the office complaining of watery, red, irritated eyes; left more than right. I have not seen this patient since last year.

HPI: Patient states that his eyes began to feel watery and irritated about five days ago. He noted that his left eye was tearing, slightly blurry, and starting to get red throughout. The eye gradually became increasingly red and irritated over the ensuing days and the patient noted increased crusting in the mornings. There was a mild "scratchy" sensation noted then, as well. Symptoms did not remit with antibiotic drops and eye continued to worsen, with early redness and watery sensation in the contralateral eye. Patient states he had an upper respiratory infection about two months prior to any ocular symptoms. He denies any medical treatment for this URI and states that it resolved on its own.

PMH/FH/POH: No previous ocular or health problems. No eye surgery, trauma, nor contact lens use.

EXAM OCULAR:
- Anterior segment: Evident crusting on lashes and watery d/c, OU. The bulbar conjunctiva is injected OS>OD. A follicular reaction is evident on the palpebral conjunctiva, especially inferiorly, OU. There is mild chemosis and palpebral edema, again L>R.
- Palpable pre-auricular lymphadenopathy (LAD), L>R

DX: Adenoviral Conjunctivitis

TREATMENT
- Patient advised to apply cool compresses and OTC artificial tears for comfort several times a day
- To prevent contagious spread, patient is given an instruction sheet on washing sheets and pillowcases, and handwashing.

Walter P. Henricks, MD

WPH/mg   D: 10/7/08 09:50:16   T: 10/9/08 12:55:01

You Code It!

What are the best, most accurate codes?

_____

_____

_____

Orthopedic surgeons are board-certified through the Board of Orthopedic Surgery, which is recognized by the American Board of Medical Specialties.

You can use these cases to practice coding diagnoses, E/M, procedures, DME, or other HCPCS Level II items, as applicable; code for the physician or the facility; code inpatient and outpatient services, as applicable:

1. Code for the physician.
2. Code for the anesthesiologist, when applicable.
3. Code for the hospital, when applicable.
4. Code for the pathology and laboratory, when applicable.
5. Code HCPCS Level II codes, when applicable.

HALVERSON ORTHOPEDIC CENTER
1212 DOG LEG ROAD • ANYTOWN, FL 32722 • 407-555-8523

PATIENT: HICKS, LOTTIE
ACCOUNT/EHR #:   HICKLO010
Date of Operation: 11/9/2008

Preoperative Diagnosis: Hallux limites, right foot
Postoperative Diagnosis: Same
Operation: Shortening, osteotomy, first metatarsal, right foot, with screw fixation and cheilectomy, first metatarsal head, right foot

Surgeon: Allen Roberston, DPM
Assistant: None
Anesthesia: IV sedation with local anesthesia

DESCRIPTION OF OPERATIVE PROCEDURE: Following the customary sterile preparation and draping the right limb was elevated approximately 5 minutes in order to facilitate circulatory drainage at which time the pneumatic cuff, which had previously been placed on her right ankle, was inflated to a pressure of 250 mmHg. The right limb was then placed in the operative position. The operative site was injected with 2% Xylocaine mixed with 0.5% Marcaine. Upon having achieved anesthesia, a curvilinear incision was created on the plantar medial aspect of the first metatarsophalangeal joint of the right foot. The incision was deepened with sharp dissection, traversing veins were cauterized. Capsule was identified on the medial and dorsomedial aspect. Capsule was longitudinally incised on the dorsomedial aspect and meticulously dissected on to expose the head of the first metatarsal into the operative site. At this point, it was noted that the cartilage of the first metatarsal head was healthy, however there was distinct irritation to the dorsal portion of the metatarsal head with an apparent flattening of the metatarsal head secondary to the hallux limites. Using a rongeur, the hypertrophic exuberant portion of the first metatarsal head was resected, and the remaining surface was rasped smooth in order to recreate a ball joint. Using an oscillating saw, an osteotomy was performed from medial to lateral in a V-shaped fashion with the apex centrally located and the dorsal arm longer than the plantar arm. A segment of bone was removed from the dorsal arm in order to shorten and plantar flex the metatarsal head. Upon having done so, two 2.0 mm screws were obliquely driven into the osteotomy site, following range of motion was noted that the osteotomy remained stable. At this point, the hallux had approximately 90 degrees of motion to the metatarsal shaft. The area was copiously irrigated with sterile saline. The capsular tissue was repaired using 4-0 Vicryl, subcutaneous tissue was repaired using 5-0 Vicryl. Operative site was injected with dexamethasone, Betadine-soaked Adaptic was applied to the incision site, sterile gauze and Kling. The pneumatic cuff was deflated. Normal color, circulation was noted to return to all digits immediately. The patient tolerated the surgery well. Vital signs remained stable throughout the entire procedure. The patient returned to the recovery room in good condition.

Allen Roberston, DPM

AR/mg   D: 11/9/08 09:50:16   T: 11/12/08 12:55:01

You Code It!

What are the best, most accurate codes?

_____

_____

_____

HALVERSON ORTHOPEDIC CENTER
1212 DOG LEG ROAD • ANYTOWN, FL 32722 • 407-555-8523

PATIENT: PETRY, MASON

ACCOUNT/EHR #:   PETRMA001

Date: 04/25/08

Attending Physician: Sandford Lockard, MD

S: Patient is a 45-year-old male seen by his regular physician after his car was struck from behind on the street near his home. Patient is complaining of severe neck pain and difficulty turning his head.

O: PE reveals tightness upon palpitation of ligaments neck and shoulders, most pronounced C3 to C5. X-rays are taken of head and neck including the cervical vertebrae. Radiological review denies any fracture.

A: Anterior longitudinal cervical sprain.

P: 1. Cervical collar to be worn during all waking hours
       2. Rx Vicodin (hydrocodone) 500mg po prn
       3. 1,000 mg aspirin q.i.d.
       4. Pt to return in 2 weeks for follow-up

Sandford Lockard, MD

SL/mg   D: 04/25/08 09:50:16   T: 04/30/08 12:55:01

You Code It!

What are the best, most accurate codes?

_____

_____

_____

HALVERSON ORTHOPEDIC CENTER
1212 DOG LEG ROAD • ANYTOWN, FL 32722 • 407-555-8523

PATIENT: WHITE, SASHA
ACCOUNT/EHR #:   WHITSA001
Date: 09/16/08

Attending Physician: Sandford Lockard, MD

S: This new Pt is a 25-year-old female who was involved in a 2 car MVA while driving on the job. She is complaining about some neck pain. She has tingling into her hand and her feet. She states that her arm hurts when she tries to pull it overhead. She apparently was told, by a friend, that she should likely need to see a spine doctor, but somehow she came to see me first. PMH is remarkable for kidney trouble. Past bronchoscopy, laparoscopy and kidney stone surgery, otherwise noncontributory as per the medical history form completed by the patient and reviewed at this visit.

O: Ht 5'5" Wt. 179 lb. R 16. Pt presented in a sling. She was told to use it by the same friend. She states if she does not use it her arm does not feel any different, so I had her remove it. On exam, the left shoulder demonstrates full passive motion. She has normal strength testing. She has no deformity. She has some tenderness over the trapezial area. The reflexes are brisk and symmetric. X-rays of her chest 2 views and C spine AP/LAT are relatively benign, as are complete x-rays of the shoulder.

A: Contusion of upper arm and shoulder

P: 1. MRI to rule/out torn ligament
      2. Rx Naprosyn.
      3. Referral to PT
      4. Referral to spine doctor

Sandford Lockard, MD

SL/mg   D: 9/16/08 09:50:16   T: 9/18/08 12:55:01

You Code It!

What are the best, most accurate codes?

_____

_____

_____

HALVERSON ORTHOPEDIC CENTER
1212 DOG LEG ROAD • ANYTOWN, FL 32722 • 407-555-8523

PATIENT: BRUTUS, JOHN
ACCOUNT/EHR #:   BRUTJO001
Date: 09/20/08

Attending Physician: Sandford Lockard, MD

S: Pt is a 27-year-old male who was involved in a fist fight at a local bar the previous evening. He complained of an ache in the area of his left eye as well as severe pain around his right ear.

O: Ht 5'10.5" Wt. 209 lb. R 19. Surface hematoma evident in the area surrounding the left eye socket reaching to the upper cheek. Head x-ray of the right side confirmed a closed fracture of the right mandible.

A: Black eye, fracture of the rt mandible, angle (closed)

P: 1. Wire right jaw
     2. NPO except liquids for three weeks
     3. Cold wet compresses on eye prn
     4. Return for follow-up in three weeks

Sandford Lockard, MD

SL/mg   D: 09/20/08 09:50:16   T: 09/22/08 12:55:01

You Code It!

What are the best, most accurate codes?

_____

_____

_____

HALVERSON ORTHOPEDIC CENTER
1212 DOG LEG ROAD • ANYTOWN, FL 32722 • 407-555-8523

PATIENT NAME: CONNOR, DENISE
MRN: CONNDE001
Date: 08/20/08

Attending Physician: Gerrard Yahnert, MD

Patient is a 79-year-old female status post MVA. Imaging studies showed a C2 fracture involving the vertebral body. Arrangements were made for placement of halo. The procedure was described in detail to the patient and her husband and consent was provided by the patient.

     The hair was shaved above both ears. The halo ring was placed. Lidocaine was used to numb the tissue. The halo was then placed in the usual manner without difficulty. A lateral cervical spine was obtained, which showed good positioning. The patient tolerated the procedure without difficulty.

Gerrard Yahnert, MD

GY/mgr   D: 08/20/08 12:33:08 PM T: 08/27/08 3:22:54 PM

You Code It!

What are the best, most accurate codes?

_____

_____

_____

HALVERSON ORTHOPEDIC CENTER
1212 DOG LEG ROAD • ANYTOWN, FL 32722 • 407-555-8523

NAME: WINGATE, SAMANTHA
PATIENT NUMBER: WINGSA001
Date of Admission: 02-20-2008

Admitting Information:

Surgeon: Martin Hande, MD
Primary Care Provider: Sandra Homacker, MD

Financial Class: Workers' Compensation (WC)
Preoperative Diagnosis: Right carpal tunnel syndrome
Postoperative Diagnosis: Same, plus flexor tenosynovitis of the palm and wrist

PROCEDURES: Multiple flexor tenosynovectomies of the palm and wrist. Decompression of the right carpal tunnel with epineurolysis of medial nerve and individual motor branch decompression.

OPERATIVE PROCEDURES AND PATHOLOGICAL FINDINGS:
This white female has had bilateral carpal tunnel syndrome, slightly greater on the left than on the right for an undetermined period of time. The patient is deaf. She also had bilateral thumb arthritis. It was elected not to address the latter problem at the present time. She had quite classic symptoms without any history of any rheumatoid type arthritis.

Nerve conduction studies showed significant prolongation of the median nerve conduction times on both sides. She also had bilateral thenar atrophy. Her more symptomatic left side was done in June. At surgery, multiple flexor tenosynovitis was found. She underwent resection of the tenosynovitis along with carpal tunnel decompression. Pathology report did not show a rheumatoid etiology for the tenosynovitis. Plan was to decompress her right side today. She has full extension of her fingers and possibly a slight diminution in flexion related to some degenerative arthritis.

DESCRIPTION OF PROCEDURE: Under satisfactory right IV block, prep and drape was performed. Using 41/2 loupe magnification, standard incision was made, which was carried down through the superficial palmar fascia. One proximal crossing branch of the median palmar cutaneous nerve was identified and preserved. Battery operated cautery was utilized to control some small bleeding points. The superficial palmar fascia and then the transverse carpal ligament were divided in a distal to proximal direction. The distal wrist fascia was decompressed. Inspection of the canal revealed a quite large median nerve with a subligamentous motor branch going into a tight hiatus. This was decompressed.

Further inspection of the canal revealed a picture reminiscent of the left side. Most of the flexor tendons were involved in the tenosynovitis. Systematic flexor tenosynovectomy was then performed down to the level of the lumbrical, removing the tenosynovium. Two of the deep flexors, namely those to the ring and little fingers, had some area of tendon erosions on them. These were excised. This involved the small portion of the tendon and no way weakened it.

The incision was extended 4 to 5 cm to allow some removal of additional tenosynovium in the wrist. After completing this, the median nerve was reinspected. There was a moderate hourglass deformity and a longitudinal epineurolysis was performed on the ulnar border.

The wound was then thoroughly irrigated with Saline. The skin was closed with interrupted 4-0 nylon suture. A Xeroform bulky gauze dressing was applied along with a volar splint out to the PIP joints, putting the wrist in a neutral position.

Continued

The tourniquet was released. Tourniquet time was a little over one hour. There was good color in the fingers. The patient tolerated the procedure quite well and was sent to the ASU for recovery.

Martin Hande, MD

DATE: 2-20-2008

You Code It!

What are the best, most accurate codes?

_____

_____

_____

HALVERSON ORTHOPEDIC CENTER
1212 DOG LEG ROAD • ANYTOWN, FL 32722 • 407-555-8523

PATIENT NAME: RUBBLE, BETTY
MRN: RUBBBE001
Date: 09/23/08

Attending Physician: Zainab Goupil, MD

Preoperative Diagnosis: C5 compression fracture
Postoperative Diagnosis: Same
Procedure: C5 corpectomy and fusion fixation with fibular strut graft and Atlantis plate
Anesthesia   General endotracheal

This is a 25-year-old female status post assault. The patient sustained a C5 compression fracture. MRI scan showed compression with evidence of posterior ligamentous injury. The patient was subsequently set up for the surgical procedure. The procedure was described in detail including the risks. The risks included but not limited to bleeding, infection, stroke, paralysis, death, cerebrospinal fluid (CSF) leak, loss of bladder and bowel control, hoarse voice, paralyzed vocal cord, death and damage to adjacent nerves and tissues. The patient understood the risks. The patient also understood that bank bone instrumentation would be used and that the bank bone could collapse and the instrumentation could fail, break or the screws could pull out. The patient provided consent.

     The patient was taken to the OR. The patient was induced. Endotracheal tube was placed. A Foley was placed. The patient was given preoperative antibiotics. The patient was placed in slight extension. The right neck was prepped and draped in the usual manner. A linear incision was made over the C5 vertebral body. The platysma was divided. Dissection was continued medial to the sternocleidomastoid to the prevertebral fascia. This was cauterized and divided. The longus colli was cauterized and elevated. The fracture was visualized. A spinal needle was used to verify location using fluoroscopy. The C5 vertebral body was drilled out. The bone was saved. The disks above and below were removed. The posterior longitudinal ligament was removed. The bone was quite collapsed and fragmented. Distraction pins were then packed with bone removed from the C5 vertebral body prior to implantation. A plate was then placed with screws in the C4 and C6 vertebral bodies. The locking screws were tightened. The wound was irrigated. Bleeding was helped with the bipolar. The retractors were removed. The incision was approximated with simple interrupted Vicryl. The subcutaneous tissue was approximated and skin edges approximated subcuticularly. Steri-Strips applied. A dressing was applied. The patient was placed back in an Aspen collar. The patient was extubated and transferred to recovery.

Zainab Goupil, MD

ZG/mgr   D: 09/23/08 12:33:08 PM   T: 09/25/08 3:22:54 PM

You Code It!

What are the best, most accurate codes?

_____

_____

_____

HALVERSON ORTHOPEDIC CENTER
1212 DOG LEG ROAD • ANYTOWN, FL 32722 • 407-555-8523

PATIENT: STARKER, SHARON
ACCOUNT/EHR #:   STARSH001
Date: 08/11/08

Attending Physician: Willard B. Reader, MD

S. Patient is a 41-year-old female, who comes in with a complaint of severe neck pain and difficulty turning her head. She states she was in a car accident two days ago, her car struck from behind when she was driving home from work.

O: PE reveals tightness upon palpitation of ligaments neck and shoulders, most pronounced C3 to C5. X-rays are taken of head and neck including the cervical vertebrae. Radiological review denies any fracture.

A.   Anterior longitudinal cervical sprain

P: 1. Applied cervical collar to be worn during all waking hours
     2. Rx Vicodin (hydrocodone) 500 mg po prn
     3. 1,000 mg aspirin q.i.d.
     4. Pt to return in 2 weeks for follow-up

_____

Willard B. Reader, MD

WBR/pw   D: 08/11/08 09:50:16   T: 08/13/08 12:55:01

You Code It!

What are the best, most accurate codes?

_____

_____

_____

HALVERSON ORTHOPEDIC CENTER
1212 DOG LEG ROAD • ANYTOWN, FL 32722 • 407-555-8523

PATIENT: AMATTI, CLIFFORD
MRN: AMATCL001
Admission Date: 9 October 2008
Discharge Date: 9 October 2008
Date: 9 October 2008

Preoperative DX: Lacerations of hand, and leg
Postoperative DX: Same
Procedure: Simple repair of leg lacerations; layered repair of hand laceration

Surgeon: Mary Lou Duncan, MD
Assistant: None
Anesthesia: General

INDICATIONS: The patient is a 9-year-old male brought to the emergency room by his father. He was helping his father hang a mirror in the bedroom when it fell and shattered. The boy suffered lacerations on his left hand and left leg.

PROCEDURE: The patient was placed on the table in supine position. Satisfactory anesthesia was obtained. The area was prepped and attention to the deeper laceration of the left palm of the hand was first. A layered repair was performed and the 5.1 cm laceration was closed successfully with sutures. The lacerations on the lower extremity, 2 cm laceration on the left leg at the base of the patella and the 3 cm laceration on the left shin, were successful closed with 4-0 Vicryl, as well. The patient tolerated the procedures well, and was transported to the recovery room.

10/9/08 11:47:39

You Code It!

What are the best, most accurate codes?

_____

_____

_____

HALVERSON ORTHOPEDIC CENTER
1212 DOG LEG ROAD • ANYTOWN, FL 32722 • 407-555-8523

PATIENT: GRANT, AMOS
ACCOUNT/EHR #:   GRANAM001
Date: 11/05/08

Attending Physician: Valerie R. Victors, MD

S: This Pt is a 15-year-old male. I have not seen this patient since last July when he came in for a certificate to play sports in school. Today he is brought in by his father after being tackled during football practice and hurting his left wrist. He is complaining of pain upon flexing and is having difficulty moving his fingers.

O: Tenderness and swelling of the wrist is observed. Pt can move his fingers slightly indicating no fracture, however, AP/lat X-rays are taken to confirm. X-ray does confirm the wrist is sprained. A conforming, non-elastic (non-sterile) bandage, 2″ x 35″, is applied.

A: Sprain, radiocarpal ligament, wrist

P: Follow-up in one week.

_____

Valerie R. Victors, MD

VRV/mg   D: 11/05/08 09:50:16   T: 11/07/08 12:55:01

You Code It!

What are the best, most accurate codes?

_____

_____

_____

HALVERSON ORTHOPEDIC CENTER
1212 DOG LEG ROAD • ANYTOWN, FL 32722 • 407-555-8523

PATIENT: FISCHER, ELVIRA
ACCOUNT/EHR #:   FISCEL001
Date: 12/09/08

Attending Physician: Gena Reynoldo, MD

Technician: Harvey Nickols

Pt is a 37-year-old female hurt during a waterskiing accident. She was performing in a ski show at Water World Adventure Park when she came off the ski jump ramp in the wrong angle and hit the water unevenly, twisting her knee. Her physician, Dr. Cipher, ordered her to use a wheelchair for the next six weeks.

    I delivered a standard wheelchair with fixed full-length arms and swing-away, detachable footrests to the patient's home. I spent twenty minutes instructing the patient on the proper way to use the chair, transfer from the chair to standard furniture and back, and transfer to other function furniture including the toilet and the bed. She was instructed on how to stop and start the chair with the least amount of strain on her upper extremities, and how to apply the brakes. Patient stated she clearly understood all instructions.

DX: Torn meniscus, lateral, knee

P: Patient given instruction booklet and technical support number

_____

Harvey Nickols

HN/mg   D: 12/09/08 09:50:16   T: 12/11/08 12:55:01

You Code It!

What are the best, most accurate codes?

_____

_____

_____

HALVERSON ORTHOPEDIC CENTER
1212 DOG LEG ROAD • ANYTOWN, FL 32722 • 407-555-8523

PATIENT: MELMANN, MICHAEL
ACCOUNT/EHR #:   MELMMI001
Date: 12/09/08

Attending Physician: Gena Reynoldo, MD

This is a 13-year-old male who presents with a chief complaint of right forearm pain. While playing soccer earlier that day, the patient fell onto his right hand and heard a snapping sound. He reports that the pain in his forearm increases with movement. It is visibly swollen and deformed.

Exam: VS are normal except for a resting tachycardia secondary to pain. He is alert and cooperative, but subdued, in moderate pain. His head, neck and torso show no signs of external trauma. Heart, lungs and abdomen are normal. Upper extremities: Swelling and deformity is observed at the right mid-forearm, corresponding to his area of greatest pain. Radial pulses and sensation are intact.

    An IV is started and he is given 3 mg of IV morphine. AP and lateral radiographs of his right forearm demonstrate displaced, angulated fractures of the radius and ulna with overriding (overlapping) ends.

    The patient is sedated and given additional analgesia. A closed reduction is performed with good alignment of the radius and ulna. Immobilization is accomplished with a fiberglass cast extending from the hand to the proximal humerus.

Gena Reynoldo, MD

GR/mg   D: 12/09/08 09:50:16   T: 12/11/08 12:55:01

You Code It!

What are the best, most accurate codes?

_____

_____

_____

HALVERSON ORTHOPEDIC CENTER
1212 DOG LEG ROAD • ANYTOWN, FL 32722 • 407-555-8523

PATIENT: O'DAY, SHANNON

ACCOUNT/EHR #:   ODAYSH001

Date: 12/09/08

Attending Physician: Gena Reynoldo, MD

This is a 7-year-old female who presents with a chief complaint of left wrist pain. She was rollerblading with several friends, and was accidentally pushed from behind. She fell forward with outstretched, pronated arms. She denies hitting her head, loss of consciousness, vomiting, and abdominal pain.

Exam: VS T37.0, P105, R20, BP 117/75. She is comfortable, alert and appears to be in no distress. Mild abrasions are noted on her left knee and palmar surfaces of both hands. No obvious puncture wounds are present. She has mild discomfort upon palpation of her left knee, but she is able walk, stand, and jump without difficulty or discomfort. Her right wrist is normal, but tenderness is elicited upon palpation of her left distal radius. Slight wrist swelling is noted, but no angular deformity is present. The remainder of her exam is unremarkable.

      Radiographs reveal a non-displaced distal radius fracture of the left wrist without angulation. She is placed in a forearm sugar tong splint, and her mother is given instructions to follow-up in three weeks.

Gena Reynoldo, MD

GR/mg   D: 12/09/08 09:50:16   T: 12/11/08 12:55:01

You Code It!

What are the best, most accurate codes?

_____

_____

_____

HALVERSON ORTHOPEDIC CENTER
1212 DOG LEG ROAD • ANYTOWN, FL 32722 • 407-555-8523

PATIENT: YAEGER, DAVID
ACCOUNT/EHR #:   YAEGDA001
Date: 12/09/08

Surgeon: Brice McArdle, MD
Anesthesiologist: Nancy Ferguson, MD

Preop Diagnosis: Osteoarthritis, right knee
Postop Diagnosis: Same
Procedure: Right total knee replacement

PATHOLOGY: The patient is a 57-year-old male with severe osteoarthritis to both knees, which has been refractory to long-term conservative treatment. He now presents for a total knee placement.

OPERATIVE FINDINGS: The patient's right knee had advanced tri-compartmental osteoarthritis.

DESCRIPTION OF PROCEDURE: General anesthesia, supine position, right above-knee tourniquet, routine sterile prep and drape of the right lower extremity, intravenous antibiotics, laminar air flow room.

    The right lower extremity was wrapped with an Esmarch and a tourniquet inflated to 300 mm Hg. An anterior incision was made over the right knee with dissection to the superficial retinaculum which was then sharply split and mobilized medially. A medial parapatellar arthrotomy was performed.

    The patella was dislocated laterally. Sharp dissection performed along the mediolateral proximal tibial plateau. The knee was flexed to expose the anterior joint. The meniscal remnants of the anterior cruciate were debrided. Osteophytes were removed from the distal femur and proximal femur using a rongeur.

    Intramedullary cutting jigs were subsequently applied to the distal femur and cuts made with an oscillating saw. The trial femur was noted to fit perfectly. The patella was then measured with the caliper and the articular surface removed with an oscillating saw. A drill hole guide was applied and drill holes created. The patella trial was noted to fit well. A lateral retinacular release was required to obtain good tracking.

    An external alignment guide was then applied to the proximal tibia and the proximal tibia transected with an oscillating saw. Trial reductions were then performed to determine the size of the tibial plate and also confirmed soft tissue balance and axial alignment. The proximal tibial was then further broached with a cruciate driver.

    All trial components were then removed and the wound thoroughly pulse lavaged. The components were then cemented in place, beginning with the tibia and patella, followed by the femur. All extraneous cement was removed. A polyethylene liner was then applied to the tibia and the knee was completed. The knee had excellent range of motion from 0 – 125 degrees with good tracking and no instability.

    The tourniquet was then deflated and hemostasis performed. A Sauvage drain was placed within the knee, existing over the anterolateral thigh. The capsule was then closed with multiple interrupted sutures of #1-0 Vicryl. The superficial retinaculum was closed with interrupted vertical mattress sutures of #3-0 nylon. A sterile compressive dressing and a knee immobilizer and PAS stockings were applied.

Continued

Estimated blood loss was 200 cc. The final sponge, instrument counts were correct. Tourniquet time was 50 minutes.

The patient was transported to recovery in stable condition. Immediate neurovascular examination of the right leg showed intact pulsation, sensation and motor. There were no complications.

Brice McArdle, MD

BM/mg   D: 12/09/08 09:50:16   T: 12/11/08 12:55:01

You Code It!

What are the best, most accurate codes?

_____

_____

_____

Otolaryngology Cases and Patient Records

INTRODUCTION

The following case studies are from an ear-nose-throat practice. In a physician's office of this type, a professional coding specialist is likely to see many different kinds of health situations, including preventive health care services.

The medical term used to identify a physician who specializes in conditions of the ears, nose, and throat (ENT) is otolaryngologist or otorhinolaryngologist.

Otolaryngologists diagnose and treat conditions and diseases that range from allergies to sleep apnea to laryngeal malignancies. These specialists care for patients with diseases such as myringitis, Ménière's disease, or suffering from nasal polyps. Allergy/immunology is a subspecialty because of the vast number of signs and symptoms that patients suffer and that affect the upper portion of the respiratory system. Another subspecialty focuses on hearing and deafness. These otolaryngologists are the surgeons who would perform a cochlear implant or excise a tumor in the ear canal.

Otolaryngologists are board-certified through the Board of Otolaryngology, which is recognized by the American Board of Medical Specialties.

You can use these cases to practice coding diagnoses, E/M, procedures, DME, or other HCPCS Level II items, as applicable; code for the physician or the facility; code inpatient and outpatient services, as applicable:

1. Code for the physician.

2. Code for the anesthesiologist, when applicable.

3. Code for the hospital, when applicable.

4. Code for the pathology and laboratory, when applicable.

5. Code HCPCS Level II codes, when applicable.

THE E.N.T. MEDICAL CENTER
Otolaryngology
321 HATCH STREET • ANYTOWN, FL 32711 • 407-555-9876

PATIENT: CAMMEN, JAN

ACCOUNT/EHR #:   CAMMJA001

Date: 10/13/08

Attending Physician: James I. Cipher, MD

This patient is a 25-year-old male with a history of recurrent sinus infections. He denies any health problems until five days before he went to his family physician's office about a year ago. He presented with fever, severe frontal headache, facial pain and runny nose. He was treated for acute sinusitis with antibiotics and pseudoephedrine (OTC) with resolution of his symptoms. Over the next six months, he had recurrent bouts of frontal and left-sided headache, fever, and nasal congestion, which always improved on oral antibiotics. Over the recent six months, he received three courses of oral antibiotics. The last course finished 10 days before this encounter. The family physician, Dr. Blanchard, referred this patient to me.

HISTORY: No known allergies. Because of recent difficulty in concentrating he asked the physician for an evaluation. Non-focal neurologic examination was performed. Tenderness over frontal and left maxillary sinuses. Afebrile.

    CT scan, taken this morning in our facility, shows opacification of both frontal and left maxillary, sphenoid sinuses and a possible large non-enhanced lesion in the brain.

    Parasagittal MRI and axial MRI show a large (7 cm) well-circumscribed epidural collection compressing the left frontal lobe.

Diagnosis: Epidural abscess with frontal lobe lesions caused by significant compression on frontal lobe.

PLAN: Recommend surgery to evacuate the large epidural abscess.

James I. Cipher, MD

JIC/mg   D: 10/13/08 09:50:16   T: 10/15/08 12:55:01

You Code It!

What are the best, most accurate codes?

_____

_____

_____

THE E.N.T. MEDICAL CENTER
Otolaryngology
321 HATCH STREET • ANYTOWN, FL 32711 • 407-555-9876

PATIENT: KRAUS, MAYNARD
ACCOUNT/EHR #:   KRAUMA001
Date: 10/13/08

Attending Physician: James I. Cipher, MD

S: This new Pt is a 35-year-old male who works in a mattress factory. He states that he has had a piercing ringing sound in his left ear that began six months ago. He noticed the ringing sound in his ear upon awakening one morning and it remains a considerable annoyance all day long, interfering with his ability to enjoy television, movies, and even conversation. Pt states he has trouble sleeping, as well.

O: Pt taken to testing suite for a bilateral tinnitus assessment: pitch (frequency) matching; loudness matching; and masking procedures are included. Findings of the testing indicate a positive determination of tinnitus. Patient is informed of the outcome, along with the recommendations for remediation therapy.

A: Acute tinnitus

P: Follow-up with masking therapy treatment plan

_____

James I. Cipher, MD

JIC/mg   D: 10/13/08 09:50:16   T: 10/15/08 12:55:01

You Code It!

What are the best, most accurate codes?

_____

_____

_____

THE E.N.T. MEDICAL CENTER
Otolaryngology
321 HATCH STREET • ANYTOWN, FL 32711 • 407-555-9876

PATIENT: ALBANNO, LOUISE
ACCOUNT/EHR #:   ALBALO001
Date: 10/13/08

Attending Physician: James I. Cipher, MD

This patient is an 81-year-old Caucasian woman referred by Dr. Stevenson due to complaints of dysphagia and dyspnea exacerbated by swallowing. She reports a three-week history of progressive dysphagia, initially for solids and subsequently for fluids leading to total dysphagia. She also reports regurgitation, cough, and hoarseness of voice.

HISTORY: The patient has a history of progressive dysphagia and the accumulation of food debris lead to mega-esophagus.

FAMILY HISTORY: There was no significant medical, family or social history.

PHYSICAL EXAMINATION: Pulse is rapid and irregular; no other cardiovascular-respiratory abnormalities are identified. Abdominal examination: unremarkable; indirect laryngoscopy shows pooling of saliva in the hypopharynx.

IMAGING: Lateral soft tissue radiograph reveals widening of the upper mediastinum and subsequent barium swallow shows achalasia with food debris filling the cervical esophagus. An electrocardiogram (ECG) showed evidence of ischaemia and atrial fibrillation with a ventricular response rate of 120–150.

LAB: Hematological and biochemical laboratory investigations were within the normal limits.

DX: Atrial fibrillation secondary to a mega-esophagus

PLAN: Patient to be admitted to hospital for resuscitation with intravenous fluids, followed by naso-esophageal leverage and removal of 300 ml of retained food debris from the cervical esophagus. A follow-up ECG is to be performed 8 hours afterwards.

James I. Cipher, MD

JIC/mg   D: 10/13/08 09:50:16   T: 10/15/08 12:55:01

You Code It!

What are the best, most accurate codes?

_____

_____

_____

THE E.N.T. MEDICAL CENTER
Otolaryngology
321 HATCH STREET • ANYTOWN, FL 32711 • 407-555-9876

PATIENT: PARMER, DIETRA
ACCOUNT/EHR #:   PARMDI001
Date: 10/13/08

Attending Physician: James I. Cipher, MD

This is a 41-year-old female who underwent routine FESS and was not packed nasally after the procedure for recurrent sinusitis.

HPI: Pre-operatively she was noted to have bilateral concha bullous on CT scan with subsequent obstruction of both osteo-meatal complexes. Attempts to control the symptoms with medication, using both steroid sprays and antibiotics, provided no relief. FESS was discussed with the patient and she opted to have the procedure.

   FESS was scheduled for early this morning. The operation was performed at the Hilltown Ambulatory Surgical Center with no facilities for in-patient care. Nasal preparation used was Otrivin 30 minutes beforehand, followed by injection of 2% lidocaine in a solution of 1:80000 adrenaline into both uncinate processes and middle turbinates. Bilateral uncinectomies with middle meatal antrostomies were performed prior to reduction of both middle turbinates. There was little bleeding noted during the procedure and also after completion of the surgery. Insertion of nasal packs was therefore not deemed to be necessary. She was transferred to the recovery room in good condition. Immediate post-operative recovery was routine.

   Six hours after the procedure she started bleeding and nasal packs were inserted. She soon developed unilateral periorbital bruising and within hours her condition had worsened so much that the viability of the left eye became questionable. The patient was then transported and admitted into the hospital. She was taken in for immediate medial and lateral canthotomies. The hematomas were evacuated surgically, particularly laterally and the tenseness of the orbit was markedly reduced. A specific bleeding point was not identifiable. She made an uneventful post-operative recovery. Post-operative CT scan revealed normal ocular anatomy, with no evidence of re-collection of hematoma. Ophthalmological opinion stated no abnormality and orthoptics were normal.

DX: Orbital complications following functional endoscopic sinus surgery (FESS)

James I. Cipher, MD

JIC/mg   D: 10/13/08 09:50:16   T: 10/15/08 12:55:01

You Code It!

What are the best, most accurate codes?

_____

_____

_____

THE E.N.T. MEDICAL CENTER
Otolaryngology
321 HATCH STREET • ANYTOWN, FL 32711 • 407-555-9876

PATIENT: PAPPIETTE, JUANITA

ACCOUNT/EHR #: PAPPJA001

Date: 10/13/08

Attending Physician: James I. Cipher, MD

The patient is a 61-year-old female with a chief complaint of involuntary movements of jaw-opening triggered mainly by talking and/or eating. She states that she has been symptomatic for the preceding three years. Her symptoms made eating difficult requiring her to bite down with effort in order to keep her mouth from opening. She wore out her regular dentures and special dentures had to be manufactured for her. Yelling would ameliorate the involuntary movements.

PERSONAL/FAMILY HISTORY: Unremarkable for other neurological disorders. The patient denies any exposure to dopamine-blocking drugs. She denies any weight loss, but admitted to eating difficulty and social embarrassment due to the jaw-opening OMD. Her neurological examination was otherwise unremarkable.

DIAGNOSIS: Oromandibular dystonia (OMD)

PLAN: BTX-A injections to her lateral pterygoids (75 units/side)

James I. Cipher, MD

JIC/mg   D: 10/13/08 09:50:16   T: 10/15/08 12:55:01

You Code It!

What are the best, most accurate codes?

_____

_____

_____

THE E.N.T. MEDICAL CENTER
Otolaryngology
321 HATCH STREET • ANYTOWN, FL 32711 • 407-555-9876

PATIENT: PAPPACCI, JUNE
ACCOUNT/EHR #:   PAPPJU002
Date: 10/13/08

Attending Physician: James I. Cipher, MD

DIAGNOSIS: Foreign body in maxillary sinus

PROCEDURE: Endoscopically assisted procedure for removal of a foreign body from the maxillary sinus

The patient is a 37-year-old female seen for chronic pain in the region of the upper first molar/right side.

HISTORY: Patient states that she had a root canal of her right upper first molar three years ago. She states that she has had previous symptoms in the last two years of maxillary sinusitis including tenderness in the left infraorbital region and nasal stuffiness.

PHYSICAL EXAM: The left upper first molar region is painful upon light pressure. Orthopantomography shows a radiopacity of the left maxillary sinus. CT scan shows the presence of a foreign body located in the superomedial aspect of the maxillary sinus, near the natural maxillary ostium. The FB appears to be a partially formed calcium deposit. A partial mucosal thickening of the sinus upon the roots of the upper first molar was also present. Videorhinoscopy shows hypertrophy of the inferior turbinates bilaterally.

PROCEDURE: Once patient is successfully under anesthesia, and draped in the usual, sterile fashion, standard surgical technique is used to create a small osteotomy in the lateral antral wall upon the roots of the upper first left molar. The antrum is examined through the endoscope and the foreign body is easily identified and gently removed. A contemporary endodontic surgical treatment of the upper first left molar roots and an endoscopic reduction of inferior turbinates is also performed.
    Patient is brought out of the anesthesia and taken to recovery. Her postoperative course was satisfactory with no evidence of sinus infection.

_____

James I. Cipher, MD

JIC/mg   D: 10/13/08 09:50:16   T: 10/15/08 12:55:01

You Code It!

What are the best, most accurate codes?

_____

_____

_____

THE E.N.T. MEDICAL CENTER
Otolaryngology
321 HATCH STREET • ANYTOWN, FL 32711 • 407-555-9876

PATIENT: APPLEMANN, DERRICK
ACCOUNT/EHR #:   APPLDE001
Date: 10/13/08

Attending Physician: James I. Cipher, MD

The patient is a 15-month-old male who presents with a mass lesion in the left post-auricle region.

HISTORY: The mass was present at birth and has gradually increased in size.

EXAM: The measurement of the mass is currently 9-5-5 cm. The skin covering it is unremarkable. The balance of ROS examination is unremarkable. A non-contrast CT - head and neck revealed the mass in the left post-auricular region. There is no intracranial involvement.

DX: Congenital alveolar rhabdomyosarcoma (RMS)

PROCEDURE: Complete excision of the mass

SURGICAL PATHOLOGY:

Gross Exam: The mass is fairly well circumscribed, multinodular with a glistening, gelatinous gray-white surface. Neither hemorrhage nor necrosis is present.

Microscopic Exam: It revealed a varying degree of cellularity with densely packed cellular areas separated by a framework of hyalinized fibrous septa. The tumor cells are non-cohesive in the center. The individual cells are large, round with darkly staining hyperchromatic nuclei, inconspicuous nucleoli, and scant indistinct cytoplasm. High mitotic rate is noticed. The tumor cells (≈40%) are positive for desmin and myogenin immunostains. The other panels of immunostains used are CD45, CD20, MIC-2, CK, Neuron specific enolase, and myeloperoxidase, all of which are negative.
    Ultrastructurally, the tumor cells show few cytoplasmic organelles and occasional bundles of thin myofilaments measuring 4–6mm in diameter. Bone marrow examination didn't reveal any metastatic deposit. A cytogenetic analysis was not performed because of technical reasons.

James I. Cipher, MD

JIC/mg   D: 10/13/08 09:50:16   T: 10/15/08 12:55:01

You Code It!

What are the best, most accurate codes?

_____

_____

_____

THE E.N.T. MEDICAL CENTER
Otolaryngology
321 HATCH STREET • ANYTOWN, FL 32711 • 407-555-9876

PATIENT: DONALDSON, KEIANNA
ACCOUNT/EHR #:   DONAKE001
Date: 10/13/08

Attending Physician: James I. Cipher, MD

The patient is a 27-year-old female who complains of right-sided hemicrania and difficult nasal breathing associated with recurrent right-sided maxillary sinusitis.

Nasal endoscopy revealed a substantial nasal obstruction on the right side that was caused by a marked hypertrophy of the turbinates and a deviated nasal septum. After shrinkage of the turbinate with a nasal decongestant, examination revealed a long septal ridge along the middle portion of the septum on the right side, which extended from anterior to posterior. The ridge was projecting into the right inferior turbinate, displacing it laterally. There was no significant obstruction on the left side of the nasal passage.

The patient is administered local anesthesia, and a longitudinal posterior-to-anterior incision was made over the ridge with a sickle knife. The superior and inferior mucosal flaps are elevated with the sharp end of a Cottle elevator. When the entire ridge is fully exposed, it is easily removed with a powered endoscopic excision. The mucosal flaps are repositioned, and a piece of Gelfoam is placed over the incision.

Patient gets through the procedure well.

_____

James I. Cipher, MD

JIC/mg   D: 10/13/08 09:50:16   T: 10/15/08 12:55:01

You Code It!

What are the best, most accurate codes?

_____

_____

_____

THE E.N.T. MEDICAL CENTER
Otolaryngology
321 HATCH STREET • ANYTOWN, FL 32711 • 407-555-9876

PATIENT: BANKS, ARTHUR
ACCOUNT/EHR #:   BANKAR001
Date: 10/13/08

Attending Physician: James I. Cipher, MD

This patient is a 39-year-old male who noted an increasing difficulty speaking audibly in noisy situations. He states that, approximately five months ago he began to experience persistent vocal fatigue after he gave a 25-minute speech. He had also experienced persistent hoarseness during the same period prior to this evaluation. The patient reported no antecedent illness or other vocal abuse. He has had several examinations by his family physician, Dr. Dominguez, and was started on a proton-pump inhibitor for laryngopharyngeal reflux. Dr. Dominguez referred this to me.

EXAMINATION: Strobovideolaryngoscopy revealed mild supraglottic hyperfunction, normal motion of the vocal folds, and a large vascular mass that was centered on the anterior third of the right vocal fold. A large varicose vessel was observed leading to the mass, and the entire right side of the vocal fold was discolored yellow and red. It is also observed that there is some thickening on the left vocal fold along the contact area as well as the presence of an anterior web. On stroboscopic examination, the right vocal fold exhibited a severely decreased amplitude and wave form.

    The patient was prescribed a brief course of voice therapy to decrease his hyperfunction and to prepare him for safe phonation following surgery.

PROCEDURE: Patient is taken for microlaryngoscopy and excision of the right vocal fold mass. After the laryngoscope was suspended, the right vocal fold was infused with saline-and-epinephrine solution. The vascular mass could not be elevated from the vocal ligament, indicating a deep fibrotic reaction attaching the mass to the vocal ligament. An incision was made along the superior surface of the mass, and the mass was carefully dissected from its deep attachments. During dissection, the vocal ligament was identified anteriorly and preserved. The remaining mucosal attachments were then incised, and the mass was sent for pathologic examination. A steroid was injected underneath the yellowish mucosa and into the region of the vocal ligament in an attempt to reduce the amount of scarring. The small anterior web was left undisturbed. Pathologic examination of the mass revealed an organized hematoma without evidence of hemangioma.

PLAN: The patient should be kept on voice rest for 10 days post-operatively. He will then be allowed to slowly increase his voice use under the close observation of a laryngologist and a speech-language pathologist.

James I. Cipher, MD

JIC/mg   D: 10/13/08 09:50:16   T: 10/15/08 12:55:01

You Code It!

What are the best, most accurate codes?

_____

_____

_____

THE E.N.T. MEDICAL CENTER
Otolaryngology
321 HATCH STREET • ANYTOWN, FL 32711 • 407-555-9876

PATIENT: HOLMES, RHODA
ACCOUNT/EHR #:   HOLMRH001
Date: 10/13/08

Attending Physician: James I. Cipher, MD

This patient is a 3-year-old female who presents with a history of congestion, runny nose, occasional cough, and fever. Her mother is concerned the cough is worsening. She states that the discharge from the child's nose is mostly clear, however, she has observed it cloudy on occasion. The child has not been wheezing per the mother. She has little exposure to ill children since her aunt takes care of her during the day. Her cousins, with ages ranging from 2 to 9 years, are rarely ill.

When asked about her ear, the child states, "My ear hurts, Mommy." Upon further questioning, her mother reveals no other symptoms. She states that her boyfriend and maternal grandmother, who both have similar symptoms, have been around the child recently.

The mother mentions that her grandmother had suggested some homemade remedies. She stated that she applied an OTC rub to the child's chest. She made some nose drops with salt and water and a bulb syringe, and that seemed to help the congestion much better than the OTC cough medicine or the OTC infant's drops. She states that she has been giving the child plenty of fluids. She states that the girl has been in good health and all of her immunizations are current. She denies any previous ear infection.

FAMILY/SOCIAL HISTORY: Positive for asthma in the maternal uncle and first cousin. The mother denies any pets or smoking at home.

PHYSICAL EXAM
General: Alert, smiling, awake, female in no acute distress

Vital Signs: Wt. 18kg Pulse 90 Temp 36.3C R 36

HEENT: Normocephalic/atraumatic, eyes normal, ears - tympanic membranes pearly white and mobile bilaterally, mouth is moist, no erythema of throat

Nodes: Posterior cervical shotty nodes, non-tender

Lungs: Normal respiratory rate, symmetrical breath sounds, some upper airway noises with no wheezes, clear

Breast: Normal

Cardiovascular: RRR, no audible heart murmur, normal pulses

Abdominal: Soft non-distended, positive bowel sounds and no palpable masses

Neurological: Grossly normal and moves all extremities, no evidence of seizures, no focal findings

DX: Viral upper respiratory infection

Continued

DX: Asthma symptoms (cough, decrease exercise tolerance) and has likely had asthma since childhood.

PLAN: A low dose inhaled steroid 2 puffs QID and albuterol 2 puffs q4hours prn. Patient is given a peak flow meter and taught how to use it and to record her daily readings.

James I. Cipher, MD

JIC/mg   D: 10/13/08 09:50:16   T: 10/15/08 12:55:01

You Code It!

What are the best, most accurate codes?

_____

_____

_____

Pathology and Laboratory Cases and Patient Records

INTRODUCTION

The following case studies are from a pathology laboratory. Labs may be located within a hospital or other health care facility or a freestanding independent facility.

Pathologists are physicians who specialize in the examination of tissue and blood samples in order to diagnose disease.

Pathologists analyze and evaluate many different types of specimens. They may receive tissues (swab, excised lesion, mole, or polyp, for example) removed from a patient during surgery or a biopsy. They also analyze blood, urine, sperm, saliva, and other bodily fluid samples. Very often, it is the results of a pathology report (test results interpreted by a pathologist) that confirm or deny a suspected diagnosis or the progress of a disease or therapeutic procedure.

A medical examiner or coroner, a pathologist who performs autopsies, is a subspecialty of pathology.

Pathologists are board-certified in a number of subspecialties through the American Board of Pathology, which is recognized by the American Board of Medical Specialties.

You can use these cases to practice coding diagnoses, E/M, procedures, DME, or other HCPCS Level II items, as applicable; code for the physician or the facility; code inpatient and outpatient services, as applicable:

1. Code for the physician.
2. Code for the anesthesiologist, when applicable.
3. Code for the hospital, when applicable.
4. Code for the pathology and laboratory, when applicable.
5. Code HCPCS Level II codes, when applicable.

AMERICAN TESTING & DIAGNOSTICS
792 TREMONT DRIVE • HAMLIN, FL 32744 • 407-555-9764

PATIENT: FRANKLIN, FRANCES
MRN: FRANFR001
Date: 17 October 2008

Procedure Performed: Comprehensive metabolic panel

Pathologist: Caryn Simonson, MD

Referring Physician: Valerie R. Victors, MD

Indications: Routine physical exam

Impressions:

Albumin	3.9
Bilirubin	Small*
Calcium	8.9
Carbon dioxide (CO2)	28
Chloride	96 L
Creatinine	1.2
Glucose	102
Phosphatase, alkaline	90
Potassium	3.9
Protein, total	30*
Sodium	138
Transferase, alanine amino (ALT)(SGPT)	30
Transferase, aspartate amino (AST)(SGOT)	29
Urea nitrogen (BUN)	18

* = Abnormal, L = Low, H = High

Caryn Simonson, MD

CS/mg D: 10/17/08 09:50:16 T: 10/20/08 12:55:01

You Code It!

What are the best, most accurate codes?

_____

_____

_____

AMERICAN TESTING & DIAGNOSTICS
792 TREMONT DRIVE • HAMLIN, FL 32744 • 407-555-9764

PATIENT: TRANSIL, BRENT
MRN: TRANBRO01
Date: 29 September 2008

Procedure Performed: Tissue, skin, head, mutation identification

Pathologist: Caryn Simonson, MD

Referring Physician: James I. Cipher, MD

Indications: Suspected melanoma

Impressions: Abnormal cells present

Molecular diagnostics; mutation identification by sequencing, single segment

Caryn Simonson, MD

CS/mg   D: 9/29/08 09:50:16   T: 9/30/08 12:55:01

You Code It!

What are the best, most accurate codes?

_____

_____

_____

PATIENT: HAVERSTROM, OLIVIA
MRN: HAVEOL001
Date: 15 November 2008

Procedure Performed: Surgical pathology, gallbladder, gross and microscopic examination

Pathologist: Caryn Simonson, MD

Referring Physician: Valerie R. Victors, MD

Indications: R/O malignancy

Impressions: All tissues unremarkable

Surgical pathology, gross and microscopic examination of gallbladder

_____

Caryn Simonson, MD

CS/mg   D: 11/15/08 09:50:16   T: 11/20/08 12:55:01

You Code It!

What are the best, most accurate codes?

_____

_____

_____

AMERICAN TESTING & DIAGNOSTICS
792 TREMONT DRIVE • HAMLIN, FL 32744 • 407-555-9764

PATIENT: FRIEDMAN, DORIS
MRN: FRIEDO001
Date: 23 September 2008

Procedure Performed: Rectal biopsies, gross and microscopic examination

Pathologist: Caryn Simonson, MD

Referring Physician: Matthew Appellet, MD

Indications: Inflammatory bowel disease

Impressions: All tissues normal

Surgical pathology, gross and microscopic examination, colon biopsy

_____

Caryn Simonson, MD

CS/mg   D: 9/23/08 09:50:16   T: 9/25/08 12:55:01

You Code It!

What are the best, most accurate codes?

_____
_____
_____

AMERICAN TESTING & DIAGNOSTICS
792 TREMONT DRIVE • HAMLIN, FL 32744 • 407-555-9764

PATIENT: FRANKS, ELMER
MRN: FRANEL001
Date: 17 June 2008

Procedure Performed: Mass (fat tissue), upper eyelid gross and microscopic examination

Pathologist: Caryn Simonson, MD

Referring Physician: Mark C. Welby, MD

Indications: Herniated orbital fat pad, OD

Impressions: Carcinoma in situ

Surgical pathology, gross and microscopic examination, soft tissue tumor, extensive resection

---

Caryn Simonson, MD

CS/mg   D: 6/17/08 09:50:16   T: 6/20/08 12:55:01

You Code It!

What are the best, most accurate codes?

_____

_____

_____

AMERICAN TESTING & DIAGNOSTICS
792 TREMONT DRIVE • HAMLIN, FL 32744 • 407-555-9764

PATIENT: BAKER, DORITTA
MRN: BAKEDO001
Date: 19 September 2008

Procedure Performed: Endocervical specimen,
                                 Intraepithelial lesion of the cervix, cytopathology smear

Pathologist: Caryn Simonson, MD

Referring Physician: Rodney L. Cohen, MD

Indications: Lesion of cervix

Impressions: Uncertain behavior neoplasm

Cytopathology, cervical, collected in preservative fluid, automated thin layer preparation; manual screening and rescreening

_____

Caryn Simonson, MD

CS/mg   D: 9/19/08 09:50:16   T: 9/23/08 12:55:01

You Code It!

What are the best, most accurate codes?

_____

_____

_____

AMERICAN TESTING & DIAGNOSTICS
792 TREMONT DRIVE • HAMLIN, FL 32744 • 407-555-9764

PATIENT: KLOTSKY, STACY
MRN: KLOTST001
Date: 5 October 2008

Procedure Performed: Bladder, biopsy gross and microscopic examination

Pathologist: Caryn Simonson, MD

Referring Physician: Leonard Dupont, MD

Indications: R/o bladder tumor

Impressions: Chronic cystitis with squamous cell metaplasia

Surgical pathology, gross and microscopic examination, urinary bladder, biopsy

_____

Caryn Simonson, MD

CS/mg   D: 10/5/08 09:50:16   T: 10/7/08 12:55:01

You Code It!

What are the best, most accurate codes?

_____

_____

_____

AMERICAN TESTING & DIAGNOSTICS
792 TREMONT DRIVE • HAMLIN, FL 32744 • 407-555-9764

PATIENT NAME: BIRRSTONE, SHIRLEY

MRN: BIRRSH001

Date: 02-20-2008

Date of Surgery: 02-20-2008

Pathologist: Allan Cantor, MD

Surgeon: Roger Torres, MD

CLINICAL DIAGNOSIS AND HISTORY:
Carpal tunnel syndrome. No history of rheumatoid arthritis.

TISSUE(S) SUBMITTED:
SYNOVIUM, right hand.

GROSS DESCRIPTION:
Specimen is received in fixative and consists of multiple yellow-tan, rubbery, irregular connective tissue fragments, 4x2x1 cm in aggregate.

MICROSCOPIC DESCRIPTION:
1 microscopic slide examined.

DIAGNOSIS:
Chronic inflammation and fibrosis, tenosynovium, clinically, right hand.

Allan Cantor, MD

AC:ygc   DD: 02-20-2008   DT: 02-22-2008

You Code It!

What are the best, most accurate codes?

_____

_____

_____

PATIENT NAME: LARMAR, CARLA
MRN: LARMCA001
Date: 02-04-2008

Date of Surgery: 02-03-2008

Pathologist: Allan Cantor, M.D.

Surgeon: Harriet Fara, M.D.

Operation: Bilateral tubal ligation
Tissue: Left and right tubes
Preop DX: Undesired fertility
Postop DX: Same

Histological Diagnosis:
    #1 and #2 segments of fallopian tube, right and left: lumen identified

Gross Description:
    Received labeled with the patient's name.

Received in formalin, labeled "right and left tubes" are grossly recognizable segment of the right and left fallopian tubes measuring 1.5 x 0.5 x 0.4 cm and 2.0 x 0.6 x 0.4 cm. The serosa is pink-tan, smooth and glistening and the cut surface is grossly unremarkable. Representative section of right and left fallopian tube is submitted in one cassette.

_____

Allan Cantor, MD

AC:ygc   DD: 02-04-2008   DT: 02-09-2008

You Code It!

What are the best, most accurate codes?

_____

_____

_____

AMERICAN TESTING & DIAGNOSTICS
792 TREMONT DRIVE • HAMLIN, FL 32744 • 407-555-9764

PATIENT NAME: COLUMBO, ENZO
MRN: COLUEN001
Date: 02-15-2008

Date of Surgery: 02-14-2008

Pathologist: Allan Cantor, MD

Surgeon: Harriet Fara, MD

Operation: Lap. Chole
Tissue: Gallbladder
Preop DX: Cholelithiasis
Postop DX: Same

Histological Diagnosis:
    Gallbladder: Chronic cholecystitis. Cholelithiasis.
    T57000, M43000, M30010

Gross Description:
    Received labeled with the patient's name.

The specimen is received in formalin in a single container labeled "gallbladder" and consists of one pink green gallbladder measuring 7 x 2.8 x 2 cm. The serosal surface is smooth and glistening. Surgical staple is removed to reveal a partially obstructed cystic duct due to a thickening of the luminal wall. The specimen is opened to reveal a smooth dark green mucosal surface that is filled with viscous green bile and multiple tan yellow gallstones measuring 1 x 0.6 x 0.8 cm up to 2.2 x 1.5 x 1.2 cm. The gallbladder wall thickness measures 0.4 cm. Representative sections of cystic duct and gallbladder wall are submitted in one cassette.

Allan Cantor, MD

AC:ygc   DD: 02-15-2008   DT: 02-23-2008

You Code It!

What are the best, most accurate codes?

_____

_____

_____

AMERICAN TESTING & DIAGNOSTICS
792 TREMONT DRIVE • HAMLIN, FL 32744 • 407-555-9764

PATIENT NAME: GONZALEZ, ANITA
MRN: GONZAN001
Date: 04-22-2008

Date of Surgery: 04-21-2008

Pathologist: Allan Cantor, MD

Surgeon: Fredrick Frankel, MD

Operation: Laparotomy, appendectomy, right salpingo-oophorectomy
Tissue: Right tube and ovary and appendix
Preop DX: Acute abdomen
Postop DX: Same

Histological Diagnosis:
1. Fibroconnective tissue with acute and chronic inflammation and micro abscess formation consistent with acute peritonitis
2. Right ovary and fallopian tube with congestion, edema, inflammation, fibrous adhesions and serositis.
3. No evidence of malignancy.

Designated right tube and ovary

Comment: Despite a meticulous search, no appendiceal tissue is identified grossly or microscopically. Case discussed with Dr. Frankel on 4/23/08.

Gross Description:
The specimen is labeled right tube, ovary, and appendix and consists of a right ovary and fallopian tube which appear adherent to one another via numerous adhesions. The entire specimen weighs 20 grams and measures 6 x 4 x 2.0 cm. The segment of fallopian tube which is present measures 6.0 cm in length. The external surface is pale tan. Sections through the tube reveals a somewhat dilated but patent lumen. The adjacent ovary measures 3.5 x 3.0 x 1.0 cm. Bisection reveals pale tan tissue with areas of hemorrhage. No grossly recognizable appendix is seen. Representative sections in six cassettes.

Microscopic Description:
This specimen has been extensively sampled. Sections of the fallopian tube show areas of vascular congestion and edema. In addition within the serosa are areas of acute and chronic inflammation associated with microabscess formation. Fibrous adhesions are also present.

    Sections of the ovary show surface adhesions, vascular congestion and corpora albicantia. The serosa of the ovary also shows areas of inflammation.

    Also present are several fragments of fibroconnective tissue with vascular congestion, acute and chronic inflammation and microabscess formation. No appendiceal tissue is identified. There is no evidence of malignancy.

Allan Cantor, MD

AC:ygc   DD: 04-22-2008   DT: 04-27-2008

You Code It!

What are the best, most accurate codes?

_____

_____

_____

AMERICAN TESTING & DIAGNOSTICS
792 TREMONT DRIVE • HAMLIN, FL 32744 • 407-555-9764

PATIENT NAME: NATRINU, HERBERT
MRN: NATRHE001
Date: 04-11-2008

Date of Surgery: 04-10-2008

Pathologist: Allan Cantor, MD

Surgeon: Allen Farina, MD

Operation: Gastroscopy
Tissue: Antrum R/O Helicobacter
Preop DX: GI Bleed
Postop DX: Same

Pathology Diagnosis:
    1. Mild chronic active gastritis
    2. No intestinal metaplasia identified
    3. Few rare Helicobacter pylori identified on the Giemsa stain
    4. No evidence of malignancy
Designated antrum

Gross Description:
The specimen is labeled antrum r/o Helicobacter and consists of a circular fragment of pale tan yellow soft tissue that measures 0.3 cm in greatest dimension. Entirely submitted in one cassette.

Microscopic Description:
All of the tissue has been submitted for microscopic examination. Multiple levels have been obtained. Sections show gastric mucosa with vascular congestion and edema. There is a mild increase in the numbers of both acute and chronic inflammatory cells within the lamina propria. No intestinal metaplasia is identified. A few Helicobacter pylori are identified on the Giemsa stain. There is no evidence of malignancy.

Allan Cantor, MD

AC:ygc   DD: 04-11-2008   DT: 04-11-2008

You Code It!

What are the best, most accurate codes?

_____

_____

_____

AMERICAN TESTING & DIAGNOSTICS
792 TREMONT DRIVE • HAMLIN, FL 32744 • 407-555-9764

PATIENT NAME: NATRINU, HERBERT
MRN: NATRHE001
Date: 04-11-2008

Date of Surgery: 04-10-2008

Pathologist: Allan Cantor, MD

Surgeon: Allen Farina, MD

Nature of specimen: Paracentesis fluid

Final diagnosis:
Abdominal fluid, aspiration
—positive for malignant cells
—consistent with adenocarcinoma

Allan Cantor, MD

AC:ygc   DD: 04-11-2008   DT: 04-11-2008

You Code It!

What are the best, most accurate codes?

_____

_____

_____

AMERICAN TESTING & DIAGNOSTICS
792 TREMONT DRIVE • HAMLIN, FL 32744 • 407-555-9764

PATIENT: DENNING, ROSE
ACCOUNT/EHR #:   DENNRO001
Date: 10/15/08

Ordering Dr: Terence Rollin, MD

Clinical Information: Emergency Room

TEST	BMP			
(136-144)	SODIUM	L	130	MEQ/L
(3.6-5.1)	POTASSIUM	4.1	MEQ/L	
(101-111)	CHLORIDE	L	97	MEQ/L
(22-32)	CO2 CONTENT	22	MEQ/L	
(08-20)	BUN	H	23	MG/DL
(74-118)	GLUCOSE	H	130	MG/DL
(0.9-1.3)	CREATININE	0.9	MG/DL	
(7.3-21.7)	BUN/CREAT RATIO	H	25.6	
(280-300)	CALCULATED OSMO	L	275	MOS/KG
(8.9-10.3)	CALCIUM	9.4	MG/DL	

Lewis Strumm, MD
Pathologist

LS/fa 10/15/08 11:47:39

You Code It!

What are the best, most accurate codes?

_____

_____

_____

AMERICAN TESTING & DIAGNOSTICS
792 TREMONT DRIVE • HAMLIN, FL 32744 • 407-555-9764

PATIENT: YAWLIN, LAWRENCE
ACCOUNT/EHR #: YAWLLA001
Date: 10/15/08

Ordering Dr: Terence Rollin, MD

PATIENT HISTORY: The patient is a 53-year-old male with a three-year history of an increasing neck mass associated with a choking feeling. The pre-op and post-op diagnoses were "left thyroid mass."

GROSS DESCRIPTION: The specimen is received fresh in one part labeled "left thyroid lobe, superior pole, marked by stitch." It consists of 8.5 x 7.0 x 4.0 cm, 125-gram thyroid lobectomy. The specimen is inked and serially sectioned revealing a single nodule involving most of the specimen, with a 0.5-cm rim of thyroid tissue superiorly. This nodule is encapsulated revealing a brown, soft, lobulated cut surface with fibrous bands, with focal areas of hemorrhage, cystic degeneration, and necrosis. Sections are frozen in bulk and OCT. A frozen section was performed. Pictures and digital images are taken.

MICROSCOPIC DESCRIPTION: Histological examination reveals an encapsulated expansile tumor which is seen to compress the normal thyroid tissue around it. The tumor is composed of nests of cells separated by fine fibrous septa. The cells are large and brightly eosinophilic, with a granular cytoplasm and a low nuclear to cytoplasmic ratio. In most areas the nuclei are rather monomorphic, with coarse chromatin features and singular prominent eosinophilic nucleoli. Focally, there is nuclear atypia suggesting aneuploidy, but mitotic figures are not easily found. There are focal areas where there seems to be invasion into the capsule, and in one region, frank breaching of the capsule is seen. The tumor appears to track along the blood vessels as they pierce the capsule. Angiolymphatic invasion is identified.

DX: Thyroid, left, lobectomy
A. Well-differentiated Hürthle cell carcinoma (8.5 cm, 125 grams) with angiolymphatic invasion, capsular invasion and focal areas of degeneration.
B. All margins of resection free of tumor.
C. Stage: T3,Nx,Mx.

Lewis Strumm, MD
Pathologist

LS/fa 10/15/08 11:47:39

You Code It!

What are the best, most accurate codes?

_____

_____

_____

AMERICAN TESTING & DIAGNOSTICS
792 TREMONT DRIVE • HAMLIN, FL 32744 • 407-555-9764

PATIENT: WALKEN, SERITA
ACCOUNT/EHR #:   WALKSE001
Date: 10/15/08

Ordering Dr: Terence Rollin, MD

HISTORY: This patient is a 25-year-old female, referred by her primary care physician, Dr. Kennison, due to complaints of abdominal discomfort and distension which she has had for about four weeks. The patient reported constipation but denied nausea, vomiting, sharp abdominal pain, and rectal bleeding. Physical examination demonstrated diffuse abdominal tenderness and firmness without guarding. A transvaginal ultrasound revealed a large, complex, cystic and solid soft tissue mass within the pelvis, extending to 2 cm above the umbilicus. A CT scan of the abdomen and pelvis showed involvement of the right adnexa. The patient underwent a right salpingo-oophorectomy.

LABORATORY DATA: Alpha-Fetoprotein (AFP) 11023 ng/mL, CA 125 93 U/mL, CA 19-9

GROSS DESCRIPTION: The right salpingo-oophorectomy specimen consisted of an unremarkable fallopian tube and a 19 x 18 x 6 cm solid and cystic ovarian mass. The serosa was intact and smooth. Serial section of the mass demonstrated multiloculated cysts containing yellow, seromucinous fluid. The interior of the cyst wall was red-tan and smooth, with focal edema and intramural hemorrhage. The solid component was fleshy and tan-pink with yellow, rubbery-to-firm stellate areas. Separate from the main solid and cystic mass was a 6.5 cm area containing hair and friable, yellow material.

MICROSCOPIC DESCRIPTION: Histologic sections of the smaller yellow, friable area showed epidermis with adnexal structures.

Sections of the larger cystic and solid mass demonstrated branching, papillary structures containing thick basement membrane material and covered with cuboidal to low columnar cells. This arrangement was best seen in a cross-section of an individual papilla. In addition to this pattern, microcystic spaces were prominent in other areas. Eosinophilic globules were present in a few sections, and were found to be PAS-positive, diastase-resistant.

IMMUNOHISTOCHEMICAL STAINS: Stains for human chorionic gonadotropin (hCG), placental alkaline phosphatase (PLAP), and epithelial membrane antigen (EMA) were negative.

FINAL DIAGNOSIS: Yolk sac tumor arising in association with mature cystic teratoma (dermoid cyst).

Lewis Strumm, MD
Pathologist

LS/fa 10/15/08 11:47:39

You Code It!

What are the best, most accurate codes?

_____

_____

_____

AMERICAN TESTING & DIAGNOSTICS
792 TREMONT DRIVE • HAMLIN, FL 32744 • 407-555-9764

PATIENT: ABATTI, BRIAN
ACCOUNT/EHR #:   ABATBR001
Date: 10/04/08

Ordering Dr: Terence Rollin, MD

DX:
1. Sepsis. Rule out pneumonitis or urinary tract infection.
2. Acute bronchitis
3. Diabetes mellitus
4. Chronic obstructive pulmonary disease

GRAM STAIN****
    Body Site: Sputum
    Gram Stain   Few epithelial cells, few WBC's, few gram positive cocci and gram positive bacilli

SPUTUM CULTURE****
    Source   Sputum
    Status   Preliminary
    Grade   +1
    Organism   Normal respiratory flora

URINE CULTURE*****
    Source   CATH
    Status   Final
    Organism   No growth 48 hr

THROAT CULTURE*****
    Source   Throat
    Body Site   Throat
    Status   Final
    Organism   Normal upper respiratory flora. No group A Beta Streptococcus isolated.

BLOOD CULTURE #1****
    Source   Blood
    Arm   Right
    Time   1550
    Status   Preliminary
    Organism   No growth 48 hr

Continued

BLOOD CULTURE #2****
Source	Blood
Arm	Left
Time	1600
Status	Preliminary
Organism	No growth 48 hr

Lewis Strumm, MD
Pathologist

LS/fa 10/04/08 11:47:39

You Code It!

What are the best, most accurate codes?

_____

_____

_____

Plastic and Reconstructive Surgery Cases and Patient Records

INTRODUCTION

The following case studies are from a plastic (reconstructive) surgical practice. In a physician's office of this type, a professional coding specialist is likely to see many different kinds of health situations. You might think that because most plastic surgery is considered cosmetic or elective surgery not typically covered by insurance, there is no need for a coder. That is not always true. The cases that you see within this chapter will, hopefully, help you gain a wider perspective.

Plastic surgeons are physicians who specialize in surgery that improves a person's appearance or functionality. Plastic surgery is not only about face-lifts and nose jobs. This health care provider performs surgery to correct congenital abnormalities, such as cleft lip and palate to enable a child to eat properly. This physician may be called in to surgically reattach a severed limb or finger, complete skin grafts to cover the scars from a severe burn, or carry out reconstruction, such as performing breast implant surgery after a mastectomy.

Plastic surgeons can subspecialize in facial reconstruction or hand surgery.

Plastic surgeons are board-certified through the Board of Plastic Surgery, which is recognized by the American Board of Medical Specialties.

You can use these cases to practice coding diagnoses, E/M, procedures, DME, or other HCPCS Level II items, as applicable; code for the physician or the facility; code inpatient and outpatient services, as applicable:

1. Code for the physician.
2. Code for the anesthesiologist, when applicable.
3. Code for the hospital, when applicable.
4. Code for the pathology and laboratory, when applicable.
5. Code HCPCS Level II codes, when applicable.

PLASTIC SURGERY ASSOCIATES
321 Newone Lane • Somewhere, FL 32811 • 407-555-9897

PATIENT:	RUDERMAN, LILLIE ANN
MRN:	RUDELI01
Admission Date:	15 October 2008
Discharge Date:	15 October 2008
Date:	15 October 2008
Preoperative DX:	Augmentation of lips
Postoperative DX:	Same
Procedure:	Collagen injections
Surgeon:	Wayne Fleeter, MD
Assistant:	None
Anesthesia:	Local

INDICATIONS: The patient is a 41-year-old female with a low self-image. She presents today for enhancement of her lips.

PROCEDURE: The patient was placed on the table in supine position. Local anesthesia was administered. As soon as patient stated a complete loss of feeling in the area, the injections were given subcutaneously - a total of 2.3 cc.

10/15/08 11:47:39

You Code It!

What are the best, most accurate codes?

_____

_____

_____

PLASTIC SURGERY ASSOCIATES
321 Newone Lane • Somewhere, FL 32811 • 407-555-9897

PATIENT: ALVAREZ, COLLEEN
MRN: ALVACO01
Date: 15 October 2008

Surgeon: Wayne Fleeter, MD

Consultation for evaluation for surgery.

This is a 2-day-old female born to a 31-year-old G3 P2 A1 mother at 38 weeks gestational age via vaginal delivery with Apgar scores of 8 and 9 at 1 and 5 minutes, who is noted to have an isolated cleft palate.

EXAM: She is alert and active in no distress. Her head shape is normal with a flat anterior fontanelle. There is no clefting of the lip. The U-shaped cleft of the palate is complete, extending across the alveolar ridge and all the way back into the palate. At this time, there do not appear to be signs of mandibular hypoplasia or glossoptosis. Her eyes and ears are normal. Her neck, heart, lungs, abdomen and extremities are normal.
    This infant has some difficulties in feeding.

PLAN: Rx written for a cleft palate nipple to aid child in feeding. Once infant begins gaining weight and is infection-free, surgical correction can be considered.

10/15/08 11:47:39

You Code It!

What are the best, most accurate codes?

_____

_____

_____

PLASTIC SURGERY ASSOCIATES
321 Newone Lane • Somewhere, FL 32811 • 407-555-9897

PATIENT: GIACOMA, ROBERTA
MRN: GIACRO01
Date: 15 October 2008

Surgeon: Wayne Fleeter, MD

This patient is a 43-year-old female who presents to discuss breast reconstruction. In October 2003, she underwent a right modified radical mastectomy for a 3.7 cm right lobular breast carcinoma. Following the mastectomy, she proceeded through both chemotherapy and radiation therapy. The prescribed plan was completed in January 2005. Due to a positive family history and abnormal mammograms, the patient chose to have a prophylactic mastectomy of her left breast. Besides the malignancy in her breast, the patient's medical history was negative.

EXAM: Patient has adequate abdominal pannus for autogenous reconstruction. After extensive discussion with the patient regarding surgical reconstruction options and risks, the patient and her husband decide to proceed with the reconstruction procedure.

PROCEDURE: Patient is brought into the surgical suite. After successful administration of general anesthesia, she is draped in the usual sterile fashion. Under high-power magnification, the pectoralis major muscle was split along its fiber over the fourth rib. The deep perichondrium was then incised and the internal mammary artery and veins identified. An elliptical incision was then made in the lower abdomen, approximately 2 cm above the umbilicus. The subcutaneous dissection was performed through the fat down to the level of the rectus abdominis fascia. Several perforators were identified and preserved as they pierced the rectus fascia. The fascia was incised and the perforators were dissected through the rectus abdominis muscle. The first flap was harvested with the right deep inferior epigastric vessels visualized as they entered the muscle, and divided at their origin. The perforator flap was brought with its vessels through the rectus abdominis muscle. No muscle was taken with this flap. The flap was transferred to the right chest and secured. A second flap was harvested from the left lower abdomen using the same technique and transferred to the left chest and secured. Dissection of both the internal mammary artery and vein was performed after flap harvest to allow for microvascular anastomosis. The abdominal donor site was closed and all surgery sites were dressed with large bulky dressings. The patient was transferred to the intensive care unit in good condition for postoperative monitoring.

The patient had little postoperative pain or discomfort.

PLAN: Nipple reconstruction will be done four months postoperatively; nipple/areolar tattooing is planned for approximately two months after successful nipple reconstruction.

10/15/08 11:47:39

You Code It!

What are the best, most accurate codes?

_____

_____

_____

PLASTIC SURGERY ASSOCIATES
321 Newone Lane • Somewhere, FL 32811 • 407-555-9897

PATIENT: BRIGGS, SHANE
MRN: BRIGSH01
Date: 15 October 2008

Surgeon: Wayne Fleeter, MD

This patient is a 19-year-old male who was hit by a car, and suffered severe head injuries. Extensive damage warrants the removal of a portion of his skull, leaving a large area of his brain exposed. Although he could be temporarily fitted with a special protective helmet, the patient would ultimately need some type of skull replacement.

Using stereolithography (SL), a custom implant for the patient was created prior to surgery. The SL master was used to create an accurate prosthesis to restore the injured man's skull.

The patient withstood the surgical procedure well and was brought into the recovery room.

10/15/08 11:47:39

You Code It!

What are the best, most accurate codes?

_____

_____

_____

PLASTIC SURGERY ASSOCIATES
321 Newone Lane • Somewhere, FL 32811 • 407-555-9897

PATIENT: RHINIER, ELBERT
MRN: RHINEL01
Date: 15 October 2008

Surgeon: Wayne Fleeter, MD

This patient is a 14-year-old male needing reconstructive rhinoplasty.

The patient was playing basketball when another player hit him across the bridge of the nose with his elbow, causing a comminuted fracture. Due to the swelling and bleeding, his parents took him to the emergency department. The ED physician notes periorbital ecchymoses and nasal displacement. Intranasal packing and an external splint were used to shape the nose.

Patient is brought into the surgical suite and given a mild sedative (conscious sedation) to lessen patient anxiety during the procedure. Using photographs provided by the parents, a reconstructive rhinoplasty is performed. An incision is made in the upper lateral cartilage and continued as an osteotomy of the medial aspect of the nasal bones. The spreader graft is placed to widen the nasal vestibule to assure that the airway is not constricted. Lateral nasal wall reconstruction is successful.

Patient withstands the procedure well and is brought into recovery.

10/15/08 11:47:39

You Code It!

What are the best, most accurate codes?

_____

_____

_____

PLASTIC SURGERY ASSOCIATES
321 Newone Lane • Somewhere, FL 32811 • 407-555-9897

PATIENT: LAWSON, MELISSA
MRN: LAWSME01
Date: 15 October 2008

Surgeon: Wayne Fleeter, MD

This patient is a 23-year-old female who was brought in by helicopter. She was driving with her best friend when she realized they had a flat tire. She pulled the car over to the shoulder of the road to assess the situation. While examining the back tire on the driver side of her vehicle, she was hit by an oncoming car. The impact severed her left leg below the knee.

She was rushed by helicopter to Backler Hospital where I was called in for a plastic surgery consultation to determine if the severed limb could be reattached. Since there were extensive injuries to the amputated leg, reattachment was not considered possible.

Assessment of the amputation stump showed marked injury to muscle tissue as well as exposed bone. Unless healthy tissue could be transferred to the site of injury the amputation level would have to be raised above the knee, sacrificing an important lower extremity joint and limiting the patient's ultimate level of rehabilitation.

Although several muscles from the patient's body could have been used as donor tissue, it was decided to utilize tissue from the amputated part. The sole of the foot was removed from the severed leg and transferred to the amputation stump with the aid of the microscope. The patient's knee joint was preserved, giving her a positive prognosis for walking again with an artificial leg.

10/15/08 11:47:39

You Code It!

What are the best, most accurate codes?

_____

_____

_____

PODIATRY ASSOCIATES OF TARSA
539 WALKING WAY • FOOTHILLS, FL 32811 • 407-555-5399

PATIENT: GRADDY, KYLE
ACCOUNT/EHR #:   GRADKY001
Date: 10/15/08

This patient is a 71-year-old male who presents with a three-day history of swelling and pain in his right lower leg. The pain worsens with walking. The patient remembers first noticing right calf pain when arising from bed the morning before yesterday. He noticed the right lower leg was swollen and red. He denies any traumatic event or recent strenuous activity. In fact, he just returned, by car, from vacation in Texas. He states the long drive gave his legs a needed rest after all the walking he did sightseeing. Patient states that the leg pain worsens with walking, especially pushing off with the toes of that foot. The pain is relieved with rest and elevation but overall, his calf continues to hurt. The pain is described by the patient to be most severe "inside his calf." He has not had this leg swelling and pain previously and has never had leg edema. He denies fever or night sweats and can't recall any reason for his skin to be infected. He recalls no bites or scrapes to his calf area.

ROS: Generally negative, and specifically the patient denies fatigue, headache, chest pain, palpitations. He claims he has no nausea nor vomiting.

Past Medical History: HTN: controlled. He has osteoarthritis.

Surgical History: Total knee replacement 2 years ago

Current Meds: Relafen 1000 mg po qday; Atenolol 50 mg qday

Allergies: Penicillin (hives)

Social History: Tobacco - 1 PPD x25 years. No alcohol use. Married, lives with wife. Retired school teacher with two sons.

Family history: Patient denies any family history of cancer, peripheral vascular disease, or hypercoagulable conditions.

Physical Exam: Patient is mildly obese, alert, oriented and in NAD.

Extremities: Right lower extremity (RLE) appears edematous and mildly erythematous distal to the knee compared to the left. The right calf is 24 cm and the left is 20 cm. There is no skin breakdown appreciated. On palpation, the right calf is warmer and firmer than the left, and the edema is nonpitting. Superficial palpation of the right calf is nontender. There is moderate tenderness to deep palpation over the calf and popliteal vein. Femoral, popliteal, posterior tibialis, and dorsalis pedis pulses are all 2+ and equal bilaterally. Homan's sign is not present. Sensation is intact bilaterally.

TESTING: In office, diagnostic duplex ultrasound of the lower extremities for suspected DVT.
    The ultrasound is positive for a DVT in the right lower extremity. Patient has a calf vein thrombi extending to the popliteal veins.

Continued

PLAN: Rx: Coumadin 5mg per day; antiembolism stockings to be worn at all times patient is erect. Bed rest whenever possible, Standing or sitting for more than 15 minutes at a time should be avoided. Schedule duplex ultrasound of lower right extremity in one week for follow-up. Patient informed that surgery may be needed.

Scott Cole, DPM

10/15/08 11:47:39

You Code It!

What are the best, most accurate codes?

_____

_____

_____

PODIATRY ASSOCIATES OF TARSA
539 WALKING WAY • FOOTHILLS, FL 32811 • 407-555-5399

PATIENT: ORTNER, HELEN
ACCOUNT/EHR #: ORTNHE001
Date: 10/15/08

This patient is a 51-year-old female who presents with an ulceration on the plantar medial aspect of the left hallux. This ulcer had been present for several months and showed no signs of healing despite regular debridement.

HISTORY OF PRESENT ILLNESS: A Jones fracture in the same foot five years ago. Two years ago, she developed an ulcer at the distal aspect of the second toe on this same foot. Subsequently an arthroplasty of the second toe allowed the ulcer to heal.

   This patient has a chronic left hallux ulcer that has been present for several months. She had previously used orthotic devices 10 years ago for plantar fasciitis. Early on in the treatment of the hallux ulcer, orthotic devices were prescribed and fabricated. When the condition resolved, the patient stopped using the orthotics.

EXAM: The patient has now developed a new hallux ulcer. She currently wears properly fitting, extra-depth footwear. The patient also has a leg length discrepancy. She has used a 1/8-inch heel lift. A 1/4-inch external shoe lift was also recommended. The thinking was that excessive pronation off the hallux during propulsion was the cause of the ulcer. However, when the patient used the orthotic devices, the ulcer actually enlarged. Since the ulcer was chronic and treatment was not helping, video/computer gait analysis was recommended.

TESTING: Gait analysis is performed in a few different situations: barefoot walking; in shoes without the heel lift; and in shoes with the heel lift. Pressure mapping software is then used to assess the patient's gait in shoes with and without orthotic devices, and in shoes with and without the heel lift.

   These gait analysis techniques revealed that the orthotic devices were actually contributing to greater pressure on the ulcer. While the goal of using the orthotics was to prevent the excessive pronation, there was actually more pressure on the hallux during propulsion. This additional friction and pressure contributed to chronic ulceration. In comparing shoes with the lift to shoes without, it was clearly evident there was less pressure on the hallux with the external shoe lift. Pressure mapping revealed that the optimal situation was having the lift on the shoe along with the regular insert that came with the shoe.

   Video assessment revealed significant differences between the patient's right and left sides both with and without the lift. Adding an external shoe lift was a necessity in this case in order to provide more symmetry and more equal pressures between her feet. The results showed that accommodative pressure relief around the hallux was the best situation along with the lift on the shoe.

   Callus is debrided, as well.

DX: Chronic Hallux Ulcer

PLAN: Patient is told to continue to use the lift, however to discontinue use of the orthotics. Periodic debridement will be necessary to keep callus to a minimum. Schedule next appointment for 30 days.

Scott Cole, DPM

10/15/08 11:47:39

You Code It!

What are the best, most accurate codes?

_____

_____

_____

PODIATRY ASSOCIATES OF TARSA
539 WALKING WAY • FOOTHILLS, FL 32811 • 407-555-5399

PATIENT: BREEDLOVE, KERRY
ACCOUNT/EHR #:   BREEKE001
Date: 10/15/08

This patient is a 59-year-old male who presents with a chronic ulcer on the plantar aspect of the right foot.

HISTORY: The patient has previously undergone a pancreas/liver transplant due to the effects of chronic diabetes mellitus. Over the years, he has developed profound diabetic peripheral neuropathy that not only affects sensation but motor function also. As a result, he wears single, upright metal AFOs on both lower extremities. In addition, he has previously undergone a complete fifth metatarsal resection of the right foot, a fourth metatarsal osteotomy, and a second metatarsal head resection because of frequent ulcerations.

This patient is conscientious in regularly coming in for podiatric care and appears to follow recommendations with regard to footwear and accommodative orthotic devices. Rocker soles were prescribed six months ago.

EXAM: A newly developed chronic ulcer inferior to the fourth metatarsal has formed. This is inferior to the area where the patient previously had an osteotomy. The patient has an elevated fourth metatarsal and does not appear to have any palpable pressure at this location. At each office visit, the patient has dried blood within the callus and a shallow ulceration. Multiple attempts to accommodate this area with his orthotic devices have failed.

TESTING: Video and computer gait analysis and pressure mapping software is used to identify pressure distribution points.
     Pressure mapping software identifies localized pressure in the region of the ulcer but the pressure was not any greater than what was found in other parts of the foot. However, the integral pressures indicated that the sustained amount of pressure in this one region was much too great. Even though the pressure may not have been an extreme amount, the duration of pressure was causing the problem.
     Video gait analysis indicated that the patient, despite wearing braces, exhibited rapid midstance. The rocker soles were prescribed to provide a smoother transition of the foot through midstance into propulsion; however, this was not the case for this patient. This pair of rocker soles was actually contributing to the rapid flatfoot and subsequently elevating the pressures on the ulcerated area. The shape of the heel was acting like a fulcrum, accelerating forefoot loading.

PLAN: Modify his rocker soles by adding a walking heel. Schedule follow-up visit in 30 days to check status.

Scott Cole, DPM

10/15/08 11:47:39

You Code It!

What are the best, most accurate codes?

_____

_____

_____

PODIATRY ASSOCIATES OF TARSA
539 WALKING WAY • FOOTHILLS, FL 32811 • 407-555-5399

PATIENT: RHINIER, ADELINA
ACCOUNT/EHR #:   RHINAD001
Date: 10/15/08

This patient is a 37-year-old female who comes in complaining of chronic plantar fasciitis in her right foot. She says she has had this pain for several months. She had a similar episode a few years prior but the use of orthotic devices and injections resolved the condition successfully. However, not only has the plantar fasciitis returned but the patient now has some complaints about her knee and hip on this right side as well. She is a runner and cyclist and likes to go for at least one two-hour run per week. This has become more difficult as the symptoms became chronic. She understands the importance of wearing good shoes and replaces them often.

EXAM: A biomechanical examination revealed asymmetry between the lower extremities. The exam noted increased external hip rotation in her left lower extremity and increased internal hip rotation in her right lower extremity. ROM in the subtalar joint is also different between the feet. During the exam, more inversion in the left foot and more eversion in the right foot is noted. The first MTP joint range of motion was also different in each foot. She had functional hallux limitus in her right foot with much less dorsiflexion than in the left foot. Existing orthotic devices fit her feet relatively well. The patient had a Morton's extension underneath the first MTP joint on each device.

TESTING: Video and computer gait analysis is performed: barefoot walking; running shoes with orthotic devices; and running shoes without orthotic devices.

    Pressure mapping results indicates significant asymmetry in the force versus time curve. This is positive for the presence of a leg length discrepancy. The patient has greater pressures on both the first metatarsal head and hallux in the asymptomatic foot. In the symptomatic foot, the mapping noted no first metatarsal head pressure but did note the occurrence of hallux pressures at peak heel strike. This indicates that a functional hallux limitus is contributing to the patient's complaint. Furthermore, her orthotic devices exacerbated the complaint. These devices are actually increasing the hallux pressures and limiting the range of motion in the first MTP joint even more.

    Video analysis shows an in-toed gait on the right side and an out-toed gait on the left. On the right side, the first MTPJ blocked propulsion. This was evident from the side camera view, which shows less hallux dorsiflexion.

DX: Chronic Plantar Fasciitis

PLAN: Existing orthotic devices are modified with dancer's pad accommodation to the right orthotic device and placed a wedge under the hallux with the thicker portion proximal and thinner part distal.

_____

Scott Cole, DPM

10/15/08 11:47:39

You Code It!

What are the best, most accurate codes?

_____

_____

_____

PODIATRY ASSOCIATES OF TARSA
539 WALKING WAY • FOOTHILLS, FL 32811 • 407-555-5399

PATIENT: LAKE, LOUISE
ACCOUNT/EHR #:   LAKELO001
Date: 10/15/08

This patient is a 69-year-old female with a 15-year history of impaired glucose tolerance. She quit smoking 16 years ago and denies the use of alcohol. The patient retired from a secretarial job three years ago.

HISTORY: Hypertension; hypercholesterolemia, both of which are treated with an angiotensin-converting enzyme inhibitor and a statin respectively. Her glucose intolerance was discovered with routine laboratory testing. She went for diabetes education, learned home glucose monitoring, and followed a diet and exercise program suggested by the diabetes educator.

    Approximately three months ago, this patient noticed a burning and tingling in both her hands and feet. The patient also felt that her sense of balance was diminished but thought it was merely a sign of aging and was reluctant to see a doctor.

ALLERGIES: NKA

EXAM: Patient is slightly overweight. Other than this, exam results are unremarkable except for some hyperesthesia of both hands and feet as well as decreased vibratory sensation. The patient has no open lesions on either foot and has intact protective sensation for both feet. Reflexes were normal and pedal pulses were palpable. A slight ataxia is noted. The patient has no clinical signs of depression. She denies fever, chills, nausea, vomiting, chest pain or shortness of breath. The patient also has no cough, vertigo or orthostatic hypotension.

    The loss of protective sensation is associated with diabetic peripheral neuropathy.

Rx: duloxetine (Cymbalta, Eli Lilly) 60 mg once daily.

___

Scott Cole, DPM

10/15/08 11:47:39

You Code It!

What are the best, most accurate codes?

_____

_____

_____

PODIATRY ASSOCIATES OF TARSA
539 WALKING WAY • FOOTHILLS, FL 32811 • 407-555-5399

PATIENT: OLDAKER, WALLACE
ACCOUNT/EHR #:   OLDAWA001
Date: 10/15/08

This patient is a 53-year-old male who presents with complaints of persistent pain in both feet, which has been going on for the last two months. He states he has had to take Tylenol #3 to help alleviate the pain.

HISTORY OF PRESENT ILLNESS: The patient denies fever, chills, nausea, vomiting, chest pain, shortness of breath, or changes to his medication. He also denies any other new symptoms. The patient also denies resting tachycardia, orthostatic lightheadedness, early satiety, early morning nausea, changes in bowel habits or post-prandial sweating. The patient stated his foot has been "asleep" for the past 5 years. The patient denies the use of alcohol and tobacco.

HISTORY: Patient was diagnosed with Type 2 diabetes at the age of 33 and has been insulin-dependent for the last five years. He has congestive heart failure, hypertension, peripheral arterial disease of bilateral lower extremity, DPN, diabetic foot ulcers, Charcot foot deformity, a partial fifth ray amputation, and a kidney transplant from a non-matched donor. The patient's glycemic control had never been optimal despite medications and a multiple-dose insulin program. His hemoglobin A1C levels have typically been in the 8 to 9 percent range.

CURRENT MEDICATIONS: The patient takes 18 different medications including two different immunosuppressive medications as well as Prednisone due to his kidney transplant. He is also taking an angiotensin-converting enzyme inhibitor for hypertension.

ALLERGIES: NKA

EXAM: Findings remain unchanged from his last visit three months ago. He is a moderately overweight (BMI 30 kg/m^2) man with a blood pressure of 131/85 mmHg with no orthostatic change and a resting pulse of 72 with no change with Valsalva maneuver.

EXTREMITIES: Decreased position sense as well as absent sensation to 10 g monofilament testing.

Rx: 5% lidocaine patch (Lidoderm, Endo Pharmaceuticals) twice daily for five weeks to treat the neuropathy because of the drug's lack of serious toxicity and drug interactions.
    Schedule next office visit for 45 days

Scott Cole, DPM

10/15/08 11:47:39

You Code It!

What are the best, most accurate codes?

_____

_____

_____

PODIATRY ASSOCIATES OF TARSA
539 WALKING WAY • FOOTHILLS, FL 32811 • 407-555-5399

PATIENT: GOLDEN, GEORGIA-ANNE
ACCOUNT/EHR #:   GOLDGE001
Date: 10/15/08

This patient is a 35-year-old female who presents with complaints of increasing burning and pain on the ball of the right foot. Over the past six months, she states she has changed her shoe styles, decreased her activity levels, and used an over-the-counter foot massager with no improvement in symptoms. Another physician had recommended neuroma surgery, however, the patient was reluctant to pursue this approach. She does believe the pain has grown worse with time.

HISTORY: Negative for contributory findings.

EXAM: Reproducible pain and radiating tingling into the third and fourth toes of the right foot with compression and direct palpation of the third intermetatarsal space.

TEST: X-rays show no abnormalities.

DIAGNOSIS: Intermetatarsal neuroma of the right foot.

PLAN: The patient is provided with a list of potential treatment options, including cortisone injection, orthotic devices, a series of alcohol sclerosing injections, or nerve surgery. I recommended a cortisone injection and orthotic devices as the first line of treatment and she was agreeable.

ADMINISTERED: 1 ml of dexamethasone plus 1 ml of local anesthetic agent is injected into the third intermetatarsal space at the point of maximum tenderness.
   Schedule examination and casting for custom orthoses for one week.

Scott Cole, DPM

10/15/08 11:47:39

You Code It!

What are the best, most accurate codes?

_____

_____

_____

PODIATRY ASSOCIATES OF TARSA
539 WALKING WAY • FOOTHILLS, FL 32811 • 407-555-5399

PATIENT: JOUDREY, CHARLOTTE
ACCOUNT/EHR #:   JOUDCH001
Date: 10/15/08

This patient is a 51-year-old female who presents complaining of burning pain in the ball of the left foot and a feeling of numbness in the middle toes.

HISTORY: Patient is an insulin-dependent diabetic who has had previously been treated with two cortisone injections and orthotic devices. When the foot problem grew worse over the last several months, the patient came in to our office.

EXAM: Patient is overweight. It is apparent the patient has a clinical neuroma of the third intermetatarsal space of the left foot with burning and numbness both reported.
   There is evidence of thinning and discoloration of the skin over the area of the previous cortisone injections.

DX: Clinical neuroma, third intermetatarsal space, left foot

TREATMENT: I discussed the options of a series of 0.5ml of 4% alcohol sclerosing injections and surgery to remove the neuroma. The patient elected to proceed with the injection series and the first injection is administered. Four additional weekly injections of 1/2 ml of 4 percent alcohol are scheduled.

Scott Cole, DPM

10/15/08 11:47:39

You Code It!

What are the best, most accurate codes?

_____

_____

_____

PODIATRY ASSOCIATES OF TARSA
539 WALKING WAY • FOOTHILLS, FL 32811 • 407-555-5399

PATIENT: NEWCOMB, CLIFFORD
ACCOUNT/EHR #:   NEWCCL001
Date: 10/15/08

This patient is a 41-year-old male who presents with a six-month history of a slowly growing, firm, well-defined, exophytic, and asymptomatic nodule measuring 1.2 cm in diameter. The lesion is on the proximal plantar surface.

HISTORY: Approximately three months prior to this encounter, the patient self-treated the lesion (which he thought was a wart) for two weeks with a topical salicylic acid 17% liquid. There was no response.

TESTING: An excisional biopsy and a deep saucerization biopsy, is done. The histologic evaluation confirms eccrine poroma.

PLAN: Surgical excision, with clear pathologic margins, is discussed and recommended to the patient.

DX: Eccrine poroma
     Patient states he wants to discuss the surgical option with his wife. He says he will call our office within 72 hours to schedule surgery.

Scott Cole, DPM

10/15/08 11:47:39

You Code It!

What are the best, most accurate codes?

_____

_____

_____

PODIATRY ASSOCIATES OF TARSA
539 WALKING WAY • FOOTHILLS, FL 32811 • 407-555-5399

PATIENT: SHANE, SHIRLEY
ACCOUNT/EHR #: SHANSH001
Date: 10/15/08

This patient is a 57-year-old female who presents with two large, erythematous scaly asymptomatic plaques on the medial surface of her leg. The patient states that the lesions started smaller and slowly expanded in radial diameter over the course of at least the last seven years.

Patient states that she tried treatment with a topical antifungal (econazole) cream for approximately one month that produced no change. Subsequent treatment with a high potency topical corticosteroid for three weeks also produced no response.

EXAM: The patient does not have any other similar lesions and there is no regional adenopathy upon palpation. The appearance of the lesion includes a sharply defined border, irregular outline of the plaques, a lack of symptomatology, pink erythema, and scattered hyperkeratotic surface change.

The surface scaling is somewhat hyperkeratotic and doesn't resemble the typical silver micaceous scaling of psoriasis. However, the recent topical corticosteroid therapy may have altered the clinical appearance of psoriasis.

TESTING: A histologic evaluation of a broad saucerization specimen confirmed this diagnosis of squamous cell carcinoma in situ.

DX: Squamous cell carcinoma in situ

TREATMENT: Options are discussed with patient. Schedule follow-up in one week.

Scott Cole, DPM

10/15/08 11:47:39

You Code It!

What are the best, most accurate codes?

_____

_____

_____

PODIATRY ASSOCIATES OF TARSA
539 WALKING WAY • FOOTHILLS, FL 32811 • 407-555-5399

PATIENT: SANDERS, JOSE
ACCOUNT/EHR #:   SANDJO001
Date: 10/15/08

This patient is a 59-year-old male who presents with a 1cm erythematous nodule on the proximal dorsum of the right foot. The nodule had grown rapidly over a period of six to eight weeks.

The clinical appearance of this erythematous nodule is highly characteristic of a melanoma with a large central nodule, possibly arising within a congenital nevus.

The patient states that the lesion has grown considerably within a preexisting dark brown "mole" which has been present for several years. The wife states that her mother-in-law told her several years ago that this mole has been present since the patient's birth. The lesion is asymptomatic.

EXAM: There is no regional adenopathy noted upon palpation. The clinical appearance is highly characteristic of a melanoma with a large central nodule, possibly arising within a congenital nevus.

TESTING: An excisional biopsy is performed here in the office and the results confirm the diagnosis. The reported histologic features were Clark's Level IV, Breslow thickness 4.5 mm with surface ulceration, no evidence of regression and no microsatellites.

DX: A contiguous melanocytic nevus consistent with a pre-existing congenital nevus

Scott Cole, DPM

10/15/08 11:47:39

You Code It!

What are the best, most accurate codes?

_____

_____

_____

PODIATRY ASSOCIATES OF TARSA
539 WALKING WAY • FOOTHILLS, FL 32811 • 407-555-5399

PATIENT: PINO, ALBERTA
ACCOUNT/EHR #:   PINOAL001
Date: 10/15/08

This patient is a 50-year-old female who presents with right heel pain of four months' duration. The patient states that her pain is at the inferior aspect of the heel at the medial tuberosity. She states the pain is worse in the morning as well as after any period of rest. She had one steroid injection several weeks ago by her family physician and feels about a 30% improvement.

EXAM: Pain is revealed with palpation at the medial tuberosity and central inferior aspect of the calcaneus. The rest of the exam is unremarkable. Radiographs are unremarkable.

TESTING: In-office musculoskeletal ultrasound imaging depicts plantar fasciosis with an abnormal central band. The upper limit of normal fascial thickness has been cited as 3 mm for the central band. Also revealed a well-formed cyst at the inferior aspect of the heel. This was not discernible clinically.

TREATMENT: Series of steroid injections to be scheduled.

Scott Cole, DPM

10/15/08 11:47:39

You Code It!

What are the best, most accurate codes?

_____

_____

_____

PODIATRY ASSOCIATES OF TARSA
539 WALKING WAY • FOOTHILLS, FL 32811 • 407-555-5399

PATIENT:	OWEN, MAXINE
ACCOUNT/EHR #:	OWENMA001
Date:	10/15/08

This patient is a 25-year-old female who presents with a nine-year history of rheumatoid arthritis and extreme pain and deformity of the forefoot. While both feet are painful, she says the right foot is more severe than the left. The patient says the pain is in the region of the lateral fourth and fifth metatarsal heads and in the metatarsophalangeal joints (MPJ) of toes two through five.

The pain has gotten worse in the past two years and she has trouble with shoes that are not soft and very cushioned. She has tried custom insoles to accommodate the plantar fourth and fifth metatarsal region without much relief. She is currently taking methotrexate and NSAIDs for her pain and rheumatoid arthritis control.

EXAM: Stable and intact neurovascular testing. The forefoot is slightly laterally deviated and there is severe hammertoe deformity of toes two through five of both feet. The main pain is located plantar to the fourth and fifth metatarsal heads with mild pain in the region of a hallux valgus deformity. The contraction of the toes is mildly reducible, yet the main deforming force occurs with dorsal contracture of the extensor tendons and skin on the dorsum of the foot. Attempting to reduce the digits relieves much of the plantar MPJ contraction and deformity yet there is continued plantar prominence of the metatarsal heads, especially on the lateral side of the foot.

There is a mild equinus deformity of the ankle with a tight Achilles tendon noted on both the straight and bent knee exam. There is a high arch with midfoot contracture yet this does not seem to be excessive and reduces well with dorsal midfoot pressure and a standing position. The patient's gait pattern reveals severe extensor substitution with dorsal pull of the extensor tendons at the associated MPJ.

TESTING: X-rays show mild MPJ dislocation with severe hammertoes and associated hallux valgus deformity of the digits. There is also some osteopenia of the metatarsal heads. Her foot alignment reveals a mild anterior cavus with excellent rearfoot alignment and no signs of degenerative joint disease.

ASSESSMENT: This patient's rearfoot is stable except for an underlying mild equinus deformity. The main part of the patient consent was for the underlying hallux valgus correction with osteotomy, hammertoe correction of all toes with extensor tendon transfer to the metatarsal heads and a V-Y lengthening of the dorsal skin contracture. The consent also included possible metatarsal osteotomies of metatarsals two through five as needed for correction of the deformity and parabola. We also discussed the possibility of an open Achilles lengthening with the patient.

Surgery to be scheduled.

Scott Cole, DPM

10/15/08 11:47:39

You Code It!

What are the best, most accurate codes?

_____

_____

_____

PODIATRY ASSOCIATES OF TARSA
539 WALKING WAY • FOOTHILLS, FL 32811 • 407-555-5399

PATIENT: CHARLSTON, ANTOINE
ACCOUNT/EHR #:   CHARAN001
Date: 03/08/08

The patient is a slightly overweight, sedentary 72-year-old male with a 15-year history of impaired glucose tolerance. He quit smoking 16 years ago and denies the use of alcohol. The patient retired from a sales job seven years ago.

PMH: Other medical problems include hypertension and hypercholesterolemia, which are treated with an angiotensin-converting enzyme inhibitor and a statin, respectively. The patient has no known drug allergies. His glucose intolerance is discovered with routine laboratory testing. He was referred for diabetes education, learned home glucose monitoring, and has been following a diet and exercise program suggested by the diabetes educator.

Approximately four months ago, patient states he noticed a burning and tingling in his hands and feet. He also felt that his sense of balance was diminished but thought it was merely a sign of aging and was reluctant to see a doctor. He denied fever, chills, nausea, vomiting, chest pain or shortness of breath. The patient also has no cough, vertigo or orthostatic hypotension.

Physical examination: Unremarkable except for some hyperesthesia of both hands and feet as well as decreased vibratory sensation. The patient has no open lesions on either foot and has intact protective sensation for both feet. Reflexes are normal and pedal pulses are palpable. There is a slight ataxia. The patient has no clinical signs of depression.

Labs revealed normal chemistries except for a fasting blood glucose of 136 mg/dl. His HbA1c is 7.6% (normal is 4.0 to 6.0%), up from 7.1% six months earlier. A complete blood count, lipid panel, liver screening and a renal profile are all normal as is a prostate-specific antigen (PSA) test. Patient's serum levels of B12, T3, T4 thyroid stimulating hormone (TSH) are within normal limits.

Rx: Duloxetine (Cymbalta) 60 mg once daily. The patient was sent for diabetic education.

Scott Cole, DPM

03/08/08 11:47:39

You Code It!

What are the best, most accurate codes?

_____

_____

_____

PODIATRY ASSOCIATES OF TARSA
539 WALKING WAY • FOOTHILLS, FL 32811 • 407-555-5399

PATIENT: WATERS, TRAVIS
ACCOUNT/EHR #: WATETR001
Date: 03/27/08

Indication: Displaced, comminuted left foot navicular

History: 29-year-old male was involved in a motorcycle racing accident, during a motocross race, sustaining the injury to his left foot.

Treatment: He was taken to the operating room, where open reduction, internal fixation of the left foot was performed, using Acutrak screws. Patient tolerated the procedure well.
    Complete operative notes dictated.

_____

Scott Cole, DPM

03/27/08 11:47:39

You Code It!

What are the best, most accurate codes?

_____

_____

_____

PODIATRY ASSOCIATES OF TARSA
539 WALKING WAY • FOOTHILLS, FL 32811 • 407-555-5399

PATIENT: ACHINSON, VANESSA
ACCOUNT/EHR #:   ACHIVA001
Date: 03/07/08

Indication: Bunion, right foot, with hallux valgus and metatarsus primus varus of the first right metatarsal

History: 41-year-old female waitress with a prominence around her metatarsal heads, with hallux valgus and a widened forefoot. She has had this for a period of many years.

Treatment: Right bunionectomy with a modified McBride procedure and proximal metatarsal dome osteotomy are performed, with fixation of the first metatarsal osteotomy using a single Acutrak screw.

Result: Postoperatively, the intermetatarsal angle is now 6 degrees with a hallux angle of 1-2 degrees. The patient has done extremely well.
    Follow-up appointment scheduled in 2 weeks.

_____

Scott Cole, DPM

03/07/08 11:47:39

You Code It!

What are the best, most accurate codes?

_____

_____

_____

_____

Psychiatric Cases and Patient Records

INTRODUCTION

The following case studies are from a mental health practice.

Psychiatrists are physicians who specialize in diagnosing and treating mental illness. These health care professionals must take into account biological, psychological, social, and cultural aspects of the patient's life. Psychotherapy, sometimes called talk therapy, may be used in addition to pharmaceutical therapies and other methodologies to help the patient recover.

Subspecialties of psychiatry include behavioral; eating disorders; forensic; industrial; learning; neuropsychiatry; psychotherapy; and posttraumatic stress disorder (PTSD), which is generally treated with cognitive therapy.

Psychologists are also health care professionals who work with patients suffering from mental disorders. The primary difference between a psychiatrist and a psychologist is education. A psychiatrist is a medical doctor who specializes in treating mental illness. A psychologist is an individual with an advanced degree (a master's degree or PhD) in clinical psychology, counseling, industrial psychology, educational psychology, or one of several other subfields and who makes professional contributions as a therapist, counselor, researcher, teacher, or consultant. A psychologist has educationally investigated matters of the mind but has not completed medical school. Only psychiatrists can write prescriptions.

Most states require both psychologists and psychiatrists to be licensed to practice legally in that individual state.

You can use these cases to practice coding diagnoses, E/M, procedures, DME, or other HCPCS Level II items, as applicable; code for the physician or the facility; code inpatient and outpatient services, as applicable:

1. Code for the physician.
2. Code for the anesthesiologist, when applicable.
3. Code for the hospital, when applicable.
4. Code for the pathology and laboratory, when applicable.
5. Code HCPCS Level II codes, when applicable.

REGO HEALTH SERVICES
753 FREUDIAN WAY • SOMEWHERE, FL 32811 • 407-555-5577

PATIENT: GONZALEZ, RENITA
ACCOUNT/EHR #:   GONZRE001
Date: 09/16/08

Attending Physician: Suzanne R. Taylor, MD

S: This new Pt is a 72-year-old female brought in by her daughter. She has been anxious, hyperventilating, labored breath, short of breath – worse since taking medication for anxiety. She is allergic to PCN, Biaxin, ASA.

    Patient has a history of asthma, tinnitus, kidney stones, and hypertension. She is retired. Patient is extremely anxious. She states her husband died 2 yrs ago and she has been having trouble. She started seeing a psychiatrist one week ago and he prescribed Zoloft 50 mg b.i.d. She is also taking Lisinopril 1 tab qd, potassium 20 mg. qd. She denies pain but has trouble breathing at times when she is anxious.

O: Wt 160 Ht 5'6" T 97.5 P 95 R 26 BP 155/83. Lungs clear. Pt calmed down with reassurance and emotional support. ECG abnormal, cardiac enzyme in normal range. Automated differential, PT, PTT, EKG shows normal sinus rhythm. Left ventricular hypertrophy with repolarization abnormality. Chest x-ray PA and Lat. x-rays show no acute intrathoracic abnormality. CBC. Glucose is elevated; sodium, potassium, and chloride are low. All other labs are unremarkable.

A: Anxiety

P: 1. Rx Xanax 1mg PO tid
      2. Follow-up in 2 weeks.

Suzanne R. Taylor, MD

SRT/pw   D: 9/16/08 09:50:16   T: 9/18/08 12:55:01

You Code It!

What are the best, most accurate codes?

_____

_____

_____

REGO HEALTH SERVICES
753 FREUDIAN WAY • SOMEWHERE, FL 32811 • 407-555-5577

PATIENT: GAYLORD, NITA
ACCOUNT/EHR #:   GAYLNI001
Date: 09/16/08

Attending Physician: Suzanne R. Taylor, MD

The patient is a 61-year-old female with a very long history of schizoaffective disorder with numerous hospitalizations who was brought in by ambulance from the YMCA where she resides for increasing paranoia, increasing arguments with other people, and in general an exacerbation of her psychotic symptoms which had been worsening over the previous two weeks.

Initially, the patient was very agitated and uncooperative. She refused medications. She wanted to leave the hospital. A 2PC was done and the patient had a court hearing that results in retention. Eventually the patient agreed to a trial of a Risperdal and then she fairly rapidly improved once she was started on Risperdal 2 mg twice daily. At the time of discharge compared to admission the patient is much improved. She is usually pleasant and cooperative with occasional difficult moments, some continuing mild paranoia. She has no hallucinations. She has no thoughts of harming herself or anyone else. She is compliant with her medication until the recently refused hydrochlorothiazide. She is irritable at times but overall she is redirectable and is considered to be at or close to her best baseline. She is considered no imminent danger to herself nor to others at this time.

Final DX: Schizoaffective disorder; hypothyroidism; hypercholesterolemia; borderline hypertension.

Prescriptions for 30-day supplies were given:
Ativan 2 mg p.o. tid; Celexa 40 mg p.o. daily; Risperdal 2 mg po bid; Synthroid 0.088 mg p.o. q.a.m.; Zocor 40 mg p.o. q.h.s

Suzanne R. Taylor, MD

SRT/pw   D: 9/16/08 09:50:16   T: 9/18/08 12:55:01

You Code It!

What are the best, most accurate codes?

_____

_____

_____

REGO HEALTH SERVICES
753 FREUDIAN WAY • SOMEWHERE, FL 32811 • 407-555-5577

PATIENT: MCDANIEL, CICI
ACCOUNT/EHR #:   MCDACI001
Date: 10/21/08

Attending Physician: Marlon Carroll, MD

Pt is a 16-year-old female recently released from a residential drug rehabilitation program and has moved back into the family home. Her therapy plan calls for a combination of individual counseling and family psychotherapy to help all members of the household understand the circumstances of her addiction and how to help her maintain a healthy, drug-free lifestyle.

　　Today is the first family psychotherapy session. Present are: Helen McDaniel, the patient's mother; Raul Esponoza, the patient's stepbrother; Jake Esponoza, the patient's stepfather; and Lucy McDaniel, the patient's paternal grandmother. The patient, Cici McDaniel, is also present.

　　The group talks openly and shows genuine concern for the patient. The session lasts 50 minutes.

P:　1. Individual session: scheduled next Monday
　　2. Next family session: two weeks

Marlon Carroll, MD

MC/mg　D: 10/21/08 09:50:16　T: 10/25/08 12:55:01

You Code It!

What are the best, most accurate codes?

_____

_____

_____

REGO HEALTH SERVICES
753 FREUDIAN WAY • SOMEWHERE, FL 32811 • 407-555-5577

PATIENT: MITCHELL, BRIDGET

ACCOUNT/EHR #:   MITCBR001

Date: 10/21/08

Attending Physician: Marlon Carroll, MD

This patient is a 33-year-old female diagnosed with schizophrenia three years ago. Pharmaceutical therapy has provided some relief from symptoms; however, the patient has been complaining of "cloudiness in her head." Several alternative treatments were discussed and she has decided to try electroshock therapy. She presents today for her first treatment.

    The patient lies on the table in the supine position. Vital signs are all normal. She is given electroshock therapy with an EKG. Patient appears to tolerate the treatment well. Due to this being her first treatment of this nature, she is kept under observation.

    Two hours after receiving the therapy, the patient has a seizure. Nurse Fletcher kept the patient safe until it passed. An EEG was performed to assure that there was no permanent damage. Anti-seizure medication is administered and the patient is sent home.

_____

Marlon Carroll, MD

MC/mg   D: 10/21/08 09:50:16   T: 10/25/08 12:55:01

You Code It!

What are the best, most accurate codes?

_____

_____

_____

REGO HEALTH SERVICES
753 FREUDIAN WAY • SOMEWHERE, FL 32811 • 407-555-5577

PATIENT: STOKES, MICHAEL
ACCOUNT/EHR #:   STOKMI001
Date: 10/21/08

Attending Physician: Marlon Carroll, MD

This patient is a 24-year-old male diagnosed with multiple personality disorder five years ago. He has been under my care since moving to this city three years ago.

Today he attends a 30-minute psychoanalysis session that I lead at the community mental health center. See tape #07211055 for complete session notes.

_____

Marlon Carroll, MD

MC/mg   D: 10/21/08 09:50:16   T: 10/25/08 12:55:01

You Code It!

What are the best, most accurate codes?

_____

_____

_____

REGO HEALTH SERVICES
753 FREUDIAN WAY • SOMEWHERE, FL 32811 • 407-555-5577

PATIENT: BECKER, NADINE
ACCOUNT/EHR #:   BECKNA001
Date: 10/21/08

Attending Physician: Marlon Carroll, MD

ALLERGIES/REACTIONS: None

CURRENT MEDICATIONS: Lithium 1,500 mg

BP: 130/80 P: 84 R:

T: WT: 265

CC: Patient states she feels well today.

PMH: Bipolar disorder, manic type.

NOTES: Veteran here for scheduled appointment. Voices no concerns.

HISTORY: Patient seen today for regular appointment. She appears relaxed, cooperative, and coherent. No evidence of recurrent manic behavior. She is 39 years old, divorced twice, Navy veteran, who served from 1991 to 1995 as a machinist mate in non-combat situation. She has been suffering from bipolar disorder, manic type, and takes medication, Lithium 1,500 mg a day, which seems effective.

    She has been employed at Alstom plant as a machinist for nine years, full time.

MENTAL STATUS EXAM: The patient has been doing very well with the current medication. No evidence of memory loss or any psychotic behavior. Her affect is appropriate, and mood is stable. Insight and judgment are good. She is not considered a danger to herself or others.

DIAGNOSIS: Bipolar disorder, manic type.

PLAN: Continue lithium 1,500 mg a day.

_____

Marlon Carroll, MD

MC/mg   D: 10/21/08 09:50:16   T: 10/25/08 12:55:01

You Code It!

What are the best, most accurate codes?

_____

_____

_____

REGO HEALTH SERVICES
753 FREUDIAN WAY • SOMEWHERE, FL 32811 • 407-555-5577

PATIENT: HOUSTON, BART
ACCOUNT/EHR #:   HOUSBA001
Date: 10/21/08

Attending Physician: Marlon Carroll, MD

This patient is a 29-year-old male, presents with complaints of fatigue and sleeplessness. He was last seen by his family physician, Dr. Crane, one year ago following a minor MVA.

PMH/PSH: Three grand mal seizures as a child—none since age 12
    ACL repair - age 19
    Appendectomy - age 26

MEDS: None prescribed

ALLERGIES: NKDA

SOCIAL HX: Married 7 years with a 5-year-old daughter, employed as a chef in a small neighborhood restaurant for the past two years, drinks a "few" beers on the weekend, smokes one pack of cigarettes per day since the age of 18, denies current or history of illicit drug use.
    Patient states that he hasn't been sleeping, he's always tired and has experienced some weight loss recently. His cousin was just diagnosed with lung cancer, and the patient is worried about getting the condition; however, not worried enough to quit smoking.

REVIEW OF SYMPTOMS: Patient denies any change in his usual morning cough and hemoptysis (helping to lower the concern for lung cancer), palpitations and heat intolerance (helping to rule out hyperthyroidism), nausea, vomiting, diarrhea, melena or hematochezia (helping to rule out GI causes of weight loss). He is not taking any medication. He is not trying to lose weight.
    Patient does acknowledge feeling depressed over the past month, stating "it just kept getting worse and worse." He has lost interest in playing on his softball team and has missed the past five games. He also says that when his daughter asks him to play, he is reluctant to do so, because he doesn't want her to see him "like this." He feels sluggish and tired, and states it all seems "worthless - like things will never get better." He denies the symptoms of mania.

PAST PSYCHIATRIC HISTORY: The patient describes passive thoughts of dying, as well as sleep disturbance and feelings of worthlessness after his appendectomy. He states these symptoms lasted "a few months" and went away after his family physician prescribed "a pill that helped me sleep." He also acknowledged depressed mood, anhedonia, and decreased energy while his wife was pregnant with their daughter. He states that he sought no treatment for these symptoms, which resolved over three or four months. He states that he has never been evaluated by a psychiatrist. He has never participated in counseling or therapy. There is no history of psychiatric hospitalizations, and he denies a history of suicide attempts.

FAMILY PSYCHIATRIC HISTORY: The patient's mother "used to take something for her nerves." There is no FHx of psychiatric hospitalizations or suicide attempts.

DX: Depression

Continued

PLAN: Begin patient with cognitive therapy. In addition, recommendation is made for family therapy to help the patient and his wife create a positive social support network.

Marlon Carroll, MD

MC/mg   D: 10/21/08 09:50:16   T: 10/25/08 12:55:01

You Code It!

What are the best, most accurate codes?

_____

_____

_____

Pulmonary and Respiratory Cases and Patient Records

INTRODUCTION

The following case studies are from a pulmonology practice.

Pulmonologists are physicians who focus on the diagnosis and treatment of diseases of the lung and lower respiratory system, such as asthma, respiratory distress syndrome, chronic obstructive pulmonary disease (COPD), and pleurisy. These health care professionals use diagnostic testing, such as pulmonary function test and arterial blood gas analysis, to assess respiratory system function. They may perform a thoracentesis or pleural biopsy to obtain samples for analysis to help determine the extent of the patient's condition and design an appropriate course of therapy.

Pulmonologists are board-certified through the Board of Internal Medicine, which is recognized by the American Board of Medical Specialties.

You can use these cases to practice coding diagnoses, E/M, procedures, DME, or other HCPCS Level II items, as applicable; code for the physician or the facility; code inpatient and outpatient services, as applicable:

1. Code for the physician.
2. Code for the anesthesiologist, when applicable.
3. Code for the hospital, when applicable.
4. Code for the pathology and laboratory, when applicable.
5. Code HCPCS Level II codes, when applicable.

PULMONOLOGY SPECIALISTS, INC.
548 BREEZE WAY • WINDER, FL 32715 • 407-555-6533

PATIENT: SCHRADER, PAULETTE
ACCOUNT/EHR #: SCHRPA001
Date: 07/16/08

Attending Physician: Suzanne R. Taylor, MD

S: This Pt is a 45-year-old female who I have not seen in eight months. She comes in today complaining of a cold that she has had for nine days. She reports that has had a dry, hacking cough and nasal congestion for the last six days and a fever for the past three days. She has also had a headache with pressure in the center of the fore-head, between the eyes. She states that she is unable to sleep due to the cough, fever, and aching. She appears to be in minor distress. Personal and family history are both negative for respiratory problems.

O: Ht 5'3.5" Wt 139 lb. R 16. T 100, BP 150/90 P93 reg. Lungs clear to percussion and auscultation. HEENT: nor-mal, mucous membranes inflamed with postnasal phlegm.

A: Frontal chronic sinusitis

P: 1. Advised to drink fluids, take aspirin as needed for pain
    2. Bed rest recommended
    3. Return if symptoms have not improved in 5 days

Suzanne R. Taylor, MD

SRT/pw   D: 7/16/08 09:50:16   T: 7/18/08 12:55:01

You Code It!

What are the best, most accurate codes?

_____

_____

_____

PULMONOLOGY SPECIALISTS, INC.
548 BREEZE WAY • WINDER, FL 32715 • 407-555-6533

PATIENT: MCLEOD, WINSTON
ACCOUNT/EHR #:   MCLEWI001
Date: 08/11/08

Attending Physician: Willard B. Reader, MD

S: Pt is a 23-month-old male who almost drowned in the swimming pool at his home two days ago. He is experiencing rapid, shallow breathing, and dyspnea.

O: Hypoxemia is apparent. Chest sounds, crackles and rhonchi indicate fluid accumulation. Tachycardia and restlessness are also evident. ABG (arterial blood gas) analysis shows respiratory acidosis; serial chest x-rays show bilateral infiltrates.

A: Acute respiratory distress

P: Oxygen hood to supply warm, humidified, oxygen-enriched gases

Willard B. Reader, MD

WBR/pw   D: 08/11/08 09:50:16   T: 08/13/08 12:55:01

You Code It!

What are the best, most accurate codes?

_____

_____

_____

PULMONOLOGY SPECIALISTS, INC.
548 BREEZE WAY • WINDER, FL 32715 • 407-555-6533

PATIENT: CUMMINGS, LINDA
ACCOUNT/EHR #:   CUMMLI001
Date: 07/16/08

Attending Physician: Suzanne R. Taylor, MD

S: This Pt is a 66-year-old female who presents today with complaints of dyspnea on exertion, and coughing. I last saw this patient one year ago.

O: Ht 5'3" Wt 157 lb. R 15. BP 145/95 P90 thready. Chest: tachycardia, tachypnea, dependent crackles. HEENT: neck vein distention. Coughing produces frothy, bloody sputum. Skin is cold, clammy, diaphoretic, and cyanotic. ABG analysis shows hypoxia. Chest x-ray shows diffuse haziness of the lung fields.

A: Acute pulmonary edema

P: 1. Administer high concentrations of oxygen by a cannula
     2. Rx Lasix

Suzanne R. Taylor, MD

SRT/pw   D: 7/16/08 09:50:16   T: 7/18/08 12:55:01

You Code It!

What are the best, most accurate codes?

_____

_____

_____

PULMONOLOGY SPECIALISTS, INC.
548 BREEZE WAY • WINDER, FL 32715 • 407-555-6533

PATIENT: CLYDE, NELSON
ACCOUNT/EHR #:   CLYDNE001
Date: 09/15/08

Attending Physician: Willard B. Reader, MD

S: This new Pt is a 23-year-old male who presents with complaints of fever and recurrent chills. He states that he has a cough producing rusty, bloody, viscous sputum (patient states "like currant jelly"). His states his breathing is difficult and shallow and he noticed that his lips and fingernails appear bluish. Pt recently moved here from Detroit. He was found to be HIV positive two years ago and is on pharmaceutical therapy.

O: HEENT: cyanosis of lips confirms hypoxemia. Chest: respirations are shallow and grunting. Chest x-ray shows consolidation in the upper lobe causing bulging of fissures; WBC count is elevated; sputum culture and gram stain show gram-negative cocci Klebsiella.

A: Pneumonia due to klebsiella, HIV positive

P: Oxygen hood to supply warm, humidified, oxygen-enriched gases

_____

Willard B. Reader, MD

WBR/pw   D: 09/15/08 09:50:16   T: 09/17/08 12:55:01

You Code It!

What are the best, most accurate codes?

_____

_____

_____

PULMONOLOGY SPECIALISTS, INC.
548 BREEZE WAY • WINDER, FL 32715 • 407-555-6533

PATIENT: CONDRON. CLARENCE
ACCOUNT/EHR #:   CONDCL001
Date: 11/25/08

Attending Physician: Willard B. Reader, MD

S: This new Pt is a 35-year-old male complaining of a cough with a foul-smelling sputum, dyspnea, excessive sweating and chills.

PMH: Patient has poor oral hygiene. Missing teeth and inflamed gums have gone untreated for years due to his fear of the dentist. He states that a few months ago, he had a bout of pneumonia. He self-medicated but hasn't felt right since then.

O: Chest: Auscultation reveals crackles and decreased breath sounds. Chest x-ray shows localized infiltrate with one clear space containing air-fluid. Blood cultures, gram stain, and sputum culture identify leukocytosis.

A: Abscess of the lung, putrid

P: Begin antibiotic therapy immediately

_____

Willard B. Reader, MD

WBR/pw   D: 11/25/08 09:50:16   T: 11/27/08 12:55:01

You Code It!

What are the best, most accurate codes?

_____

_____

_____

PULMONOLOGY SPECIALISTS, INC.
548 BREEZE WAY • WINDER, FL 32715 • 407-555-6533

PATIENT: POTTER, FRED
ACCOUNT/EHR #:   POTTFR001
Date: 11/25/08

Attending Physician: Willard B. Reader, MD

CC: Wheezing

History: The patient is a 57-year-old male who was admitted to the hospital on November 24 with complaints of generalized weakness. The patient has a history of chronic lower extremity edema for which he has been evaluated, but no cause has been discovered. Over the past several days, the left lower extremity has become quite erythematous. On admission, the patient was found to have gram-positive cocci in the blood, and he is currently being treated by infectious disease for cellulites with secondary bacteremia. While in the hospital, he has also been noted to have some dry cough without any significant sputum production, and some intermittent wheezing. Currently, the patient is resting comfortably in bed. He is a poor historian, but denies any specific complaints.

PMH: Hypertension, benign prostatic hypertrophy, chronic left lower extremity edema.

Past Surgical History: The patient denies any prior surgeries.

Allergies: No known drug allergies.

Medications: Cardura, Lovenox, HydroDIURIL, Prednisone 30 mg. q.d., Prevacid, and Penicillin G.

Social History: The patient is married and lives with his wife. He is a lifelong nonsmoker. He does not drink alcohol. He is a retired accountant, with no occupational exposures to any lung irritants or carcinogens.

Family History: No history of lung disease in the family.

ROS:

General: Denies any change in appetite or weight. Denies fevers, chills, or sweats.

HEENT: Denies any change in vision or hearing. Denies nasal congestion or sore throat.

Cardiovascular: Denies chest pain or palpitations.

Respiratory: Has some dry cough, but no sputum production, and no hemoptysis. He has been noted to have occasional wheezing and has a questionable history of childhood asthma. He denies shortness of breath at present.

Gastrointestinal: Denies any change in bowel habits or reflux. Denies nausea, vomiting, or abdominal pain.

Genitourinary: Denies urinary frequency or dysuria.

Musculoskeletal: Denies joint pain or swelling.

Skin: Denies any rashes. He does have erythema secondary to cellulites over the left lower extremity.

PE:

Vital signs: Temperature 99.1; heart rate 74, respiratory rate 20, blood pressure 143/86.

General: Middle-aged male resting in bed in no acute distress.

Skin: Warm, dry, no rashes.

HEENT: Pupils equal, round, and reactive to light. Throat clear, no erythema or exudates.

Continued

Neck: No adenopathy, no JVD, no thyromegaly.

Heart: Regular rate and rhythm, normal S1, S2.

Lungs: Diminished breath sounds and expiratory wheezes. No rhonchi, no dullness to percussion.

Abdomen: Soft, nontender, not distended, positive bowel sounds, no organomegaly.

Extremities: Left lower extremity 2+ edema and erythema.

Neuro: Alert and oriented x3, grossly intact motor exam.

I reviewed his chest x-ray that showed some basilar effusions and/or atelectasis. I also reviewed his CT scan of the abdomen that did confirm bilateral pleural effusions, small on the right and tiny on the left side. There was also some secondary atelectasis of the right lower lobe. He had lower extremity Dopplers that were negative for DVT.

WBC 7.5; hemoglobin 9.4, hematocrit 26.7, platelets 304,000. Sodium 142, potassium 3.7, chloride 103, bicarbonate 28, BUN 23, creatinine 1.0.

IMPRESSIONS:
1. Bronchospasm
2. Tracheobronchitis
3. Right pleural effusion
4. Cellulites with bacteremia

RECOMMENDATIONS:
I discussed the case with the patient and his wife, who was at his bedside. He appears to be having an episode of asthmatic bronchitis. I will temporarily increase his steroids to Decadron 4 mg every 8 hours. Will also continue him on Albuterol and Atrovent nebulizers. He has been started on Zithromax by infectious disease for treatment of bronchitis. I am also concerned over the possibility of aspiration in this patient with bronchitis and right lower lobe consolidation. I will request a bedside swallow evaluation. Finally, in regards to his pleural effusion, we will obtain an ultrasound of the chest. If there is significant fluid, will go ahead with a diagnostic thoracentesis. I discussed this with his wife, who is in agreement.

_____

Willard B. Reader, MD

WBR/pw   D: 11/25/08 09:50:16   T: 11/27/08 12:55:01

You Code It!

What are the best, most accurate codes?

_____

_____

_____

PULMONOLOGY SPECIALISTS, INC.
548 BREEZE WAY • WINDER, FL 32715 • 407-555-6533

PATIENT: PROCTOR, CLYDE
ACCOUNT/EHR #:   PROCL001
Date: 11/25/08

Attending Physician: Willard B. Reader, MD

This 41-year-old male was referred to me by Dr. Hernandez for the evaluation of hemoptysis. Dr. Hernandez, his primary care physician, had followed him for the past year for chronic cough. When questioned further he reported that this cough had been increasingly productive of thick material that was "strange tasting" and seemed almost tissue-like as opposed to sputum he had experienced in the past. He reported streaky hemoptysis over two weeks time, a 9 lb. weight loss over 2 months, but denied fever, denied chills, denied dyspnea on exertion. Pt had been treated off and on with inhalers over the past year with no benefit.

PAST HISTORY: The patient denies ever smoking and drinks alcohol rarely. He currently takes no medications and has no allergies.

FAMILY HISTORY: Significant for colon carcinoma in his mother and coronary artery and mitral valvular disease in his father.

PHYSICAL EXAM: Significant for markedly reduced breath sounds posteriorly on the left.

CXR showed tracheal deviation to the left and left lower lobe collapse as well as an opacification in the subcarinal area.
     Chest CT performed subsequently showed an approx. 4 cm mass in the subcarinal area extending around the left mainstem bronchus to the hilar region with probable impingement and growth into the left mainstem bronchus. There is subsequent LLL collapse. No effusions or lymphadenopathy are appreciated.
     Bronchoscopy was performed and a mass arising in the left mainstem bronchus 3 cm from the carina was noted. The mass nearly occluded the LLL bronchus. The carina was minimally widened. Biopsies of the mass were adenoid cystic carcinoma. Carinal biopsies were also consistent with adenoid cystic despite its near normal appearance. Tracheal biopsies were negative.

DX: Adenoid cystic carcinoma

PLAN: The mass is considered inoperable due to the carinal involvement. The patient is referred to Radiation Oncology.

_____

Willard B. Reader, MD

WBR/pw   D: 11/25/08 09:50:16   T: 11/27/08 12:55:01

You Code It!

What are the best, most accurate codes?

_____

_____

_____

PULMONOLOGY SPECIALISTS, INC.
548 BREEZE WAY • WINDER, FL 32715 • 407-555-6533

PATIENT: KRAJSA, REBECCA
ACCOUNT/EHR #:   KRAJRE001
Date: 11/25/08

Attending Physician: Willard B. Reader, MD

This is a 19-year-old female with a history of atopy and mild lung disease secondary to cystic fibrosis presented with a three-week history of increased sputum production, dyspnea and wheezing.

The patient's genotype was Delta F508/2789+5 G-T. She was pancreatic sufficient and had never required therapy with intravenous antibiotics. The patient had previously undergone allergy testing and had received immunotherapy for allergies to pet dander. She attributed this recent illness to an exacerbation of her allergies as a result of exposure to a dog while visiting relatives.

PAST HISTORY: Pancreatitis at age 15 requiring hospitalization, and major depression for which she had received treatment with sertraline in the past.

PHYSICAL EXAM: Significant for crackles in the mid lung fields, and a prolonged expiratory phase with diffuse wheezing.

LAB: WBC 14,400 with 0.9% eosinophils and an elevated serum IgE level of 2840 IU. Spirometry performed pre-bronchodilator revealed an FEV1 of 3.15 liters (69% of predicted). Post-bronchodilator the FEV1 increased to 3.55 liters (77% of predicted). Chest x-ray revealed a patchy infiltrate in the superior segment of the right lower lobe. Based on this presentation, a further evaluation for allergic bronchopulmonary aspergillosis was performed.

An intracutaneous skin test using aspergillus antigen produced a wheal of 5 mm and a flare of 11mm. Serum was sent for examination for antibodies to A. fumigatus. Serum IgE for A. fumigatus was 9.21 and serum IgG was 2.39.

DX: Allergic bronchopulmonary aspergillosis

PLAN: The patient to start therapy with Itraconazole 100 mg per day and a lower dose of Prednisone (10 mg) per day.

_____

Willard B. Reader, MD

WBR/pw   D: 11/25/08 09:50:16   T: 11/27/08 12:55:01

You Code It!

What are the best, most accurate codes?

_____

_____

_____

PULMONOLOGY SPECIALISTS, INC.
548 BREEZE WAY • WINDER, FL 32715 • 407-555-6533

PATIENT: WATCHORN, MARISA
ACCOUNT/EHR #:   WATCMA001
Date: 11/25/08

Attending Physician: Willard B. Reader, MD

The patient is a 29-year-old female with end stage lung disease secondary to cystic fibrosis (CF). She had frequent hospitalizations prior to lung transplantation due to exacerbations of her bronchiectasis. Sputum cultures
had revealed Stenotrophomonas maltophilia and Mycobacterium abscessus. Her pre-transplantation course was
also complicated by persistent gastrocutaneous fistula after removal of a gastric feeding tube. She underwent
bilateral lung transplantation and subsequently takedown of her persistent gastrocutaneous fistula. Both donor
and patient were cytomegalovirus (CMV) seropositive and the patient was Epstein-Barr virus (EBV) seronega-
tive. Her post-operative course was uncomplicated except for a persistent small right pleural effusion. She was
discharged home doing fairly well.

   Five weeks after transplantation, she developed a fever and a significant fall in spirometry. A bronchoscopy
was performed. Bronchoalveolar lavage fluid analysis was normal (differential count, N=20%; L=4%), with
negative microbiologic stains and cultures. Transbronchial biopsy specimens showed acute, minimal (AI) rejection. She was treated with high dose methylprednisolone and showed clinical improvement. Two weeks later,
she redeveloped fever of 39C and right pleuritic chest pain. A chest x-ray, and subsequent CT scan of the chest
revealed accumulation of bilateral pleural effusions, left greater than right. There was enhancement of both pleural layers on the right and bibasilar atelectasis. There was also a question of a nodular infiltrate at the left base
but this was not definite given the atelectasis. Bilateral thoracenteses showed uncomplicated exudative fluid. Her
port-a-cath was removed and its tip culture grew coagulase negative methicillin-resistant Staphylococcus. She
was treated with a 14-day course of vancomycin with resolution of her clinical symptoms. Soon after she was
discharged, the left pleural fluid culture turned positive with a rapid growing mycobacterium. A repeat CT scan
obtained 10 days after the initial study showed slight interval increase in size of the left effusion, improved atelectasis, and multiple new pleural-based nodular densities throughout both lungs. A thoracoscopic lung biopsy
was performed. Lung tissue cultures were negative. Light microscopic examination showed no viral cytopathic
changes but revealed large angiocentric nodules with sheets of atypical large lymphocytes and plasma cells, and
central coagulative necrosis consistent with polymorphous post-transplant lymphoproliferative disorder (PTLD).
Immunoglobulin light chain staining showed polyclonality. In situ hybridization for EBV encoding region (EBER)
RNA was positive. Her EBV titers remained negative. The nontuberculous mycobacterium was subsequently identified as Mycobacterium abscessus.

DX: Polymorphous post-transplant lymphoproliferative disorder (PTLD)

_____

Willard B. Reader, MD

WBR/pw   D: 11/25/08 09:50:16   T: 11/27/08 12:55:01

You Code It!

What are the best, most accurate codes?

_____

_____

_____

PULMONOLOGY SPECIALISTS, INC.
548 BREEZE WAY • WINDER, FL 32715 • 407-555-6533

PATIENT: BOLANOS, KIRK
ACCOUNT/EHR #:   BOLAKI001
Date: 11/25/08

Attending Physician: Willard B. Reader, MD

This patient is a 23-year-old male who was brought into the Emergency Room with a sharp right-sided chest pain and shortness of breath of one-day duration. The patient was in excellent health until yesterday. He was awakened from his sleep by sharp right-sided chest pain. The pain worsened with motion and deep breathing. The pain has been progressively increasing in severity and he now has severe right shoulder pain. He complains of shortness of breath and is very apprehensive about dying. He denies any cough, fever, sputum production or hemoptysis.

PFH/PSH: The patient is married and has one child. Review of systems is negative. He denies any past history of venous problems. He reveals having a similar transitory minor episode of chest pain approximately one year ago while he was vacationing in California.

He works as an IT manager. He smokes one pack of cigarettes a day for the past ten years. He considers himself a social drinker.

PHYSICAL EXAM: BP 114/80; pulse 118; T 37.0 (oral)

The patient appears to be in moderate respiratory distress. He is well developed and nourished. Pertinent findings include a respiratory rate of 30 and shallow breathing. There is dullness, decreased chest expansion and decreased breath sounds in the right base. There is egophony in the right base. There were no rales or rubs.

HEART: PMI in the 5th intercostal space in MCL. The pulmonic component of the second sound is accentuated.

ABDOMEN, PELVIC AND RECTAL EXAMS: Unremarkable

EXTREMITIES: No evidence of edema, cyanosis or clubbing.

Patient has negative Homan's Sign.

Joint exam reveals shoulder movements complete in range. No warmth or tenderness noted. The rest of the patient's joints are normal.

Decubitus reveals a small amount of fluid in the left pleural space.

LAB: CBC: Hgb 15.0; Hct 43; WBC 11,500; 83 polys, 1 band and 14 lymphs; SMA-12: Normal; Arterial blood gases: FIO2 .21; pH 7.39; PCO2 30; HCO2 20; PO2 80; SO2 95%

IMAGING: EKG: sinus tachycardia and non-specific S-T-T wave changes axis + 80.

CXR: A small pleural effusion in the left base. The right diaphragm is elevated.

Shoulder x-ray is normal. Lung scan revealed a defect corresponding to the area of pleural effusion. Pleural tap revealed yellow fluid; protein 3.5 grams; glucose 64 and pH 7.4. Doppler exam revealed deep vein thrombosis of the left lung.

Continued

DX: Pulmonary Embolism

Willard B. Reader, MD

WBR/pw   D: 11/25/08 09:50:16   T: 11/27/08 12:55:01

You Code It!

What are the best, most accurate codes?

_____

_____

_____

PULMONOLOGY SPECIALISTS, INC.
548 BREEZE WAY • WINDER, FL 32715 • 407-555-6533

PATIENT: HOLDERFIELD, NATHAN
ACCOUNT/EHR #: HOLDNA001
Date: 11/25/08

Attending Physician: Willard B. Reader, MD

This patient is a 71-year-old male, who comes in with complaints of increased SOB. He states he has also noted a change in the quantity and color of his sputum over the past week. The sputum is usually scant and clear. However, recently it has become yellow and continues all day. He has had trouble raising sputum in the past year. He has become progressively short of breath over the last three years. He is now dyspneic at rest.

HISTORY: Patient denies asthma, childhood respiratory problems, allergies and any occupational exposures.

PHYSICAL EXAM: T 99.5; BP 140/90; pulse 110; respiratory rate 28. Patient is in obvious respiratory distress with prominent use of accessory muscles.

HEAD/NECK: Distended neck veins throughout expiration.

CHEST: Increased A-P diameter; reduced chest wall excursion; lungs hyperresonant to percussion; diaphragms low and immobile; auscultation reveals a prolonged expiratory phase with diminished breath sounds and generalized rhonchi.

HEART: PMI in epigastrium; heart sounds distant with regular rhythm and no murmurs.

EXTREMITIES: Trace pitting edema of the lower extremities.

CXR: Hyperinflation of lungs with an increase in the retrosternal space; low, flattened diaphragms; hyperlucent lung fields with paucity of vascular markings in the periphery but prominent hila and narrow heart silhouette.

EKG: Low voltage; right axis; peaked P waves and clockwise rotation.

LAB: WBC 8,500 with normal differential and Hgb 14.7 gm, ABG's:

DX: COPD

_____

Willard B. Reader, MD

WBR/pw   D: 11/25/08 09:50:16   T: 11/27/08 12:55:01

You Code It!

What are the best, most accurate codes?

_____

_____

_____

PULMONOLOGY SPECIALISTS, INC.
548 BREEZE WAY • WINDER, FL 32715 • 407-555-6533

PATIENT: FABER, CLAYTON
ACCOUNT/EHR #:   FABECL001
Date: 11/25/08

Attending Physician: Willard B. Reader, MD

This patient is a 31-year-old male who comes in stating that 10 days ago he woke up in the middle of the night with sudden onset left sided chest pain described "like a knife" in quality, aggravated by deep inspiration, accompanied by mild dyspnea.

HPI: He denies history of recent trauma, fever, chills nor sweats. Pain went away after taking Tylenol and rest. The next day, he was seen by a chiropractor and after some chiropractic maneuvers he felt better. Pain continued to occur intermittently until, eight days PTA while bowling, the pain recurred.

ROS: No headaches, blurred vision, nor seizures; no earaches, nor tinnitus; no cough, nor colds; no abdominal pains, melena, hematochezia, nor change in bowel habits; no dysuria, urgency, frequency, nor hematuria; and no bleeding tendencies.

MEDICATIONS: Atenolol, Ceftin, Tylenol #3

Allergies: NKDA

PMH: HTN x 17 years; S/P MVA-laparotomy; S/P laryngeal polypectomy; S/P R shoulder surgery

FAMILY HX: Father 62 y/o CVA, 3 uncles CVA, brother CVA 10 y/o

SOCIAL AND OCCUPATIONAL HX: Non-smoker, no alcohol, or illicit drug use; married with one son; works as a real estate agent

PHYSICAL EXAM
VITALS: BP=110/70 HR=88 RR=24 T=36.7

HEENT: Review palpebral conjunctiva

NECK: Supple, no LAD

RESP: Good air entry, minimal lagging on R with deep inhalation, decreased breath sounds R base, + egophony, occasional inspiratory crackles, no wheezes

CVS: RRR S1 and S2 audible no murmur

Abd: Obese, good BS, soft, non-tender, no bruit, no organomegaly, + laparotomy scar

CNS: Normal

Rectal: OB negative brown stools

Ext: No C/C/E, ++ pedal pulses

Skin: Review chest, warm dry

Other systems are unremarkable.

Labs
CBC: WBC 5,600   Hgb 12.5   Hct 36.5 MCV 85   Plt 360,000

Chemistry:
BUN 10   Creat 0.8   K 4.6 Na 142   Cl 108 Co2 24   ABG 7.45/36/94/25

Continued

Thoracentesis showed: bloody fluid.
WBC=4,400 RBC=3,850,000 Lymphocytes=7%
Mesothelial cells=4% Macrophage=4%
PF LDH=46% Glucose=Less than 10 LDH=2,050
PF Protein Less than 2
CXR shows pleural effusion.

DX: Hemothorax

_____

Willard B. Reader, MD

WBR/pw   D: 11/25/08 09:50:16   T: 11/27/08 12:55:01

You Code It!

What are the best, most accurate codes?

_____

_____

_____

PULMONOLOGY SPECIALISTS, INC.
548 BREEZE WAY • WINDER, FL 32715 • 407-555-6533

PATIENT: PERSI, CHRISTINA
ACCOUNT/EHR #:   PERSCH001
Date: 11/25/08

Attending Physician: Willard B. Reader, MD

Patient is a 23-year-old female who come in with a cough, productive of yellow/green sputum with fever to 100.1F, and complaints of pain in the "back" on the right side for a duration of one week.

HPI: Patient has a history of cystic fibrosis and underwent a bilateral sequential single lung transplant six years ago with subsequent chronic rejection and progressively incapacitating obliterative bronchiolitis. She received a repeat BSLTx two years later with the post-operative period complicated by intrathoracic bleeding, that twice required mediastinal exploration, and was finally discharged more than two weeks later. Bronchoscopic biopsies one month after re-transplant revealed grade A0B0 (not significantly acute) rejection and she had been well until the above symptoms developed three weeks after biopsy. Her respiratory function by spirometry was stable, and she denied any additional symptoms such as prior fever, dysuria, nausea, headache, vomiting or diarrhea. During the last bronchoscopy, the question of silent aspiration was raised and on close questioning at the time of this admission, some difficulty in swallowing was acknowledged.

MEDICATIONS: Tacrolimus 1 mg BID, itraconazole 400 mg daily, prednisone 20 mg daily, flunisolide MDI 2 p BID, dapsone 100 mg TID, digoxin 0.125 mg daily, diltiazem 60 mg TID, erythropoietin MWF, ganciclovir 1 g TID, famotidine 40 mg daily, albuterol MDI TID, Pancrease, Vit C, Vit D, MVI.

ALLERGIES: Sulfa, ciprofloxacin, pentoxifylline, amox/clav, codeine

PMH: Left vocal cord paresis, S. aureus sepsis, pulmonary embolism with IVC filter. Lung transplant, donor CMV negative, recipient positive; repeat transplant donor positive.

SOCIAL AND OCCUPATIONAL HX: G1 P0010, non-contributory, no tobacco or alcohol. Travel history and pets and hobbies: none.

PHYSICAL EXAM

VITALS: BP=100/60 RR=22 HR=104 T=37.4 Wt=37 kg

HEENT: Minimal oral thrush but no other oral lesions or erythema, no sinus tenderness; no evidence of otitis

RESP: Coarse breath sounds bilaterally, no wheezes, rales, rhonchi; no dullness or egophony described; mild use of accessory muscles in respiration

CVS: Tachycardia with normal heart sounds, no murmurs, rubs, S3 or S4

ABD: Flat, soft abdomen with normal bowel sounds; no tenderness, guarding or rigidity; no significant hepato-splenomegaly

CNS: Alert to person, place and time; coherent speech and thought process; no evident asymmetry in muscle or neurological function; mild generalized muscle weakness. Cranial nerve exam unremarkable.

EXT: Mild lower extremity pitting edema, greater on the right; clubbing but no acrocyanosis; no erythema or tenderness

LYMPH: No lymphadenopathy

SKIN: Pale and thin skin, no rashes, ecchymoses on forearms and hands

OTHER SYSTEMS: Unremarkable

Continued

HOSPITAL COURSE:

After admission, cultures of urine, sputum and blood were obtained. High flow oxygen and empiric antibiotics consisting of ceftazidime, tobramycin and clindamycin were started. Sputum cultures identified MRSA, Serratia marcescens, and Pseudomonas aeruginosa. Blood cultures demonstrated Serratia.

On the third hospital day the patient underwent surgical placement of a percutaneous jejunal feeding tube as well as a left subclavian tunneled central catheter. On the fifth hospital day, after an elevation in temperature, cultures were again obtained and grew candida albicans. Fluconazole was started.

By the eighth day, a progressively downward trend in white blood cell and platelet counts continued despite minimizing her medication profile and significant epistaxis occurred, requiring blood component transfusion and ICU monitoring. The chest radiograph that day revealed a worsening bilateral infiltrate and elective intubation and bronchoscopy was performed in the face of increasing and unaccountable hypoxemia. Bronchoalveolar lavage fluid cultures revealed only candida and tissue biopsies were not obtainable. The recently placed tunneled catheter was finally removed as a possible source of fungemia. By this time her antibiotic regimen was broadened to include foscarnet and CMV Ig. Transfusions were required daily to support hemoglobin and platelet levels.

High flow O2 and empiric antibiotics consisting of ceftazidime, tobramycin and clindamycin were started. MRSA, Serratia marcescens and Pseudomonas aeruginosa in sputum and serratia in blood. On 5th day candida albicans grew and Fluconazole was started. By 8th day, a progressively downward trend in WBC PLT counts continued. Transfusions were given. CXR was repeated.

DX: Progressive respiratory failure post-lung transplant

Willard B. Reader, MD

WBR/pw   D: 11/25/08 09:50:16   T: 11/27/08 12:55:01

You Code It!

What are the best, most accurate codes?

_____

_____

_____

PULMONOLOGY SPECIALISTS, INC.
548 BREEZE WAY • WINDER, FL 32715 • 407-555-6533

PATIENT: DETRICK, PATRICK
ACCOUNT/EHR #:   DETRPA001
Date: 02/11/08

Attending Physician: Willard B. Reader, MD

This patient is a 23-year-old man serving a 10-20 year sentence for armed robbery. He has been incarcerated at the state prison for 18 months, mainly without incident. However, over the last month he has lost 18 pounds (in part due to anorexia and relatively poor oral intake), had fever and rigors as well as night sweats. In the last few weeks he has developed a paroxysmal, nonproductive cough, for which he was given a prescription for an antibiotic (clarithromycin), which he took for one week.

The patient has had a significant history of intravenous drug abuse, most recently with heroin. Five years ago he tested positive for antibody to the Human Immunodeficiency Virus (HIV). He is a lifelong resident of this area. His profession is that of a plumber, but he has not worked at this for >5 years. There is no history of travel outside of the state in the last five years.

He has no history of taking antiretroviral therapy, although when he went to the Veteran's Administration Medical Center, it was been suggested to him that it would be wise to initiate such therapy. He is currently on no medications. He has no known drug allergies. He admits to drinking alcohol quite often prior to incarceration. Physical examination revealed a thin, chronically ill-appearing male. R: 24; P: 96 at rest; BP 110/75; T 100.6° F. His skin is normal with the exception of several tattoos on his arms and trunk. HEENT: No abnormalities. There is no adenopathy. Auscultation of the chest revealed bibasilar rales. Cardiac exam is within normal limits, as is the abdominal exam, the skeletal, and neurologic exam.

Laboratory: Hct 37, WBC 8900/mm^3 (62% polys, 5% eos, 26% lymphs, 7% monos), platelet count of 160,000/mm^3, and a negative urinalysis. Blood chemistry: BUN 18, creatinine 1.2, sodium 140, potassium 4.7, carbon dioxide 21, chloride 96, and normal liver function tests. Viral load measurements: HIV of 100,000 copies per ml. His CD4 count is 96/mm^3.

DX: Bibasilar pneumonia, Pneumocystis carinii

PLAN: Fiberoptic bronchoscopy with bronchoalveolar lavage +/- transbronchial biopsy. Initiation of trimethoprim-sulfamethoxazole therapy, while awaiting results of biopsy.

Willard B. Reader, MD

WBR/pw   D: 02/11/08 09:50:16   T: 02/15/08 12:55:01

You Code It!

What are the best, most accurate codes?

_____

_____

_____

PULMONOLOGY SPECIALISTS, INC.
548 BREEZE WAY • WINDER, FL 32715 • 407-555-6533

PATIENT: NORTON, ANITA
ACCOUNT/EHR #:   NORTAN001
Date: 02/27/08

Attending Physician: Willard B. Reader, MD

This is a 47-year-old female who was referred to our office after changes were noted on a chest x-ray.

Pt presented to her oncologist, Dr. Nevis, for follow-up after a recent right segmental mastectomy for a grade I infiltrating ductal breast carcinoma. Initial staging work-up had revealed degenerative changes at the L5 level on the nuclear bone scan and no evidence of metastatic disease on radiographs of the chest or on the CT scan of the abdomen, but there were changes on a repeat chest radiograph. The patient was scheduled for radiation and chemotherapy.

Review of symptoms reveals no history of weight loss, loss of appetite, fatigue, cough, dyspnea, palpitations, chest pain, headaches, syncope, seizures, or any abdominal symptoms.

Past medical history: The patient had a history of endometriosis. She was not on any medications. Past surgical history included removal of a lipoma from the back and a tonsillectomy at age 6.

Menstrual and obstetric history: Menarche at age 12, G1P1A0, with first childbirth at age 31. The patient is premenopausal and has been on oral contraceptives for 5 years.

Family history: The patient's mother had breast cancer, diagnosed at age 95. Her grandmother and two of her uncles had colon cancer. The patient does not have any known allergies.

Social history: The patient denies smoking and only occasionally uses alcohol. There is no history of exposure to dusts, toxins, or household pets, or any recent history of foreign travel. She is employed as a librarian.

DX: Pulmonary Sarcoidosis

_____

Willard B. Reader, MD

WBR/pw   D: 02/27/08 09:50:16   T: 02/27/08 12:55:01

You Code It!

What are the best, most accurate codes?

_____

_____

_____

Radiology and Nuclear Medicine Cases and Patient Records

INTRODUCTION

The following case studies are from an imaging center. In an imaging center, a professional coding specialist is likely to see many different types of health situations.

Radiologists are physicians who specialize in performing and interpreting diagnostic imaging tests. They provide supervision and interpretation of diagnostic tests, including radiological imaging; ultrasounds; dual-energy x-ray absorptiometry (DEXA), or bone density, tests; computed tomography (CT) scans; positron emission tomography (PET) scans; and magnetic resonance imaging (MRI). In addition, they may provide fluoroscopic or ultrasonic guidance, radiation oncology treatments, nuclear medicine including the placement of radiopharmaceuticals, and other radiopharmaceutical therapies.

Radiologists also supervise technicians who perform special tests, such as barium enemas or computed tomography (CT) scans.

The Board of Radiology offers board certification for radiologists. The American Board of Medical Specialties recognizes this board.

You can use these cases to practice coding diagnoses, E/M, procedures, DME, or other HCPCS Level II items, as applicable; code for the physician or the facility; code inpatient and outpatient services, as applicable:

1. Code for the physician.
2. Code for the anesthesiologist, when applicable.
3. Code for the hospital, when applicable.
4. Code for the pathology and laboratory, when applicable.
5. Code HCPCS Level II codes, when applicable.

BROADMORE IMAGING CENTER
234 DOPPLER ROAD • ANYTOWN, FL 32711 • 407-555-5977

PATIENT: BUSCH, JAKE
MRN: BUSJA01
Date: 29 September 2008

Procedure Performed: Carotid artery angiography

Radiologist: Keith Robbins, MD
Referring Physician: James I. Cipher, MD

Indications: Dementia

Impressions: Angiography, cerebral carotid, bilateral
                         Supervision and interpretation only
                         Negative for blockage

Keith Robbins, MD

KR/mg   D: 9/29/08 09:50:16   T: 9/30/08 12:55:01

You Code It!

What are the best, most accurate codes?

_____

_____

_____

BROADMORE IMAGING CENTER
234 DOPPLER ROAD • ANYTOWN, FL 32711 • 407-555-5977

PATIENT: KLEMPTER, BRANDY
MRN: KLEBR01
Date: 29 September 2008

Indication: Stenosis brachiocephalic artery
Procedure Title: Arch aortogram, right brachiocephalic arteriogram, angioplasty, and stent right brachiocephalic

PROCEDURE: The patient was informed of risks associated with the procedure, including stroke, and agreed to the procedure. The patient's right groin was sterilely prepped and draped in the usual fashion.

Via retrograde right femoral arterial approach, 4Fr vascular sheath was inserted. 5Fr pigtail catheter was then advanced into the ascending aorta. An arch aortogram was then performed in the left anterior oblique projection. The arch aortogram demonstrated a high-grade stenosis present at the origin of the right brachiocephalic artery. A Simmons II catheter was inserted and the catheter was reformed in the ascending aorta.

The right brachiocephalic was selectively catheterized. Supracore guide was advanced into the right subclavian artery, and the catheter was positioned within the subclavian artery. The guide wire was advanced into the axillary artery. The catheter was then removed and a 7 Fr shuttle sheath was advanced to the origin of the right brachiocephalic artery. 8 mm x 2 cm long angioplasty balloon was then inserted. The patient received 3,000 units of heparin intravenously. The area of stenosis was then balloon-dilated.

A repeat arteriogram was obtained demonstrating marked residual stenosis. A 12 mm x 30 mm long LUMINEXX stent was then inserted and deployed in the usual fashion across the area of stenosis. A 10 mm x 2 cm long angioplasty balloon was then inserted and the stent was further balloon-dilated to a 10 mm diameter.

A repeat arteriogram was obtained demonstrating good angiographic result with no significant residual stenosis identified. The catheter and sheath were then removed and hemostasis was obtained with Perclose suture device.

IMPRESSION: High-grade stenosis origin of the right greater cephalic artery. This was successfully angioplastied and stented to a 10 mm diameter as described above.

_____

Keith Robbins, MD

KR/mg   D: 9/29/08 09:50:16   T: 9/30/08 12:55:01

You Code It!

What are the best, most accurate codes?

_____

_____

_____

BROADMORE IMAGING CENTER
234 DOPPLER ROAD • ANYTOWN, FL 32711 • 407-555-5977

PATIENT: EVANS, ELAINE

MRN: EVAEL01

Date: 13 October 2008

Indication: Low Oxygen Saturation

Procedure: Chest x-ray; Fluoroscopic feeding tube placement

PROCEDURE: Fluoro Procedure; chest 1 view, inspiration

INDICATION: Low oxygen saturation

A progress portable examination of the chest is obtained and compared to one dated 20 March 2000. There is some infiltrate developing in the right lower lobe which was not present on the previous study and is very worrisome for pneumonia. Patchy areas of atelectasis are seen in the left lower and left mid-lung. The heart is normal in size. There is a soft tissue density behind the heart consistent with hiatal hernia.

Impression: Interval change in the appearance of the chest. There are areas of pneumonia developing in the right lower lobe.

FLUOROSCOPIC FEEDING TUBE PLACEMENT: Indication: Need for nourishment in unresponsive patient.

Attempts to place a feeding tube fluoroscopically were unsuccessful. There is a prominent hiatal hernia. The distal stomach extends ventrally to pass the through the esophageal hiatus. Because these are not steerable or directable tubes, it is not possible to actually place the tip of the catheter where one would like. Multiple attempts at advancing the catheter beyond the hiatus into the distal stomach or duodenum were unsuccessful utilizing gravity technique, etc. The procedure was terminated.

IMPRESSION: Unsuccessful attempt at feeding tube placement.

Keith Robbins, MD

KR/mg   D: 10/13/08 09:50:16   T: 10/19/08 12:55:01

You Code It!

What are the best, most accurate codes?

_____

_____

_____

BROADMORE IMAGING CENTER
234 DOPPLER ROAD • ANYTOWN, FL 32711 • 407-555-5977

PATIENT: WOZNIACK, SURI
MRN: WOZSU01
Date: 14 October 2008

Indication: Mental status change. Brain tumor. Status post radiation therapy with recent change in mental status.
Procedure: MRI Brain S/ & C/contrast

PROCEDURE: MRI of the brain with and without contrast

COMPARISON: 2-2-00

Multiplanarmultisequence imaging of the brain was performed preceding and following gadolinium contrast administration.

A large irregular enhancing abnormality of the right frontal and temporal regions seen on preceding CT scan shows a marked interval decrease in size with decreasing mass effect upon the right lateral ventricles. There is a new focal area of increased signal on T2 and proton weighted images that are also intense on T1 post gadolinium images. This may reflect specific regeneration along the tumor margin or para stages of focal hemorrhage. There is a new region of increased signal on T2 weighted images within the left basal ganglia that do not possess contrast enhancement. The appearance is most typical of focal basal ganglionic infarct on the left. Again, this is a new finding since prior exam. There is generalized increased signal abnormality throughout the periventricular white matter, not significantly changed from prior exam and likely reflects chronic change of small vessel disease.

IMPRESSION:
1. Reduction in the size and mass effect of right frontotemporal enhancing tumor.
2. New abnormality left basal ganglia, likely ischemic in nature.

Stable background of ischemic white matter changes in periventricular distribution.

Keith Robbins, MD

KR/mg   D: 10/14/08 09:50:16   T: 10/15/08 12:55:01

You Code It!

What are the best, most accurate codes?

_____

_____

_____

BROADMORE IMAGING CENTER
234 DOPPLER ROAD • ANYTOWN, FL 32711 • 407-555-5977

PATIENT: PADUA, RAUL
MRN: PADRA01
Date: 21 October 2008

Indication: Mental status change. Brain tumor.
Procedure: Non-Invasive Vascular Study

PROCEDURE: Carotid Study

An 84-year-old male with mental status changes and cerebral malignancy. The patient is studied at this time to rule out transient ischemic attack.

Color duplex scanning bilaterally shows no evidence of mural plaquing. There is no luminal stenosis. Flow parameters are normal. Vertebral flow is forward bilaterally.

IMPRESSION:
1. There is no evidence of hemodynamically significant stenosis within the cervical carotid segments.
2. Vertebral flow is forward bilaterally.

Keith Robbins, MD

KR/mg   D: 10/21/08 09:50:16   T: 10/25/08 12:55:01

You Code It!

What are the best, most accurate codes?

_____

_____

_____

BROADMORE IMAGING CENTER
234 DOPPLER ROAD • ANYTOWN, FL 32711 • 407-555-5977

PATIENT: ONTARI, MICHAEL
MRN: ONTMI01
Date: 21 October 2008

Indication: Rule out endocarditis
Procedure: Echocardiogram

DESCRIPTION: This is only a fair quality exam with limited information available.

On two-dimensional view, left ventricular chamber size and wall motion appear satisfactory and there is no pericardial effusion. LV appears thickened, typical of LV concentric hypertrophy.

Mitral valve structures are fairly well seen, and no mitral annulus calcification seen, and only trace mitral regurgitations noted. The LA chamber is mildly dilated at 4.4 cm. The valve does not suggest mitral stenosis or mitral valve prolapse, and there are no unusual echo densities suspicious of a vegetative process.

The proximal aortic root is normal in size at 3.6 cm. The valve leaflets are calcified, and there appears to be decreased opening. Peak velocity across the aortic valve is approximately 2.0 m/sec, with max instantaneous gradient of 16.2 mmHg, and a mean gradient of 10.6 mmHg. This probably represents only mild aortic stenosis. Again, no unusual echo densities are seen suspicious of a vegetative process. The right heart chambers are not significantly dilated and only mild tricuspid regurgitation is seen.

CONCLUSIONS:
1. Mild aortic stenosis, with no significant aortic regurgitation.
2. Trace mitral regurgitation, mild LA (left atrial) chamber dilation.
3. Grossly normal left ventricular chamber size, and normal left ventricular systolic function.
4. LVH (Left ventricular hypertrophy) appears prominent by 2D (two-dimensional) view.
5. Mild tricuspid regurgitation.
6. No unusual echo densities seen suspicious of a vegetative process, but if clinically indicated, consider TEE (transesophageal echocardiogram).

Keith Robbins, MD

KR/mg   D: 10/21/08 09:50:16   T: 10/25/08 12:55:01

You Code It!

What are the best, most accurate codes?

_____

_____

_____

BROADMORE IMAGING CENTER
234 DOPPLER ROAD • ANYTOWN, FL 32711 • 407-555-5977

PATIENT: YAMAGUCHI, HIRO
MRN: YAMHI01
Date: 21 October 2008

Indication: BP shunt placement, right lower quadrant pain
Procedure: X-ray abdomen (KUB), 1 view

INTERPRETATION: Flat plate KUB shows a ventricular peritoneal catheter terminating in the pelvis in the left. The catheter from the level of lower ribs is intact. There are no large displacing abdominal masses and the bowel gas pattern is unremarkable. There is a calcification present in the lateral pelvis and below the femoral heads, consistent with arteriosclerotic calcification. Degenerative disco-vertebral changes are seen in the upper lumbar levels. Note is made of short ribs on T12.

CONCLUSIONS:
1. Intact abdominopelvic VP-shunt catheter segment. Normal bowel gas pattern.
2. Degenerative disco-vertebral changes and arteriosclerotic calcification of the iliac and common femoral arteries.

Keith Robbins, MD

KR/mg   D: 10/21/08 09:50:16   T: 10/25/08 12:55:01

You Code It!

What are the best, most accurate codes?

_____

_____

_____

BROADMORE IMAGING CENTER
234 DOPPLER ROAD • ANYTOWN, FL 32711 • 407-555-5977

PATIENT: PEACOCK, VANESSA
MRN: PEAVA01
Date: 8 November 2008

Indication: Pleural effusion
Procedure: Ultrasound

PROCEDURE: Ultrasound right hemothorax for pleural fluid localization

Sonography of the right hemothorax demonstrates right basal pleural effusion. The skin surface marking at the sight of the maximum depth of the pleural fluid identified sonographically was marked on the dorsal skin surface with a magic marker.

IMPRESSION: Chest marking accomplished.

Keith Robbins, MD

KR/mg   D: 11/08/08 09:50:16   T: 11/12/08 12:55:01

You Code It!

What are the best, most accurate codes?

_____

_____

_____

BROADMORE IMAGING CENTER
234 DOPPLER ROAD • ANYTOWN, FL 32711 • 407-555-5977

PATIENT: LIPTON, PAUL
MRN: LIPPA01
Date: 8 November 2008

Indication: Possible benign prostatic hypertrophy
Procedure: CT pelvis, with contrast

PROCEDURE: CT Scan of the pelvis with contrast

    Oral contrast media was given. 7mm helical sections were obtained during intravenous nonionic contrast administration.

    The examination shows no evidence of pelvic mass or adenopathy. There is a small amount of pelvic ascites. There is no bowel dilation or bowel wall thickening seen. The prostate gland is enlarged. The venous structures are unremarkable.

IMPRESSION: Small amount of pelvic ascites. Enlarged prostate gland.

___

Keith Robbins, MD

KR/mg   D: 11/08/08 09:50:16   T: 11/12/08 12:55:01

You Code It!

What are the best, most accurate codes?

___

___

___

BROADMORE IMAGING CENTER
234 DOPPLER ROAD • ANYTOWN, FL 32711 • 407-555-5977

PATIENT: VOLBRECHT, CHRISTOPHER
MRN: VOLCH01
Date: 19 November 2008

Indication: Pleural effusion
Procedure: CT Upper ABD w/Contrast

PROCEDURE: CT Scan abdomen

Serial axial images of the abdomen are obtained with intravenous contrast.

Bilateral pleural effusions, right greater than left, are seen with adjacent compressive atelectatic change. There are no focal lesions seen within the liver. The pancreas, spleen, adrenal glands are unremarkable. The kidneys are within normal limits without evidence of hydronephrosis. There is no significant retroperitoneal adenopathy, free fluid, or bowel obstruction. Inferior vena cava is normal in caliber.

IMPRESSION: Bilateral pleural effusions with adjacent compressive atelectatic changes. No other significant abnormality noted.

Keith Robbins, MD

KR/mg   D: 11/19/08 09:50:16   T: 11/27/08 12:55:01

You Code It!

What are the best, most accurate codes?

_____

_____

_____

BROADMORE IMAGING CENTER
234 DOPPLER ROAD • ANYTOWN, FL 32711 • 407-555-5977

PATIENT: LAVENDER, GRACE
MRN: LAVGR01
Date: 8 November 2008

PROCEDURE: Fluoro Procedure; Chest 1 view

Fluoro Procedure
No films taken. No dictation rendered.
One View chest.
Clinical history: Post op
Comparison film: 4-21-00

Left Port-A-Cath is seen with the tip in the SVC. No pneumothorax is evident. There does appear to be a mild kinking noted in the proximal Port-A-Cath line near the insertion site. Lungs are clear. The heart is upper limits of normal in size.

There is a prominence of the right hilum with a rounded density noted inferior to the right hilum, suspicious for mass. I understand recent chest computed tomography showed two pulmonary parenchymal lesions. There is a suggestion of focal rounded density noted in the right lung base also.

IMPRESSION: Status post left Port-A-Cath placement with tip in superior vena cava. No pneumothorax.

Mild kinking at the insertion site noted.

Keith Robbins, MD

KR/mg   D: 11/08/08 09:50:16   T: 11/12/08 12:55:01

You Code It!

What are the best, most accurate codes?

_____

_____

_____

BROADMORE IMAGING CENTER
234 DOPPLER ROAD • ANYTOWN, FL 32711 • 407-555-5977

PATIENT: QUINONESS, ROBERTO
MRN: QUIRO01
Date: 8 November 2008

Clinical history: Malignant pleural effusion

Portable chest: 11/7/08
      Current study is compared to previous one of 10/29/08
      There is a right-sided chest tube in place, the right pleural effusion is decreased. There is residual effusion present in the right hemithorax.
      No pleural effusions are seen on the left side. Recommend follow-up studies.

Keith Robbins, MD

KR/mg   D: 11/08/08 09:50:16   T: 11/12/08 12:55:01

You Code It!

What are the best, most accurate codes?

_____

_____

_____

BROADMORE IMAGING CENTER
234 DOPPLER ROAD • ANYTOWN, FL 32711 • 407-555-5977

PATIENT: WATERMAN, JASON
MRN: WATJA01
Date: 8 November 2008

Clinical history: Status post chest tube

Portable chest:
The current exam is from 5:45 a.m. dated 11-08-07.
   The right pleural effusion and possible infiltrate in the right lung appear largely unchanged since yesterday's examination. No pneumothorax is seen and the right chest tube is stable in position. There appear to be diffuse interstitial changes in the left lung which are also unchanged.

IMPRESSION:
No significant change since yesterday's exam.

Keith Robbins, MD

KR/mg   D: 11/08/08 09:50:16   T: 11/12/08 12:55:01

You Code It!

What are the best, most accurate codes?

_____

_____

_____

BROADMORE IMAGING CENTER
234 DOPPLER ROAD • ANYTOWN, FL 32711 • 407-555-5977

PATIENT: BALDUCCI, MIRANDA
MRN: BALMI01
Date: 17 September 2008

Clinical history: Ascites

Paracentesis under ultrasound guidance:
Under ultrasound guidance, a large pocket of ascites was localized in the right flank. Using sterile technique and local anesthesia, a catheter was placed within the localized pocket of ascites and 4 liters of amber fluid were obtained. The patient tolerated the procedure well without complication. The fluid was sent to cytology for evaluation.

_____

Keith Robbins, MD

KR/mg   D: 9/17/08 09:50:16   T: 9/20/08 12:55:01

You Code It!

What are the best, most accurate codes?

_____

_____

_____

BROADMORE IMAGING CENTER
234 DOPPLER ROAD • ANYTOWN, FL 32711 • 407-555-5977

PATIENT: SAINT JOHNS, VANESSA
MRN: SAIVA01
Date: 20 October 2008

Indication: Abdominal Pain
Procedure: X-rays: Chest x2; Abdomen x2

TWO VIEWS OF THE CHEST: 10/18/08

FINDINGS: Two views of the chest demonstrate the lungs to be clear. There is no evidence of pleural effusions or pneumothorax. Heart size is normal. The pulmonary vascularity is normal. Mild hypertrophic changes are identified within the thoracic spine.

IMPRESSION: No acute pulmonary disease

SUPINE AND ERECT VIEWS OF THE ABDOMEN:

HISTORY: Abdominal pain

FINDINGS: Views of the abdomen demonstrate residual radiopaque contrast within the colon and urinary bladder. The bowel gas pattern is unremarkable. There is no evidence of free intraperitoneal air. Lung bases are clear.

IMPRESSION: Negative supine and erect abdomen.

Keith Robbins, MD

KR/mg   D: 10/20/08 09:50:16   T: 10/25/08 12:55:01

You Code It!

What are the best, most accurate codes?

_____

_____

_____

BROADMORE IMAGING CENTER
234 DOPPLER ROAD • ANYTOWN, FL 32711 • 407-555-5977

PATIENT: ABBOTT, ALICIA
MRN: ABBAL01
Date: 21 October 2008

Indication: Abdominal Pain
Procedure: CT abd w/wo contrast; CT pelvis w/contrast; CT abd w/contrast

CT SCAN OF THE ABDOMEN AND PELVIS WITH AND WITHOUT IV CONTRAST

CLINICAL HISTORY: Abdominal pain

CT of the abdomen was performed from the lung bases to the pubic symphysis, bilateral adrenals and bilateral kidneys are normal in appearance. There is extensive wall thickening of the cecum and proximal ascending colon. There is a 4 cm fluid collection with several pockets of air immediately adjacent to the cecum and there is a 5 mm calcification visualized within the fluid collection (images #58 and 59).

      There are multiple calcifications in the region of the uterus presumably related to degenerative leiomyomas. The bladder appears unremarkable.

IMPRESSION: Pericecal fluid and air collection with corresponding extensive wall thickening of the cecum and proximal right colon. These findings are suggestive of a perforated appendix with a periappendiceal abscess and an appendicular. Other differential considerations are cecal malignancy with associated abscess, right-sided tubo-ovarian abscess and right ovarian malignancy.

      Another consideration would be a right-sided diverticulitis with associated abscess. Recommend clinical correlation and further work-up as clinically indicated.

      Probable fibroid uterus. Pelvic ultrasound may be useful in further evaluation if clinically indicated.

Keith Robbins, MD

KR/mg   D: 10/21/08 09:50:16   T: 10/25/08 12:55:01

You Code It!

What are the best, most accurate codes?

_____

_____

_____

BROADMORE IMAGING CENTER
234 DOPPLER ROAD • ANYTOWN, FL 32711 • 407-555-5977

PATIENT: WITTNER, MARCUS
MRN: WITMA01
Date: 21 October 2008

Indication: ACUTE ONSET OF GLOBAL AMNESIA
Procedure: ELECTROENCEPHALOGRAM

CLINICAL HISTORY: The patient is a 71-year-old male with prior left hemispheric cerebrovascular accident, admitted for the possibility of transient global amnesia/transient ischemic attack.

ELECTROENCEPHALOGRAM REPORT: The electroencephalogram is recorded. The patient is awake throughout this study. There is well-regulated Alpha activity at 9 to 10 Hz, low to medium voltage, asymmetric in appearance in the posterior quadrants, less well defined on the left as compared to the right. There is 15-20 Hz low voltage beta activity anteriorly, roughly symmetrical on both sides.

There is continuous arrhythmic low voltage slow activity seen in most areas of the left hemisphere, but particularly pronounced at the F7, C3, P3, T3, and T5.

At times, the amplitude increases to medium levels. There are no epileptiform discharges in the area of focal slowing.

Photic driving response in the occipital regions is also asymmetric, less well defined on the left than on the right.

ELECTROENCEPHALOGRAM CLASSIFICATION: Abnormal significance III (awake).
1. Continuous slow, focal, left hemisphere, more pronounced at the frontal-central-parietal-mid and posterior temporal areas.
2. Background asymmetry, diminished Alpha in the left posterior quadrant.
3. Asymmetric photic driving response, diminished, left occipital region.

ELECTROENCEPHALOGRAM INTERPRETATION: Abnormal electroencephalogram, with the findings consistent with the clinical information of previous left hemisphere stroke.

It cannot be determined from this single electroencephalogram whether the changes are the result of the remote stroke or the more recent ischemic event. If clinically appropriate, follow-up recordings may be useful in determining the significance of the above-described abnormalities.

Keith Robbins, MD

KR/mg   D: 10/21/08 09:50:16   T: 10/25/08 12:55:01

You Code It!

What are the best, most accurate codes?

_____

_____

_____

BROADMORE IMAGING CENTER
234 DOPPLER ROAD • ANYTOWN, FL 32711 • 407-555-5977

PATIENT: ALEVY, FIONA
MRN: ALEFI01
Date: 21 October 2008

Indication: BILATERAL LE ANGIO

Procedure: RUNOFF ARTERIOGRAM OF THE LOWER EXTREMITIES INCLUDING FLUSH ABDOMINAL AORTOGRAM

CLINICAL HISTORY: Claudication left leg, history of atrial fibrillation

The procedure performed via a right transfemoral artery route utilizing local anesthesia and sterile technique with a 5 French omni catheter passed to just above the level of the renal arteries. The abdominal aorta shows a single and widely patent renal arteries bilaterally and no aneurysm or other vascular lesions seen in the lower abdominal aorta.

RUNOFF ARTERIOGRAM REPORT: Runoff arteriogram is performed with a catheter in the distal abdominal aorta with injection of non-ionic contrast material and DSA steptable filming. Contrast injected at the rate of 10 cc a second for a total of 80 cc.

   Widely patent iliac and common femoral arteries. The right superficial femoral arteries are also widely patent with only mild stenosis of the distal right SFA no greater than 30 to 40% and therefore doubtful significance. On the left side, the superficial femoral artery is completely occluded at the mid-thigh level. Numerous collateral arteries especially from the deep femoral artery are noted to reconstitute flow into the distal left superficial femoral artery near the adductor canal region. Reconstituted popliteal artery is widely patent. Runoff below the knees is predominately via large and widely patent anterior tibial arteries bilaterally with occlusion of the peroneal and posterior tibial arteries bilaterally, although small collateral arteries are also seen in the calves bilaterally.

CONCLUSION: Complete occlusion of the left superficial femoral artery at the mid-thigh level with collateral reconstitution of the distal left SFA just above the adductor canal region.

   Occlusion of both peroneal and posterior tibial arteries although there are large and widely patent anterior tibial arteries seen all the way to the foot bilaterally including smaller collateral arteries.

Brian Masters, MD

BM/mg   D: 10/21/08 09:50:16   T: 10/25/08 12:55:01

You Code It!

What are the best, most accurate codes?

_____

_____

_____

BROADMORE IMAGING CENTER
234 DOPPLER ROAD • ANYTOWN, FL 32711 • 407-555-5977

PATIENT: FEATHERS, MAURY
MRN: FEAMA01
Date: 21 October 2008

Indication: RULE OUT DVT
Procedure: UNILATERAL RIGHT LOWER EXTREMITY DUPLEX VENOUS ULTRA-SOUND/PORTABLE CHEST X

CLINICAL HISTORY: Rule out DVT

UNILATERAL RIGHT LOWER EXTREMITY DUPLEX VENOUS ULTRASOUND
    The right common femoral, superficial femoral, and popliteal veins were studied. There is normal compressibility, augmentation, and phasicity. There is no filling defect or color flow abnormality to suggest deep vein thrombosis.

IMPRESSION: Normal study and negative for DVT

PORTABLE CHEST ON 10/20/08
    Pacemaker is present with lead tips in the region of the right atrium and right ventricle. Atherosclerotic calcification is present in the aorta. There is mild-to-moderate cardiomegaly with prominence of the left ventricle. The pulmonary vascularity is normal. There is blunting of the right costophrenic angle by a small pleural effusion. Subsegmental atelectasis is noted at the bases. No definite infiltrate is present.

IMPRESSION: Mild cardiomegaly and small right pleural effusion. Incidental note is made of osteopenia and arthritis in the shoulders. Since the previous x-ray of 11/22/06, the right pleural effusion has developed and the atelectasis is new. At that time, healed rib fractures were more noticeable in the right ribs.

Brian Masters, MD

BM/mg   D: 10/21/08 09:50:16   T: 10/25/08 12:55:01

You Code It!

What are the best, most accurate codes?

_____

_____

_____

BROADMORE IMAGING CENTER
234 DOPPLER ROAD • ANYTOWN, FL 32711 • 407-555-5977

PATIENT: QUINTINE, WARREN
MRN: QUIWA01
Date: 21 October 2008

Indication: POPLITEAL ANEURYSM
Procedure: AORTOGRAM AND RUNOFF

CLINICAL HISTORY: Popliteal aneurysm

AORTOGRAM AND RUNOFF: Initially, a right femoral puncture was performed and a 5 French pigtail catheter placed in the abdominal aorta. Following this, a selective catheter was placed into the proximal left common femoral artery from the right approach. After filming of the left lower extremity, the catheter was withdrawn and contrast injected through the sheath in the right external iliac artery.

    The abdominal aorta appears to be upper limits of normal in size measuring up to 3 cm. There is no significant stenosis at the origin of either renal artery. Both common and external iliac arteries are large. The common iliacs measure up to 1.5 cm in size. The external iliacs measure about 1.2 cm in size.

    Both superficial femoral and deep femoral arteries are patent. Both vessels are slightly large.

    There are bilateral popliteal artery aneurysms present. The aneurysms appear to begin above the knee joint and extend down below the knee joint to the trifurcation. The luminal diameter measures approximately 1.5 cm on the right and approximately 1 cm on the left. Aneurysm on the right extends for about 8 cm, on the left it extends for approximately 10 cm. Both anterior tibial arteries are small vessels. The peroneals bilaterally are patent. They appear to reconstitute the posterior tibial in the distal leg.

IMPRESSION:
1. Arteriomegaly
2. Bilateral popliteal aneurysms which extend down to the trifurcation. Primarily single vessel runoff which is a good-sized peroneal artery which supplies the distal posterior tibials.

Brian Masters, MD

BM/mg   D: 10/21/08 09:50:16   T: 10/25/08 12:55:01

You Code It!

What are the best, most accurate codes?

_____

_____

_____

Urology, Nephrology, and Men's Health Cases and Patient Records

INTRODUCTION

The following case studies are from a urology and nephrology practice. In a physician's office of this type, a professional coding specialist is likely to see many different kinds of health situations, including preventive health care services.

Urologists are physicians who specialize in the diagnosis and treatment of urinary system conditions affecting both men and women as well as disorders of the male reproductive system.

Urologists can prescribe medications, perform surgery, and treat diseases and conditions of the urinary system, including the kidneys and the bladder. These health care professionals care for patients with such conditions as polycystic kidney disease, acute renal failure, and urinary tract infections (UTI).

They treat problems of the male reproductive system as well, focusing on conditions such as erectile dysfunction or benign prostatic hyperplasia (BPH).

Subspecialties in urology include urogynecology, which focuses on treating urinary problems in women, and pediatric urology, which narrows the scope to diagnosing and treating urinary problems in infants and children. Nephrologists are urologists whose subspecialty is the diagnosis and management of kidney disease.

Urologists are board-certified through the American Board of Urology, which is recognized by the American Board of Medical Specialties.

You can use these cases to practice coding diagnoses, E/M, procedures, DME, or other HCPCS Level II items, as applicable; code for the physician or the facility; code inpatient and outpatient services, as applicable:

1. Code for the physician.
2. Code for the anesthesiologist, when applicable.
3. Code for the hospital, when applicable.
4. Code for the pathology and laboratory, when applicable.
5. Code HCPCS Level II codes, when applicable.

WASSERMAN UROLOGY CENTER
233 STREAMLINE DRIVE • MAZE, FL 32811 • 407-555-6591

PATIENT: KLOTSKY, STACY
MRN: KLOTST01
Admission Date: 5 October 2008
Discharge Date: 5 October 2008

Date: 5 October 2008
Preoperative DX: Rule out bladder tumor
Postoperative DX: Same
Procedure: Cystoscopy, biopsy, and fulguration of bladder

Surgeon: Leonard Dupont, MD
Assistant: None
Anesthesia: Spinal

INDICATIONS: The patient is a 73-year-old female with a history of grade II superficial transitional cell carcinoma of the bladder. Cystoscopy showed a suspicious erythematous area on the right trigone. She presented today for cystoscopy, biopsy, and fulguration. Findings: The urethra was normal, the bladder was 1+ trabeculated, the mid and right trigone areas were slightly erythematous and hypervascular. No papillary tumors were noted, no mucosal abnormalities were noted.

PROCEDURE: The patient was placed on the table in supine position. Satisfactory spinal anesthesia was obtained. She was placed in dorsal lithotomy position. She was prepped sterilely with Hibiclens and draped in the usual manner. A #22 French cystoscopy sheath was passed per urethra in Atraumatic fashion. The bladder was resected with the 70-degree lens with findings as noted above. Cup biopsy forceps were placed and three biopsies were taken of the suspicious areas of the trigone. These areas were fulgurated with the Bugby electrode; no active bleeding was seen. The scope was removed, the patient was returned to recovery having tolerated the procedure well. Estimated blood loss was minimal.

PATHOLOGY REPORT: Chronic cystitis (cystica) with squamous cell metaplasia.

10/5/08 11:47:39

You Code It!

What are the best, most accurate codes?

_____

_____

_____

WASSERMAN UROLOGY CENTER
233 STREAMLINE DRIVE • MAZE, FL 32811 • 407-555-6591

PATIENT: DENNISON, DANIEL
MRN: DENNDA01
Date: 23 November 2008

Procedure Performed: Vasectomy

Physician: Sunil Kaladuwa, MD

Indications: Elective sterilization

Procedure: The patient was given Versed for anxiety, and local anesthesia was administered. Removal of a segment of the deferent duct was accomplished bilaterally. Patient tolerated the procedure well.

Impression: Successful outcome

Plan: Postoperative semen examination is scheduled for one week.

_____

Sunil Kaladuwa, MD

SK/mg   D: 11/23/08 09:50:16   T: 11/25/08 12:55:01

You Code It!

What are the best, most accurate codes?

_____

_____

_____

WASSERMAN UROLOGY CENTER
233 STREAMLINE DRIVE • MAZE, FL 32811 • 407-555-6591

PATIENT:	FALLON, WILLA
ACCOUNT/EHR #:	FALLWI01
Date:	07/16/08

Attending Physician: Suzanne R. Taylor, MD

S: This Pt is a 26-year-old female who I have not seen since last September when she came in for a UTI. She presents today with burning upon urination and lower back pain. She stated that the symptoms began 2-3 days ago. She had been on vacation in Mexico and arrived back home yesterday.

O: Ht 5′7″ Wt 169 lb. R 19. HEENT: unremarkable. Abdomen is tender. I ordered an automated urinalysis with microscopy, which was analyzed in our laboratory on the second floor. After the UA showed the presence of white blood cells in the urine, I ordered a culture and sensitivity test, which was positive for E. coli.

A: Urinary tract infection – cystitis, due to E. coli

P: 1. Rx. Broad-spectrum antibiotics
      2. Return prn

_____

Suzanne R. Taylor, MD

SRT/pw   D: 7/16/08 09:50:16   T: 7/18/08 12:55:01

You Code It!

What are the best, most accurate codes?

_____

_____

_____

WASSERMAN UROLOGY CENTER
233 STREAMLINE DRIVE • MAZE, FL 32811 • 407-555-6591

PATIENT: FERNANDEZ, OLIVIA

ACCOUNT/EHR #:   FERNOL01

Date: 7/16/08

Attending Physician: Laverne Aspiras, MD

CLINICAL HISTORY: This patient, a 5-year-old Hispanic female who had been previously healthy, was admitted to the hospital five days ago with bloody diarrhea and dehydration. She was treated with bowel rest and intravenous fluids. Her diarrhea seemed to be improving, however, this morning she experienced a prolonged generalized convulsion and she was transferred emergently.

    Upon arrival to the PICU, she appeared quite ill. She was extremely irritable and quite pale. A blood coagulation test is performed.

IMPRESSION: Hemolytic uremic syndrome caused by E. coli H:0157.

PLAN: Dialysis is ordered.

Laverne Aspiras, MD

LA/pw   D: 7/16/08 09:50:16   T: 7/18/08 12:55:01

You Code It!

What are the best, most accurate codes?

_____

_____

_____

WASSERMAN UROLOGY CENTER
233 STREAMLINE DRIVE • MAZE, FL 32811 • 407-555-6591

PATIENT: BEETER, KYLE
ACCOUNT/EHR #:   BEETKY01
Date: 9/30/08

Attending Physician: Laverne Aspiras, MD

INDICATIONS: This new Pt is a 9-year-old male with end-stage renal disease, here for dialysis, monitoring, assessment, and counseling with parents.

PROCEDURE: Dialysis services for month of September – 30 days

Laverne Aspiras, MD

LA/mg   D: 9/30/08 09:50:16   T: 9/30/08 12:55:01

You Code It!

What are the best, most accurate codes?

_____

_____

_____

WASSERMAN UROLOGY CENTER
233 STREAMLINE DRIVE • MAZE, FL 32811 • 407-555-6591

PATIENT: GORDON, LOU ANNE

MRN: GORDLO01

Date: 23 November 2008

Procedure Performed: Cystoscopy and left double J stent removal

Physician: Sunil Kaladuwa, MD

Indications: Left hydronephrosis

Procedure: The patient was brought to the cystoscopy suite and placed on the table in the supine position. The patient was prepared and draped in the usual sterile fashion. A flexible cystoscope was inserted. Stent was grasped with alligator forceps and removed. The patient tolerated the procedure well. The patient will return to the office for IVP.

_____

Sunil Kaladuwa, MD

SK/mg   D: 11/23/08 09:50:16   T: 11/25/08 12:55:01

You Code It!

What are the best, most accurate codes?

_____

_____

_____

WASSERMAN UROLOGY CENTER
233 STREAMLINE DRIVE • MAZE, FL 32811 • 407-555-6591

PATIENT: FLYMAN, DONALD
MRN: FLYMDO01
Date: 23 November 2008

Physician: Sunil Kaladuwa, MD

This is a 9-year-old male who was referred by his pediatrician, Dr. Southwell, with the chief complaint of dark "cola colored" urine, facial puffiness, and abdominal pain for the past three days.

HPI: The mother states that he had been in his usual state of good health until two weeks ago when he developed a sore throat and fever. His sore throat and fever resolved. He was not seen by a physician at that time. Over the past 2 days facial puffiness has been noted, but no swelling of his hands or feet. He has had some nonspecific abdominal pain that comes and goes which does not seem to be related to eating or bowel movements. There is no nausea or vomiting. His urine is dark brown and he has not been voiding as much as usual—only 2 times in the past 24 hr. There is no urinary frequency, urgency, dysuria, or foul smell to the urine. His appetite has been poor although he is still drinking fluids well. He is also complaining of some back pain in the flank area that he describes as a dull pain that comes and goes and does not seem to be related to activity. His energy level is down and he has not felt up to going to school for the past 2 days. He is also complaining of a dull generalized headache that has not been relieved with acetaminophen.

REVIEW OF SYSTEMS: Negative for recent skin infection, skin rash, cough, rhinorrhea, seizure activity, fever, arthralgia or weight loss.

PMH/FH/SH: Unremarkable.

EXAM: VS T 37, P 100, RR 20, BP 120/75, oxygen saturation 100% in RA. Height and weight at 50th %tile. He appears tired but in no acute distress. Pupils are equal and reactive. Optic disc margins are sharp. Sclera are white and conjunctiva are clear. Mild periorbital edema is noted. TMs are normal. Throat, oral mucosa and nose are normal. His neck is supple without lymphadenopathy. Heart is regular without murmurs. Lungs are clear. Abdomen is diffusely tender (mild), without guarding or rebound. Bowel sounds are normal. No organomegaly is noted. Mild CVA tenderness is present. His extremities are warm, with strong pulses. Capillary refill is less than 2 seconds. No edema is noted in his legs, feet or hands. No skin rashes or impetigo scars are noted. His genitalia are normal. No scrotal edema is present. Neurologic exam is normal.

LAB: His urine is tea colored. UA shows an increased specific gravity. A dipstick is positive for a large amount of blood and moderate protein. RBCs are too numerous to count. 5-10 WBCs per HPF. RBC casts are present. CBC with diff is normal. Throat swab is sent for culture. ASO titer is elevated. Serum complement C3 level is low. Serum electrolytes are normal. BUN 23 and Cr 0.8.

Continued

DX: Acute poststreptococcal glomerulonephritis

CLINICAL COURSE: Admission to hospital for treatment of oliguria/volume overload with furosemide, and monitoring of his modest hypertension.

Sunil Kaladuwa, MD

SK/mg   D: 11/23/08 09:50:16   T: 11/25/08 12:55:01

You Code It!

What are the best, most accurate codes?

_____

_____

_____

WASSERMAN UROLOGY CENTER
233 STREAMLINE DRIVE • MAZE, FL 32811 • 407-555-6591

PATIENT: DE MATTEIS, ASHLIE
MRN: DEMAAS01
Date: 23 November 2008

Physician: Sunil Kaladuwa, MD

This patient is a 1-month-old female, brought in by her mother. She is referred by Dr. Nozetti, her pediatrician, with concerns about an abdominal mass. Her mother noticed the mass earlier in the week and immediately made an appointment to see the pediatrician. The mother also notes that the infant has been frequently wetting her diapers.

HPI: There is no history of fever, vomiting or diarrhea. The infant's perinatal and birth history are unremarkable (spontaneous vaginal delivery at term with a birth weight of 2765 grams).

FAMILY HISTORY: There is a family history of cystic kidneys in the infant's 12-year-old sister. The infant's two other siblings do not have any renal disease and both parents deny a history of renal disease.

EXAM: VS T 37.5, P 110, R 26, BP 115/85, Weight 3.32 kg (10th percentile). She is alert and active, in no distress. Her physical exam is unremarkable except for a nontender 6 cm by 7 cm right-sided abdominal mass.

LAB: Urinalysis reveals cloudy urine, positive for leukocyte esterase and nitrites. A renal ultrasound is performed and reveals bilateral enlargement of her kidneys with diffuse echogenicity and microcysts. A hepatic ultrasound reveals periportal fibrosis.

DX: Autosomal-recessive polycystic kidney disease and a possible urinary tract infection.

PLAN: Admit to hospital for antibiotic treatment and further evaluation.

Sunil Kaladuwa, MD

SK/mg   D: 11/23/08 09:50:16   T: 11/25/08 12:55:01

You Code It!

What are the best, most accurate codes?

_____

_____

_____

WASSERMAN UROLOGY CENTER
233 STREAMLINE DRIVE • MAZE, FL 32811 • 407-555-6591

PATIENT: RAPINO, ELIAS
MRN: RAPIEL01
Date: 23 November 2008

Physician: Sunil Kaladuwa, MD

This patient is a 5-year-old male who is brought in by his mother when she noted bloody diarrhea earlier in the day. Dr. Tribinni, his pediatrician, referred them to me by phone.

HPI: There is no fever, ill contacts, or recent exposures to children with diarrhea. His family attended a birthday party a week ago where the child had consumed hot dogs and hamburgers.

EXAM: VS T 37.7, P 150, R 28, BP 100/45, oxygen saturation 100% in RA. Weight 33 kg (75%ile). He is alert but fussy, pale, and non-toxic appearing. His conjunctiva are pale. His TMs are normal. He has no nasal flaring or palatal petechiae. His oral mucosa is moist and his tongue is pale. His neck is supple without adenopathy. His heart has a regular rhythm with tachycardia and a grade III/VI vibratory systolic ejection murmur at the left sternal border without radiation. No heaves, lifts, thrills, rubs, or gallops are present. His lungs are clear with good aeration. His abdomen is flat, soft, and non-tender, with the liver edge palpable 3cm below the RCM. The spleen is non-palpable. His genitalia and anus are normal (no rectal prolapse). His pulses and perfusion are good. There is no edema, rash, or petechiae.

LABS: CBC: WBC 16,000 with 56% segs, 12% bands, 27% lymphs, 3% eos, 2% basos, hemoglobin 8 mg/dL, hematocrit 24.6, platelet count 75,000; peripheral smear shows schistocytes, helmet cells, and polychromasia. Na 133, K 5.9, Cl 96, bicarbonate 16, BUN 45, creatinine 1.3, glucose 145 mg/dL, Ca 7.8, PO4 7.1, uric acid 7.3, and LDH 300. Coagulation studies are normal.

DX: Hemolytic Uremic Syndrome

Tx: Mother instructed to keep him home and push fluids. If no improvement is seen in the next 48 hours, she is instructed to return immediately.

Sunil Kaladuwa, MD

SK/mg   D: 11/23/08 09:50:16   T: 11/25/08 12:55:01

You Code It!

What are the best, most accurate codes?

_____

_____

_____

WASSERMAN UROLOGY CENTER
233 STREAMLINE DRIVE • MAZE, FL 32811 • 407-555-6591

PATIENT: TOUCHTON, ZENA
MRN: TOUCZE01
Date: 23 November 2008

Physician: Sunil Kaladuwa, MD

This is a 31-year-old female who presents to the office with a chief complaint of fever, vomiting, and loose stools. Referred by Dr. Wellman, her primary care physician, she has had tactile fever for 3 days, and had 5-6 episodes of emesis on the first day of illness. Stools were liquid on the first and second days of illness. She was seen at Dr. Wellman's office 2 days ago, where the impression was gastroenteritis. No labs or x-rays were done at that time. She comes to our office now because of persistent fever. Vomiting and diarrhea have resolved, but her appetite is lower than usual. She notes that her urine seems "strong" and that she is not as energetic as usual. She has had no known ill contacts. She has no cough, URI symptoms, or rash. Past history is unremarkable and she is on no medications.

EXAM: VS T 38.9, P 164, R 40, Wt 135 lb – 5 lb less than one week ago. She is alert, not toxic, and in no apparent distress. HEENT: Her eyes and ENT exams are unremarkable. Her oral mucosa is moist. Her neck is supple. Heart rate is regular without murmurs. Lungs are clear and her respirations are non-labored. ABDOMEN: flat, soft, non-tender, without hepatosplenomegaly or masses. Her external genitalia are normal. SKIN: warm and well perfused, with no rash. BACK EXAM: no deformities or cutaneous defects NEURO: normal tone, strength, and activity.

LAB: A urine specimen yields a small amount of cloudy urine, which is positive for leukocyte esterase and nitrite tests. This is sent for culture. Her CBC shows a WBC 9.4, H/H 9.3/27.5, platelets 389,000, 51% neutrophils, 44% lymphocytes, 3% monocytes, 2% eosinophils. She is given 250mg of ceftriaxone intramuscularly.

Urine culture is positive for greater than 100,000 colonies/ml of a non-lactose fermenting organism, with identification and sensitivities pending and identifies E. coli. Ceftriaxone is repeated at the same dose.

DX: Urinary tract infection

PLAN: She is started on oral trimethoprim-sulfamethoxazole (TMP-SMZ) to complete 10 days of antibiotic therapy.

Sunil Kaladuwa, MD

SK/mg   D: 11/23/08 09:50:16   T: 11/25/08 12:55:01

You Code It!

What are the best, most accurate codes?

_____

_____

_____

WASSERMAN UROLOGY CENTER
233 STREAMLINE DRIVE • MAZE, FL 32811 • 407-555-6591

PATIENT: OVERTOLL, BRYANT
MRN: OVERBR01
Date: 23 November 2008

Physician: Sunil Kaladuwa, MD

This patient is a 13-year-old male who comes at the referral of his pediatrician, Dr. Cozgrove, requesting a circumcision.

HPI: He was a full-term male infant with a normal penis (no evidence of hypospadias or penile chordee). Testes are descended bilaterally and normal to palpation. At the time, his parents did not want their child to be circumcised.

    Since the majority of his male friends are circumcised, he now desires circumcision.

    This is performed, under anesthesia, in the operating room at the Maze Ambulatory Surgical Center. He recovers without any complications.

___

Sunil Kaladuwa, MD

SK/mg   D: 11/23/08 09:50:16   T: 11/25/08 12:55:01

You Code It!

What are the best, most accurate codes?

_____

_____

_____

WASSERMAN UROLOGY CENTER
233 STREAMLINE DRIVE • MAZE, FL 32811 • 407-555-6591

PATIENT: DESIMINI, LANCE

MRN: DESILA01

Date: 23 November 2008

Physician: Sunil Kaladuwa, MD

This is a 7-year-old male who presents to the office with his mother with a chief complaint of bed-wetting twice a week. Essentially he is healthy except for an occasional cough and fever that the mother attributes to exposure to other children with colds. Urinary discharge occurs at night only and he therefore has to wear diapers to bed. His mother is worried since his brothers and sisters were all toilet trained by this age. There is no history of dysuria, intermittent daytime wetness, polyuria, or polydipsia.

PAST MEDICAL HISTORY: Unremarkable.

FAMILY HISTORY: Significant for his father being a bed-wetter. His child development is normal.

EXAM: VS T 37, P 110, R 20, BP 107/64, Ht 102 cm (25th percentile), Wt 16.2 kg (25th percentile). He is alert and active, in no distress. His appearance is non-toxic. HEENT and neck exams are negative. His lungs are clear bilaterally. His heart has a normal rate and rhythm, normal S1 and S2, and no murmurs or rubs. No masses, organomegaly, or tenderness are appreciated on exam of his abdomen. Bowel sounds are present. He has no inguinal hernias. He has a circumcised penis of normal size. The meatus is normally placed, without discharge. No phimosis is present. His testes are descended bilaterally and are of normal size (Tanner stage 1). His back is straight with normal posture with no scoliosis or tenderness, or midline defects. His extremities and muscle tone are normal. His gait is normal. His speech and behavior are age appropriate.

DX: Enuresis

PLAN: Mother is told that bladder control is usually attained between the ages of 1 and 5 years and bed-wetting becomes less frequent with each passing year. I recommend that she be supportive of her son's dry nights and avoid criticism of wet nights. I also recommend avoiding excessive fluid intake two hours before bedtime and emptying his bladder at bedtime.

Sunil Kaladuwa, MD

SK/mg   D: 11/23/08 09:50:16   T: 11/25/08 12:55:01

You Code It!

What are the best, most accurate codes?

_____

_____

_____

WASSERMAN UROLOGY CENTER
233 STREAMLINE DRIVE • MAZE, FL 32811 • 407-555-6591

PATIENT: GOLDSBERRY, IVEY
MRN: GOLDIV01
Date: 23 November 2008

Physician: Sunil Kaladuwa, MD

This patient is a 33-year-old female who has been referred by Dr. Inmann, her gynecologist, due to complaints of pain when she urinates. She is a single mother of three children - ages 5, 9, and 11. She admits to having multiple sexual partners. She has not used any form of birth control since undergoing tubal ligation after the birth of her last child. She is not sure when her last menstrual period was because her menses have always been irregular. She thinks it was 6 weeks ago. Other than a recent URI, she states that she has been in good health. She has no other complaints.

HPI: Patient admits to having mild pelvic pain. She also states that she feels like she "always has to go." She has been waking up 4-5 times at night to urinate for the last five nights. Although she has not taken her temperature, she has felt warm now and then over the past week but she dismisses this as part of her recent cold symptoms. She denies blood in her urine or chills. She denies ever having a urinary tract infection. She admits that she has been feeling fatigued and run down lately. Her job is becomingly increasingly stressful as she takes on more responsibility. When asked about her sexual history, she states that since she broke up with her last boyfriend, she has been seeing a few guys she met in local clubs. She refers to this as "sowing her wild oats." She says she had children at such a young age that she missed out on a lot of the experiences other women her age have already enjoyed. She loves her children but finds them overwhelming when they "act like little devils."

PAST MEDICAL HISTORY: Asthma, allergic rhinitis

PAST SURGICAL HISTORY: Appendectomy age 13. Tubal ligation after the birth of her last child.

MEDICATIONS: Albuterol inhaler and Claritin, as often as she can get samples from the city clinic

SOCIAL HISTORY: She works full time as a receptionist at an insurance office. Only recently has she begun receiving health insurance benefits. She has not had regular annual gynecological exams or received any consistent health care. She drinks 2-3 beers per day, usually more on the weekends to help her deal with the stress of her children. She denies tobacco or illicit drug use.

FAMILY HISTORY: Mother has diabetes type 2 and hypertension. Father died last year of an MI at age 60.

VITALS: Temp 99.0, Pulse 82, BP 127/84, Resp 16/min

HEENT: Head normocephalic. PERRL. EOMI. Oropharynx and TMs clear.

NECK: Some nodal enlargement in the anterior cervical chain. Non-tender.

CV: S1, S2, RRR. No murmurs, rubs, or gallops appreciated.

CHEST: Good air exchange. Slight expiratory wheezes over upper lung fields. No crackles. No CVA tenderness.

ABDOMEN: +BS. soft, ND. Diffuse lower quadrant tenderness. Marked suprapubic tenderness. No rebound or guarding.

EXTREMITIES: Peripheral pulses strong and equal bilaterally. DTRs 2+ upper and lower extremities.

RECTAL: Not performed

GYNECOLOGICAL: Normal external genitalia without lesions. Cervix and vaginal wall appeared normal. No bacteria or fungus were seen on KOH prep and wet mount. GC and chlamydia cultures sent. Bimanual exam shows normal size uterus, no cervical motion tenderness, and no adnexal masses or tenderness.

Continued

UA: A dipstick analysis is performed in the office. The results are:
* 2+ leukocyte esterase * 1+ nitrites * pH 7.4 * negative blood * ketones * glucose * protein * bilirubin

No further tests are performed.

DX: UTI

Tx: Rx: TMP-SMX for 3 days. Patient told to return if her symptoms do not resolve or if she experiences fever, CVA tenderness, or a worsening of symptoms. I also discuss with her the importance of using condoms for disease prevention.

Sunil Kaladuwa, MD

SK/mg   D: 11/23/08 09:50:16   T: 11/25/08 12:55:01

You Code It!

What are the best, most accurate codes?

_____

_____

_____

WASSERMAN UROLOGY CENTER
233 STREAMLINE DRIVE • MAZE, FL 32811 • 407-555-6591

PATIENT: ROCKPORT, ANISHA
MRN: ROCKAN01
Date: 12/15/08

HISTORY: A 31-year-old female transplant recipient presents in our office with diffuse lymph node adenopathy. She developed end-stage renal failure in the context of a Lupus Erythematosus Disseminatus, which was diagnosed in 2007. After evolving into lupus nephritis, morphologically typed as membrano-proliferative glomerulonephritis, she needed dialysis first in 2004 and received a successful kidney graft in early 2005. Shortly after the transplantation, she developed a ureteral leak, for which the ureter of the transplant kidney was connected to her own left ureter, after nephrectomy of her own left kidney. In that removed kidney, a hypernephroma was found accidentally upon routine morphological examination, apparently without further sequel, in spite of intense follow-up. In 2005, a vascular stent was positioned in the renal artery of the transplant kidney because of stenosis. After that, the patient's history was uneventful until 2007.

RECENT HISTORY: In February 2007, corticosteroid immunosuppressive therapy was completely stopped, after gradual tapering. In September 2007, the patient developed skin lesions on the legs which were similar to the lesions developed many years previously during flares of her lupus. The lupoid nature of the lesions was confirmed by skin biopsy. Corticosteroids were then restarted again for a short 2-week period while azathioprine (Imuran) was replaced by mofetil mycophenolate (CellCept). The third immunosuppressive agent (Neoral) was maintained all the time at the same dose and the same adequate serum levels.

In October 2007, the patient developed multiple palpable cervical, supraclavicular and occipital lymph nodes; they were not painful, and some of these nodes had a diameter > 0.5 cm. This evolution was accompanied by a subfebrile status, weight loss, night sweats, general malaise and resistance to erythropoietin.

The patient was hospitalized, and upon admission, body temperature was 37°4C. Blood pressure was 150/100 mmHg. Pulmonary and cardiac auscultation were normal. Upon abdominal palpation, no hepatosplenomegaly could be registered. The patient showed no edema. Palpable, non-painful lymph nodes were present as described above.

In the three months that followed the diagnosis, the lymph nodes grew bigger and the patient showed a body weight loss by 10 kg. She remained subfebrile, and CRP rose to 18 mg/dL. Lymphocyte counts fell to an absolute minimum of 60 cells/mm³. In the meanwhile, the results of the antibiogram became available, and it appeared that the infective Mycobacterium was resistant to ethambutol and ofloxacin. These two agents were replaced by rifabutin and clofazimine.

Kidney function has deteriorated, forcing the start of hemodialysis. As inflammation persists and the general condition continues to deteriorate, the association of aminoglycosides is considered and the recommendation is to remove the transplanted kidney.

DX: Organ rejection, kidney

PLAN: Begin hemodialysis.

Sunil Kaladuwa, MD

12/15/08 11:47:39

You Code It!

What are the best, most accurate codes?

_____

_____

_____

Alternative Medicine: Acupuncture, Chiropractics, and Physical Therapy Cases and Patient Records

INTRODUCTION

The following case studies are from an alternative health practice. These services are more commonly covered by insurance now, so professional coders are needed in these types of health care facilities. The term "conventional medicine" is typically used for health care practices provided by professionals with the training that leads to being a medical doctor (MD) or a doctor of osteopathy (DO) degree. *Alternative medicine*, sometimes referred to as *complementary and alternative medicine (CAM)*, includes the practicing of theories and principles that are not considered a part of conventional medicine, at this time.

This chapter concentrates on three types of alternative medicine: acupuncture, chiropractics, and physical therapy.

An acupuncture practitioner is a licensed and credentialed health care professional who combines acupuncture points with herbal formulas, cupping, heat, and moxibustion to relieve pain and treat illness.

Traditional Chinese medicine practitioners believe acupuncture unblocks and balances the energy (*chi* or *qi*—pronounced "chee"), which flows through the body along pathways called *meridians*. Western health care practitioners speculate that acupuncture reduces pain through physiological processes, perhaps involving stimulus of the hypothalamus and pituitary glands, as well as modifications in neurotransmitters, hormones, and/or immune function.

Acupuncturists may have many different credentials, including doctor of oriental medicine (DOM). Acupuncturists are usually licensed by their state's board of medical examiners, which, in most cases, require an educational background in traditional Chinese medicine (TCM) theory, clinical training, as well as Western medicine including pharmacology, physical examination, Western diagnosis, psychiatry, imaging, anatomy, and physiology. In addition, they must also successfully complete a national certification exam given by the National Commission for the Certification of Acupuncture and Oriental Medicine (NCCAOM).

Chiropractors are health care professionals who specialize in the diagnosis and treatment of health care problems that affect the musculoskeletal system. They use a variety of techniques to adjust the spinal column to prevent, as well as remedy, muscle, joint, and ligament problems.

Chiropractors believe the spinal and musculoskeletal system must be aligned for the body to function properly. They examine the spinal column, nervous system, and circulatory system and consider lifestyle choices, such as eating and exercise habits, when treating illness. Chiropractors can also provide muscle massage and ultrasound stimulation of tissue and may order tests, such as x-rays, but they generally do not prescribe medications.

Chiropractors must complete a minimum of two to three years of college, with coursework in anatomy, physiology, and chemistry, and followed by four years at a chiropractic school. Upon graduation, they must successfully complete a national examination and be licensed by the state in which they practice. Licensure is required in all 50 states and the District of Columbia. The Council on Chiropractic Education is the accrediting agency for chiropractic colleges in the United States.

A physical therapist (PT) is a health care professional who provides evaluation and treatment in order to increase healthy physical function. A physical therapist will first examine the patient so a treatment plan can be developed that will enable normal movement of joints and muscles, reduce pain, prevent disability, and restore and improve function. They instruct in, and assist the patient with, exercises to help heal and strengthen the body. The application of heat and/or cold, electrical stimulation, massage, and ultrasound therapeutic procedures may be used to improve circulation.

Some physical therapists treat a wide range of disorders; others concentrate in such specific areas as pediatrics, geriatrics, orthopedics, sports medicine, neurology, or cardiopulmonology. PTs work in many different types of health care facilities, including hospitals, nursing homes, rehabilitation facilities, schools, and patients' homes.

While the specifics may change from state to state, most require that physical therapists must graduate from an accredited physical therapist educational program, complete a period of clinical work, and pass a national examination. All states require physical therapists to pass a licensure test before they can practice.

You can use these cases to practice coding diagnoses, E/M, procedures, DME, or other HCPCS Level II items, as applicable; code for the physician or the facility; code inpatient and outpatient services, as applicable:

1. Code for the physician.
2. Code for the anesthesiologist, when applicable.
3. Code for the hospital, when applicable.
4. Code for the pathology and laboratory, when applicable.
5. Code HCPCS Level II codes, when applicable.

ALTERNATIVE MEDICAL SERVICES
517 DIVERGENT WAY • HARRIS, FL 32811 • 407-555-9999

PATIENT: ATTRIDGE, CHELSEA
ACCOUNT/EHR #: ATTRCH001
Date: 10/15/08

This patient is a 34-year-old female who came in complaining of severe headaches and lower back pain. She states that she has tried over-the-counter medications and nothing seemed to work. Her friend recommended that she try acupuncture.

PMH: Patient has a history of environmental allergies (hayfever) and childhood asthma. No current medications other than birth control.

PROCEDURE: 20 needles with electrical stimulation for 45 minutes. Re-insertion of the needles is included.

Josine Kini, DOM

10/15/08 11:47:39

You Code It!

What are the best, most accurate codes?

_____

_____

_____

ALTERNATIVE MEDICAL SERVICES
517 DIVERGENT WAY • HARRIS, FL 32811 • 407-555-9999

PATIENT: WILLIAMSON, BELINDA
ACCOUNT/EHR #:   WILLIBE001
Date: 10/15/08

Attending Physician: Rhonda E. Beardall, MD

Referring Physician: James I. Cipher, MD

Pt is a 75-year-old female who recently had a stroke. She is here on referral from Dr. Cipher for an assessment of her aphasia.

Assessment of expressive and receptive speech and language function; language comprehension, speech production ability, reading, spelling, writing, using Boston Diagnostic Aphasia Examination.

Interpretation and report to follow.
    Total time: 60 minutes

_____

Rhonda E. Beardall, MD

REB/mg   D: 10/15/08 09:50:16   T: 10/17/08 12:55:01

You Code It!

What are the best, most accurate codes?

_____

_____

_____

ALTERNATIVE MEDICAL SERVICES
517 DIVERGENT WAY • HARRIS, FL 32811 • 407-555-9999

PATIENT: DEPARI, WILLARD
ACCOUNT/EHR #:   DEPAWI001
Date: 08/11/08

Physical Therapist: Donata R. Chen, MPT

Attending Physician: Willard B. Reader, MD

DX. Old bucket handle tear of medial meniscus, right knee

Order for physical therapy:
    Moist heat, cryotherapy, muscle stimulation, whirlpool, massage
    ROM: active, active assistive, passive
    Exercise: isometric, isotonic
    Ambulation training, as tolerated 3x a week for 6 weeks

Session# 3/6:   Pain Level: 4/10
    Pt states pain shooting down right medial lower leg and numbness in toes.

Total time: 35 minutes
    10 min. Cold pack/right knee
    25 min. Therapeutic exercise . . . to increase strength and ROM

Symptoms began to return in right lower leg toward the end of the exercise. No new exercises added.

Donata R. Chen, MPT

DRC/pw   D: 08/11/08 09:50:16   T: 08/13/08 12:55:01

You Code It!

What are the best, most accurate codes?

_____

_____

_____

ALTERNATIVE MEDICAL SERVICES
517 DIVERGENT WAY • HARRIS, FL 32811 • 407-555-9999

PATIENT: HANEY, RANI
ACCOUNT/EHR #:   HANERA001
Date: 10/15/08

Location: Patient's home
Procedure: New patient evaluation

Patient is a 93-year-old female who had hip surgery 90 days ago. She was discharged from the hospital to Harris Rehabilitation Center where she spent these last three months getting physical and occupational therapies to help her regain functional mobility on her own.

    She is being evaluated for any supportive needs since she came home from the rehabilitation center.

Recommendation: A four-wheel rolling walker; twice-weekly in-home exercise therapies.

Johanna Logan, LPT

You Code It!

What are the best, most accurate codes?

_____

_____

_____

ALTERNATIVE MEDICAL SERVICES
517 DIVERGENT WAY • HARRIS, FL 32811 • 407-555-9999

PATIENT: MATHESON, ROGER
ACCOUNT/EHR #: MATHRO001
Date: 10/15/08

Location: Patient's home
Procedure: Muscle strength rebuild

Patient is a 21-year-old male who is a professional basketball player. Patient is recovering from knee surgery and requires exercise to rebuild muscle strength.

One hour: climbing stair machine.

_____

Mark Caine, physical therapist

You Code It!

What are the best, most accurate codes?

_____

_____

_____

ALTERNATIVE MEDICAL SERVICES
517 DIVERGENT WAY • HARRIS, FL 32811 • 407-555-9999

PATIENT: FINNEALE, JEREMY
ACCOUNT/EHR #: FINNJE001
Date: 10/15/08

Patient is a 63-year-old male referred to the audiology department by the hospital speech-language pathologist following a post-CVA assessment. On May 6th, the patient suffered a left anterior CVA, resulting in right hemiparesis, expressive language problems consistent with Broca's aphasia, and mild receptive language difficulties. Previous audiometric results and relevant auditory history have not been obtained from his family physician. His daughter, who is present at this assessment, reported that her father has no known hearing problems. The patient speaks with his daughter regularly on the telephone without difficulty.

EXAM: Pure tone air and bone conduction thresholds are conducted with fair reliability and indicated a mild bilateral sensorineural hearing loss, with further decreased sensitivity in the high frequencies. Speech detection thresholds were obtained with fair reliability and indicated a slight loss of sensitivity. Discriminating testing was not attempted.

Cursory otoscopic examination is essentially unremarkable. Acoustic immittance procedures indicated normal middle ear function bilaterally. Acoustic stapedial reflexes are present at normal levels bilaterally on both ipsi- and contralateral stimulation.

Tone decay measures and acoustic reflex decay measurement are also conducted. These tests are negative, suggesting no evidence of eighth nerve pathology.

ASSESSMENT: Test results indicate a mild loss of hearing sensitivity bilaterally sufficient to cause communicative difficulty in normal conversational situations and considerable difficulty in noisy or reverberant conditions. These results are consistent with the speech-language pathologist's report of mild receptive problems and reports of communication problems with health care personnel in the hospital.

Recommendations: Strategic plan for communications, necessitated by hearing loss, is discussed with patient and his daughter. It is suggested that the patient use an assistive listening device to reduce stress of trying to communicate with others, particularly strangers.

PLAN: Return for further assessment in three months.

_____

Harris Mulhaney, Audiologist

You Code It!

What are the best, most accurate codes?

_____

_____

_____

ALTERNATIVE MEDICAL SERVICES
517 DIVERGENT WAY • HARRIS, FL 32811 • 407-555-9999

PATIENT: BRIGGS, MICHAEL
ACCOUNT/EHR #:   BRIGMI001
Date: 10/15/08

TREATMENT PLAN FOR OCCUPATIONAL THERAPY
Patient is a 59-year-old male who suffered a L CVA with R hemiparesis one week ago.

ADL (Activities of Daily Living)
- Feeds self independently once tray prepared
- No swallowing difficulties noted
- Washes self independently once set up in chair at bedside, except requires assistance of one staff member to stand for peri-care
- Requires assistance for most aspects of dressing; do buttons, put on and fasten shoes and socks, to stand, to pull up pants

Mobility
- Transfers with assist of one staff member
- Able to propel wheelchair short distances
- Ambulates with assistance of a therapist
- Sitting balance poor, needs chair with armrests and supervision to reach down to feet
- Standing balance poor, needs light assistance to ambulate

Upper Extremity Mobility
- R hand is swollen, passive flexion of interphalangeal (IP) joints limited
- R arm Brunnstrom stage 1

Psychosocial Issues
- Becomes frustrated over expressive communication problems
- Comprehension seems inconsistent
- Expresses concerns about his health and future
- He has two grown children
- Speaks with daughter every week or ten days by telephone
- Calls son weekly, but he is not always in and rarely returns calls, so he speaks with him approximately every two weeks and sees him monthly (invites him to dinner)
- Has a number of friends and neighbors whom he says he could ask for assistance, but he prefers to be independent or to offer help to others

Client Goals
1. He wants to return to living alone in two-story house (laundry in basement, powder room ground floor, bedroom and full bathroom on second floor).
2. He wants to continue driving.
3. He wishes to continue leisure interest in woodworking.

Continued

Plan
1. See him 30-45 minutes daily on an individual basis in OT
2. See him twice weekly in the morning for activities of daily living (ADL) training

Suzanne Koss, LPT

You Code It!

What are the best, most accurate codes?

_____

_____

_____

ALTERNATIVE MEDICAL SERVICES
517 DIVERGENT WAY • HARRIS, FL 32811 • 407-555-9999

PATIENT: ANDREWS, GRACE
ACCOUNT/EHR #: ANDRGR001
Date: 10/15/08
Physical Therapy

Assessment of physical and functional status

This patient is a 71-year-old female who is seen for the first time today in the acute stage of her illness in the physical therapy suite of Harris Hospital.

ASSESSMENT: Patient demonstrates significant weakness in the right limb muscles. The upper limb shows flaccidity due to the paresis present - with an inability to resist gravity. The lower limb is not capable of full weight-bearing and there is a flexed knee posture present. For the trunk, strength of forward flexion is impaired.

Balance in upright standing is also impaired with an asymmetrical stance to the non-affected side; the patient requires a wheelchair for effective mobility. Trunk stability is poor in the anterior/posterior direction.

There is complaint of pain in the right shoulder area. Due to the swollen, flaccid nature of the right upper limb, there is some evidence of developing subluxation of the glenohumeral joint.

CLIENT GOALS
1. Use of affected limbs, as much as future muscle tone allows
2. Regain standing balance, and walking ability
3. Reduce shoulder discomfort

PLAN
1. See her one-hour daily on an individual basis
2. Massage therapy: focus on shoulder and legs

Suzanne Koss, LPT

You Code It!

What are the best, most accurate codes?

_____

_____

_____

ALTERNATIVE MEDICAL SERVICES
517 DIVERGENT WAY • HARRIS, FL 32811 • 407-555-9999

PATIENT: HARBOUR, HARRIS
ACCOUNT/EHR #:   HARBHA001
Date: 10/15/08
Physical Therapy

Assessment of Speech-Language Pathology
    Patient is a 67-year-old male seen for assessment in the acute stage of his illness, three days after his admission. He was visited first in his room for a preliminary bedside examination. He is seen in the speech-language pathologist's office for three, 1.5 hour assessment sessions over the next three days.

ASSESSMENT: Standardized and non-standardized speech and language assessment tools are administered to identify the nature of his speech and language problems and to help establish goals for therapy. These included the:

- Western Aphasia Battery
- Revised Token Test
- Boston Naming Test
- Action Naming Test
- Apraxia Battery for Adults
- Functional Assessment of Communication Skills of Adults
- Bedside speech and language examination (non-standardized)
- Oral peripheral examination

The results from the detailed language and speech assessment revealed that the patient exhibits a mild-to-moderate Broca's aphasia, moderate apraxia of speech (i.e., verbal apraxia), and moderate oral apraxia (non-verbal apraxia). His expressive language skills (i.e., spoken and written) are more impaired relative to his mildly impaired receptive language skills (i.e., listening and reading comprehension).
    The patient also shows difficulty speaking as a result of his apraxia of speech. He spoke in short, poorly articulated phrases, which contained mostly nouns, verbs, adjectives, and adverbs (i.e., content words). He made several attempts to produce words and phrases correctly, often exhibiting errors in which sounds were substituted, distorted, or omitted on an irregular basis (i.e., paraphasic error). He gets frustrated by his inability to say words clearly, as well as by the inconsistency in the accuracy of his speaking.

Client Goals:
    1. Patient wants to be able to speak more clearly on a regular basis.
    2. Patient wants to be able to use more words in his sentences.
    3. Patient wants to use words more accurately in his sentences.

Eloise Mason, Chief of Speech/Language Pathology

You Code It!

What are the best, most accurate codes?

_____

_____

_____

ALTERNATIVE MEDICAL SERVICES
517 DIVERGENT WAY • HARRIS, FL 32811 • 407-555-9999

PATIENT: WALKMAN, JOYCE
ACCOUNT/EHR #:   WALKJO001
Date: 10/15/08

ASSESSMENT OF OCCUPATIONAL AND PHYSICAL THERAPY

Patient is a 59-year-old female, seen twice daily during her stay in the Neuro-Rehabilitation Unit. She suffered a right hemisphere stroke that resulted in:

MOTOR IMPAIRMENT:
- L leg paresis
- Some active hip flexion in synergy
- Little spasticity at rest
- L arm hemiparesis
- Marked flexor synergy with attempted elbow flexion
- Moderate spasticity at rest
- Hand held flexed/fisted, especially at night
- Bobath Stage 1

FUNCTIONAL IMPAIRMENT:
- Assist of one staff member for all ADL (washing, dressing, preparing tray)
- Able to feed self, but tone in arm decreased so this was discouraged
- Assist of two staff members for transfers and standing
- One staff member needed to assist for mobility

PERCEPTUAL IMPAIRMENT:
- Difficulty dressing
- Constructional apraxia
- Right-left discrimination problems

COGNITIVE IMPAIRMENT:
- Impaired insight
- Impulsivity
- Poor problem solving
- Poor safety judgment
- Distractible

INTERVENTIONS
MOTOR:
- Neurodevelopmental treatment (NDT)
- Attempts to normalize tone
- Positioning in RIPs in chair and bed
- Foam finger spreader for night

FUNCTIONAL:
- Rented wheelchair and cushion

PERCEPTUAL:
- Transfer of training approach
- Peg board puzzles
- Block designs
- Mirrored movements

Continued

Patient has shown some response to therapy, though it was difficult to estimate prognosis for functional out-come.

Patient is being transferred to a rehabilitation center closer to the home of her daughter.

Walter R. Korinne, LPT

You Code It!

What are the best, most accurate codes?

_____

_____

_____

ALTERNATIVE MEDICAL SERVICES
517 DIVERGENT WAY • HARRIS, FL 32811 • 407-555-9999

PATIENT: QUAHOG, OWEN
ACCOUNT/EHR #:   QUAHOW001
Date: 10/15/08

ASSESSMENT

This patient is a 63-year-old male who is transferred from a stroke rehabilitation center. He suffered an embolic right hemisphere CVA four weeks ago.

ADMISSION ASSESSMENT: Patient has left upper and lower limb paresis, Brunnstrom Stage 3 and 4, respectively. Perceptual testing reveals similar results to those reported at the rehab center, difficulty dressing and constructional apraxia and right-left discrimination problems as well as mild-moderate unilateral neglect of left side of space and body.

The patient states that his goal is to return home. He seems unconcerned about his inability to wash and dress himself but says he would like to get rid of the wheelchair, stating that it is very ugly.

RECOMMENDATIONS FOR TREATMENT:
 • Carr and Shepherd's motor relearning program (MRP)
 • Functional approach to perceptual retraining

PLAN: Begin MRP Monday morning

Yancy Leadante, LPT

You Code It!

What are the best, most accurate codes?

_____

_____

_____

ALTERNATIVE MEDICAL SERVICES
517 DIVERGENT WAY • HARRIS, FL 32811 • 407-555-9999

PATIENT: BARTLETT, PETER
ACCOUNT/EHR #:   BARTPE001
Date: 10/07/08

This patient is a 45-year-old male complaining of neck pain and lower back pain which have become increasingly more difficult since an MVA two weeks ago.

Patient states he was driving down Main Street and struck from behind by another driver. He states that the pain has been constant since about 2 hours after the accident. He describes the pain as pressure, "pulling, aching" in his neck and constant aching in his lower back. The sharpness of the pain increases with movement, and subsides when he lies still. It is painful to bend or walk. He said that he went to see his family physician, Dr. Farina, last week, who referred him to our office.

X-rays: Cervical x-rays (PA-Lat) show multiple subluxations of the cervical vertebrae with pain on movement. Dens and spinous process are intact. No breaks or fracture noted. Lumbar spine x-rays (PA-Lat) is intact with no breaks or fractures.

Treatment Plan: Spinal manipulations at neck and lower back 2 – 3x per week for approximately 3 months, followed by moist heat to release spasm and pain and increase circulation. This will be followed by cryotherapy for the reduction of swelling and pain. Ice/heat: prn.

Prognosis: Good with no permanent impairment expected.

Diagnosis: Cervical hyperflexion; dislocation of multiple cervical vertebrae; lumbar sprain/strain, after 2-car MVA.
Therapeutic treatments provided during this visit: Chiropractic adjustment 3-4 regions; traction; hot/cold pack therapy.

Natalie Crystalis, DC

You Code It!

What are the best, most accurate codes?

_____

_____

_____

ALTERNATIVE MEDICAL SERVICES
517 DIVERGENT WAY • HARRIS, FL 32811 • 407-555-9999

PATIENT: SYMAN, SIMONE
ACCOUNT/EHR #:   SYMASI001
Date: 05/19/08

This patient is a 39-year-old female complaining of lower back pain which began one month ago. Patient states that she is constantly achy and stiff. She states that the pain radiates from her right outside thigh into her abdomen. She says it feels worse first thing in the morning, and at night, after she exercises.

   She was seen in this office previously, about five years ago.

X-rays: Lumbar spine x-rays (PA-Lat) show lumbar stenosis of the 2-5 vertebrae with sciatica down the right leg into toes. Patient presents with full spine MS that are rope-like on static palpation. Patient is unable to extend trunk and has limited ROM in lumbar spine.

Treatment Plan: Spinal manipulations of lower back 2 – 3x per week for ten weeks. In between office visits, it is recommended that the patient apply moist heat to release spasm and pain and increase circulation, followed by cryotherapy for the reduction of swelling and pain. Ice/heat: prn.

Prognosis: Guarded

Diagnosis: Lumbar stenosis, sciatica, muscle spasm, restricted range of motion

Therapeutic treatments provided during this visit: Chiropractic adjustment 3-4 regions

Natalie Crystalis, DC

You Code It!

What are the best, most accurate codes?

_____

_____

_____

Credits

Frontmatter

Chapter Openers